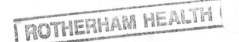

Transient
Ischemic
Attacks

Dedication

To my family, Seema, Nikhil, Kavya, and parents Rama and Veena
To my mentors, Marc Fisher, Vladimir Hachinski, and Henry Barnett
S.C.

To my family, Joanne, Aaron, David, and Aliza, and parents Elaine and Hal
To my mentors, Sid Gilman and K.M.A. Welch
S.R.L.

To our patients who have taught us about TIAs
To our readers, who will hopefully practice what is preached here or
at least be stimulated to think critically about TIAs
And to all of our colleagues, whose sense of inquiry, knowledge,
wisdom, and understanding are also contained in this book

Transient Ischemic Attacks

EDITED BY

Seemant Chaturvedi, MD

Associate Professor of Neurology
Wayne State University School of Medicine
Director
Wayne State University/Detroit Medical Center Stroke Program
Detroit, Michigan

AND

Steven R. Levine, MD

Professor of Neurology
Director, Cerebrovascular Education
Stroke Program
The Mount Sinai School of Medicine
New York City, New York

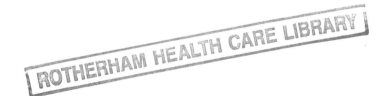
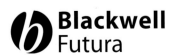
Blackwell
Futura

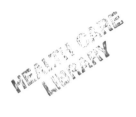

© 2004 by Futura, an imprint of Blackwell Publishing
Blackwell Publishing, Inc., 350 Main Street, Malden, Massachusetts 02148-5020, USA
Blackwell Publishing Ltd, 9600 Garsington Road, Oxford OX4 2DQ, UK
Blackwell Science Asia Pty Ltd, 550 Swanston Street, Carlton, Victoria 3053, Australia

04 05 06 07 5 4 3 2 1

ISBN: 1-4051-2059-2

Library of Congress Cataloging-in-Publication Data

Transient ischemic attacks / edited by Seemant Chaturvedi and Steven R. Levine.
        p. ; cm.
    Includes bibliographical references and index.
    ISBN 1-4051-2059-2
    1. Cerebral ischemia.
    [DNLM: 1. Ischemic Attack, Transient.   WL 355 T7724 2004]   I. Chaturvedi, Seemant.
II. Levine, Steven R.
    RC388.5.T672 2004
    616.8'1—dc22

                                                                        2004005408

A catalogue record for this title is available from the British Library

Acquisitions: Steve Korn
Production: Julie Elliott
Typesetter: Graphicraft Limited, Hong Kong, in 10/12 Meridien
Printed and bound by Edwards Brothers, Ann Arbor, MI (USA)

For further information on Blackwell Publishing, visit our website:
www.Blackwellfutura.com

The publisher's policy is to use permanent paper from mills that operate a sustainable forestry
policy, and which has been manufactured from pulp processed using acid-free and elementary
chlorine-free practices. Furthermore, the publisher ensures that the text paper and cover board
used have met acceptable environmental accreditation standards.

Notice: The indications and dosages of all drugs in this book have been recommended in the medical
literature and conform to the practices of the general community. The medications described do not
necessarily have specific approval by the Food and Drug Administration for use in the diseases and
dosages for which they are recommended. The package insert for each drug should be consulted for
use and dosage as approved by the FDA. Because standards for usage change, it is advisable to keep
abreast of revised recommendations, particularly those concerning new drugs.

Contents

Contents

Part IV Surgical and Interventional Treatments and Cost-Effectiveness

List of Contributors

Alex Abou-Chebl, MD
Department of Neurology, The Cleveland Clinic
Foundation, Cleveland, OH

Fadi Al-Khayer, MD
Fellow, Division of Endocrinology, Metabolism
and Hypertension, Department of Internal
Medicine, Wayne State University School of
Medicine, Detroit, MI

James Bichsel, MD
Department of Neurology
Emory University School of Medicine
Atlanta, GA

Robert D. Brown, Jr., MD
Consultant, Division of Cerebrovascular Diseases
and Department of Neurology, Mayo Clinic,
Rochester, Minnesota; Associate Professor of
Neurology, Mayo Medical School, Rochester, MN

Louis R. Caplan, MD
Department of Neurology, Division of
Cerebrovascular Diseases, Beth Israel Deaconess
Medical Center, Harvard Medical School,
Boston, MA

Mar Castellanos, MD
Stroke Fellow
Comprehensive Stroke Program
Department of Neurology
Wayne State University School of Medicine

Richard K.T. Chan, MBBS
Associate Professor of Neurology
University of Western Ontario
London, ON, Canada

Seemant Chaturvedi, MD
Associate Professor of Neurology
Wayne State University School of Medicine
Director, Wayne State University/Detroit Medical
Center Stroke Program
Detroit, MI

Colin P. Derdeyn, MD
Associate Professor of Radiology, Program
Director, Endovascular Surgical Neuroradiology,

Mallinckrodt Institute of Radiology, Washington
University Medical School, St. Louis, MO

Marco R. Di Tullio, MD
Columbia University
New York, NY

John M. Flack, MD, MPH
Division of Endocrinology, Metabolism, and
Hypertension and the Cardiovascular
Epidemiology and Clinical Applications Program,
Department of Internal Medicine, Wayne State
University, Detroit, MI

Matthew L. Flaherty, MD
Mayo Graduate School of Medicine and Department
of Neurology, Mayo Clinic, Rochester, MN

Michael R. Frankel, MD
Associate Professor of Neurology, Emory
University School of Medicine
Chief of Neurology, Grady Health System
Atlanta, GA

Karen Furie, MD, MPH,
Harvard Medical School
Massachusetts General Hospital
Boston, MA

Larry B. Goldstein, MD
Director, Duke Center for Cerebrovascular Disease
Head, Stroke Policy Program, Center for Clinical
Health Policy Research
Duke University; Durham VA Medical Center,
Durham, NC

George Grunberger, MD
Clinical Professor, Department of Internal
Medicine, Center for Molecular Medicine and
Genetics; Medical Director, Morris J. Hood
Comprehensive Diabetes Center, Wayne State
University School of Medicine, Detroit, MI

Susan L. Hickenbottom, MD, MS
Clinical Assistant Professor
Director, Stroke Program
University of Michigan Health System
Ann Arbor, MI

List of Contributors

Shunichi Homma, MD
Columbia University
New York, NY

Chung Y. Hsu, MD, PhD
Professor, The Stroke Center and Department of
Neurology, Washington University School of
Medicine, St. Louis, MO

Bradley S. Jacobs, MD, MS
Assistant Professor
Comprehensive Stroke Program
Department of Neurology
Wayne State University School of Medicine

Peter J. Kelly, MB, BCh, MMedSc
Harvard Medical School
Massachusetts General Hospital
Boston, MA

Chelsea S. Kidwell, MD
UCLA Stroke Center and Department of
Neurology, UCLA Medical Center, Los
Angeles, CA

J. Philip Kistler, MD
Harvard Medical School
Massachusetts General Hospital
Boston, MA

Sandeep Kumar, MD
Department of Neurology, Division of
Cerebrovascular Diseases, Beth Israel Deaconess
Medical Center, Harvard Medical School, Boston,
MA

Jin-Moo Lee, MD, PhD
Assistant Professor, The Stroke Center and
Department of Neurology, Washington
University School of Medicine, St. Louis, MO

Steven R. Levine, MD
Professor of Neurology,
Director, Cerebrovascular Education
Stroke Program, Mount Sinai School of Medicine,
New York City, NY

Ramesh Madhavan, MD
Stroke Fellow
Comprehensive Stroke Program
Department of Neurology
Wayne State University School of Medicine

Vishal Mehra, MD
Division of General Internal Medicine and the
Academic Hospitalist Program, Department of
Internal Medicine, Wayne State University,
Detroit ,MI

James F. Meschia, MD
Assistant Professor
Department of Neurology
Mayo Clinic
Jacksonville, L

Samar Nasser, PAC
Cardiovascular Epidemiology and Clinical
Applications Program, Department of Internal
Medicine, Wayne State Univesity, Detroit, MI

Abdullah M. Nassief, MD
Assistant Professor, The Stroke Center and
Department of Neurology, Washington
University School of Medicine, St. Louis, MO

Neel Patel, MD
Department of Internal Medicine, Wayne State
University, Detroit, MI

William J. Powers, MD
Professor of Neurology, Radiology, and
Neurosurgery, Co-Director, Cerebrovascular
Section, Department of Neurology, Washington
University Medical School, St. Louis, MO

Patrick Pullicino, MD, PhD
Professor of Neurology
Chairman, Department of Neurosciences,
New Jersey Medical School, University of
Medicine and Dentistry of New Jersey, Newark, NJ

Jeffrey L. Saver, MD
UCLA Stroke Center and Department of
Neurology, UCLA Medical Center, Los Angeles, CA

Michael J. Schneck, MD
Associate Professor of Neurology
Department of Neurology
Loyola University Chicago
Chicago, IL

Gregory P. Van Stavern, MD
Assistant Professor, Departments of
Ophthalmology and Neurology
Kresge Eye Institute, Wayne State University,
Detroit, MI

Janet L. Wilterdink, MD
Associate Professor, Department of Clinical
Neurosciences
Brown Medical School, Providence, RI

Jay S. Yadav, MD
Director, Vascular Intervention
Department of Cardiovascular Medicine
The Cleveland Clinic Foundation
Cleveland, OH

Foreword

Transient ischemic attacks (TIA) may be transient, but the threat that they signal is not. Increasingly we realize that about one-fifth of patients with TIA will suffer a stroke within 3 months, about half occurring in the first week! Thus it becomes imperative that both the public and physicians become familiar with the symptoms and what needs to be done about them. Physicians have a one stop means of doing so, through this volume.

First they will learn about the epidemiology and pathophysiology of TIAs and will become familiar with the diverse cerebral and ocular syndromes. Then they will appreciate the advantages and limitations of different diagnostic modalities. Brain imaging occupies a deservedly prominent place, beside the less used but uniquely and selective, helpful single photon emission computer tomography (SPECT) and positron emission tomography (PET). Cerebrovascular ultrasonography, cardiac diagnostic and coagulation studies are evaluated with equanimous objectivity.

Subsequently the reader becomes acquainted with the indications and controversies surrounding the use of antiplatelet agents. The role of anticoagulants is well justified, while heparin and related compounds are put into proper perspective, given the continuing triumph of hope over evidence. Diabetes treatment while essential, does not have the obvious beneficial effects of antihypertensive therapy. Other medical therapies are also discussed, as well as thrombolysis for TIA and mild stroke.

Next the indications for surgery in stroke prevention and the role of angioplasty and stenting are weighed. Cost effectiveness issues merit a whole chapter and the book ends with a flourish of clinical vignettes.

Throughout, editors and authors strive to base their conclusions on evidence where it exists, and on pragmatism and common sense where it does not. At a time of rising awareness of the peril and opportunities for prevention posed by TIAs, this is a most timely book.

Vladimir Hachinski, MD, FRCPC, DSc
Professor of Neurology
Department of Clinical Neurological Sciences
Western University
London, Ontario, Canada

Preface

This book was born from the synthesis of the rapidly proliferating field of cerebrovascular disease research, excitement about effective new imaging and therapeutic strategies, and the need to timely educate clinicians about the changing playing field for a common, serious, and expensive syndrome —transient ischemic attacks (TIA). TIAs can now stand on their own as an important and, at times, unique aspect of symptomatic cerebrovascular disease, distinct enough to warrant a textbook in its own right. With new information on a worrisome and serious natural history, growing knowledge of risk factors and their management, sophisticated neuroimaging techniques, and a broadening armamentarium of therapeutic approaches, the clinician is now faced with multiple levels of decision making. Does one admit the patient with a recent TIA to the hospital? What are the optimal imaging and diagnostic strategies? Which antiplatelet agent to use? What is the role for surgery and interventional techniques? How do I optimally control associated risk factors? This book serves to provide the most current information to help guide clinicians through the best decisions to care for their patients, using evidence-based recommendations when available and expert opinion when no good data exist.

Having initiated (SRL with Dr. Lawrence Brass of Yale University), directed, and taught (SRL and SC) the course on TIAs at the annual American Academy of Neurology meeting for the past several years, it has become clear that clinicians are keen on the latest synthesized data and approaches to the problem of transient cerebral ischemia. They require cutting edge analyses, and express concerns over the lack of consensus in several important areas. Diagnosis and management of TIAs continues to perplex even the most seasoned clinicians. Further impetus for providing this book includes response to the issues raised over the years at the TIA course, our own clinical and research experience (and those of our colleagues who have generously contributed their expertise to this team effort), the need to handle the TIA patient differently in some regards from the patients with a severe neurological deficit having a similar underlying pathophysiologic mechanism, and the need to bring TIA to its own place in the field of cerebrovascular disease.

This book is intended to be a one-volume, highly readable source of current, accurate information for the clinician and clinical stroke researcher, that can readily answer questions that arise, provide guidance in patient care, and establish quickly what we do and do not know in the field. We have chosen esteemed colleagues from the field to address all of the important topics that serve as chapters. They have each helped create a perspective that will provide the clinician important and useful information in a readily available format. Our wish is that patients will directly benefit from the knowledge imparted such that they will never suffer from the consequences of a disabling stroke.

Steven R. Levine, MD
New York City, New York

Seemant Chaturvedi, MD
Detroit, Michigan

PART I

Clinical Background

CHAPTER 1

The Epidemiology of Transient Ischemic Attacks

Matthew L. Flaherty, Robert D. Brown, Jr

Introduction

A transient ischemic attack (TIA) can be defined as a sudden focal loss of neurological function with complete recovery within 24 h, caused by inadequate perfusion in the partial or complete distribution of the carotid or vertebrobasilar arteries [1]. TIAs may involve either the brain or the retina. Transient monocular blindness (TMB) caused by retinal ischemia has also historically been known as amaurosis fugax and the terms are often used synonymously [2]. Nonspecific neurological complaints such as dizziness, isolated vertigo, presyncope, syncope, or confusion should not be considered TIAs without other substantiating evidence.

The maximal duration of symptoms caused by a TIA has been arbitrarily set at 24 h, although most last less than 30 min [3]. Deficits caused by cerebral ischemia lasting more than 24 h but less than 3 weeks are sometimes called a reversible ischemic neurological deficit (RIND), but contemporary cross-sectional brain imaging studies have shown these to represent minor strokes and this terminology is now infrequently used. Computed tomography (CT) studies and particularly diffusion weighted (DWI) magnetic resonance imaging (MRI) have also shown that many symptoms clinically suggestive of TIA are actually minor ischemic strokes (or cerebral infarctions). Although some data suggest that TIAs of longer duration are more likely to correspond to infarction on imaging, other investigators have been unable to distinguish clinically TIAs with and without infarction [4–7].

The question thus arises whether TIAs should continue to be defined clinically or only in conjunction with neuroimaging studies which fail to show infarction. CT scanning, though easily obtainable, lacks sensitivity and specificity for both the presence and timing of infarction. Diffusion weighted MRI would be more useful. Imaging all TIA patients with MRI would be cumbersome, expensive, and logistically impossible in many clinical situations. Therefore, the compelling reason to redefine TIAs based upon MRI findings would be prognostic differences between TIAs (more strictly defined) and minor ischemic strokes.

An analogous question concerns the practical usefulness of distinguishing clinically between minor ischemic stroke and TIA. Several community and hospital-based studies suggest that the stroke risk of patients with clinically diagnosed TIA is comparable to those with RIND or minor stroke, especially if patients with amaurosis fugax are excluded [8–10]. Treatment trials often include TIA and minor ischemic stroke patients under this assumption, and terms such as 'reversible ischemic attacks' have been proposed to cover both categories, although the traditional categories of TIA and minor stroke have also been defended as useful in both differential diagnosis and case–control studies [2]. A very small number of minor strokes and symptoms suggesting TIA are caused by intracerebral hemorrhage. These small hemorrhages are readily identified by CT imaging, which is important given that they differ in etiology, prevention, and optimal management.

TIA incidence, prevalence, and risk factors

The incidence of TIA is defined as the proportion of a population experiencing a first TIA in a given period of time (usually a year). The point prevalence of TIA is the number of people in a defined population, at a given point in time, who have ever experienced a TIA. In each instance individuals who have suffered a stroke are usually excluded. Both definitions may also be modified in rather complex ways which can vary between studies and (presumably) influence outcome. For example, incidence studies may 'count' TIAs which occur prior to a study period and bring the patient to a physician, while ignoring prior TIAs which did not prompt medical evaluation [11]. Many studies do not explicitly define the inclusion criteria used.

Several factors make TIA incidence and prevalence studies challenging. The symptoms of TIAs, being transient by definition, may not prompt an affected individual to seek medical attention. The diagnosis of a TIA is strictly clinical, and historical details may become blurred with time. There are also many nonspecific symptoms common in the elderly (such as dizziness, vertigo, syncope, confusion, and gait disturbance) which may be mistaken for a TIA. Hospital dismissal summaries and medical records used to identify stroke (and by reasonable inference TIA) are liable to error [12]. Finally, interobserver reliability in the diagnosis of TIA, even amongst neurologists, has proven less than ideal [13,14].

With these limitations, a number of studies of varying design have reported the incidence and prevalence of TIAs. In theory the best approach would utilize a population-based, observational study of individuals with easy access to medical care and a demographic mix allowing conclusions to be drawn about groups of different age, race, gender, and socioeconomic status. No single study satisfies all of these criteria.

Incidence

In Rochester, Minnesota, the Rochester Epidemiology Project Medical Records Linkage System allows retrospective identification of nearly all cases of stroke and TIA that occur in a defined population. The most recent study of TIA epidemiology in Rochester produced a crude TIA incidence rate of 68 per 100 000 persons per year for the years 1985–1989 after age and sex adjustment to the 1980 US white population [15]. As expected, age-specific rates showed increasing incidence with increasing age to a maximum of 584 events per 100 000 persons 75–84 years old, after which age the rate declined slightly. This 'incidence decline' in the 'oldest old' has been noted in other studies and may be explained by several issues. While the incidence may truly decline in those people who have survived to age 85 and beyond, other explanations include lack of complete case ascertainment in the oldest members of the population, in this relatively small population [11,16,17]. While the age-adjusted incidence rate for TIA in Rochester was slightly higher for men than for women (76 vs. 62 per 100 000), the difference was not statistically significant. This is in accordance with other studies which show roughly equivalent rates between sexes, although women tend to be older at the time of the incident event [11,16,17].

TIA incidence data from Rochester for 1985–1989 are summarized in Table 1.1. Comparison of data from the Rochester linkage system for the years 1955–1969 with the more recent data reveals some discrepancy, with crude age and sex-adjusted incidence rates rising from 33 per 100 000 to 68 per 100 000 [18,19]. The lower incidence rates in the earlier study have been attributed to methodological issues in case ascertainment. This is supported by a cohort study from 1960 to 1972 (without such methodological issues) that produced incidence rates comparable to the recent data [20].

Crude age and sex-adjusted incidence rates from other population-based studies cluster around those of the earlier Rochester report [11,21–25] (Table 1.2). While actual differences in TIA incidence are possible, this would seem an unlikely explanation, especially as stroke incidence in Rochester is not significantly higher than at other sites (discussed under epidemiology of cerebral infarction). Differences in population type, methods of case ascertainment, and incomplete case ascertainment would be more plausible.

A breakdown of TIA incidence by arterial distribution in the Rochester population is shown in Table 1.3 [15]. The high percentage of carotid

Table 1.1 Average annual age- and sex-specific incidence rates* of transient ischemic attack in Rochester, Minnesota, 1985–1989

Age group	Men		Women		Total	
	Rate	No.	Rate	No.	Rate	No.
45–54	54	8	57	9	56	17
55–64	128	14	96	12	111	26
65–74	323	24	277	30	296	54
75–84	687	26	539	47	584	73
≥ 85	498	6	467	20	474	26
All†	76		62		68	

*Per 100 000 population.
†Rates are age-adjusted or age- and sex-adjusted to 1980 US white population.
Adapted from: Brown RD *et al*. Incidence of transient ischemic attack in Rochester, Minnesota, 1985–1989. *Stroke* 1998; 29: 2109–13, with permission.

territory events is similar to TIA distribution in Russia and western Europe; a small Japanese study with only 18 total events found a more even balance between anterior and posterior circulations [11,22,24,25].

Rates of amaurosis fugax have not been commonly reported in TIA studies. The age and sex-adjusted incidence of amaurosis fugax in Rochester from 1985 to 1989 was 13/100 000, accounting for 18% of TIAs [15]. A prospective Danish study found an incidence of 7/100 000, but estimated the 'true' incidence to be 14/100 000 based upon poor case ascertainment in the elderly [26]. In Oxfordshire, England, and Umbria, Italy, amaurosis fugax accounted for 17% and 5.3% of all TIAs, respectively [11,17]. In Segovia, Spain, only one of 103 TIAs recorded was isolated amaurosis fugax [16].

While nonspecific transient neurological symptoms such as dizziness and visual disturbance seem ubiquitous in the elderly population, one study found the prevalence of 'transient neurological attacks' (TNAs) to be similar to that of typical TIA in older persons (1.6%) [27]. 'Atypical TIAs' have been found to carry a lower risk of future stroke and a higher risk of future cardiac events compared with 'typical' TIAs [28].

Although there is limited longitudinal data regarding TIA incidence, and comparisons between studies suffer from differences in case ascertainment and statistical methods, data from Rochester and other sites suggests that the TIA incidence rates have been stable over time [15,25,29]. This contrasts with an apparent decline in the incidence of stroke from the 1950s through the mid early 1980s, with the subsequent end of the decline in the 1980s and early 1990s (see epidemiology of cerebral infarction).

Table 1.2 Comparison of incidence of transient ischemic attack (TIA) reported from sites throughout the World

Location	Time period	Study type	Case no.	Incidence rate (crude, unadjusted by age, per 100 000)			Age/sex-adjusted incidence rate*
				Men	Women	Total	
Rochester, USA [15]	1985–1989	Population-based, retrospective registry	202	68	54	6	68
	1955–1969		198	31	31	31	33
Novosibirsk, Russia [25]	1987–1988	Population-based, prospective registry	122	17	15	16	18
	1996–1997		89	25	32	29	31
Dijon, France [24]	1990–1994	Population-based, prospective registry	258	37	33	36	NR
Oxfordshire, England [11]	1981–1986	Population-based, prospective registry	184	39	31	35	36
Söderhamn, Sweden [21]	1975–1978	Population-based, prospective registry	44	43	48	NR	33
	1983–1986		53	56	45	NR	38
Hisayma, Japan [22]	1961–1982	Population-based, prospective cohort study	18	78	38	56	22
Estonia, USSR [23]	1970–1973	Population-based, retrospective registry	119	36	33	33	37

*Age- and sex-adjusted to 1980 US white population, per 100 000 population. NR, Not reported.
Adapted from Brown RD et al. Incidence of transient ischemic attack in Rochester, Minnesota, 1985–198. Stroke 1998; 29: 2109–13, with permission.

Table 1.3 Average annual incidence rates of transient ischemic attack subtypes in Rochester, MN, 1985–1989

Subtype	Men* Rate	Men* No.	Women* Rate	Women* No.	Total† Rate	Total† No.	% of total
Carotid distribution (excluding AF)	41	45	37	75	38	120	59
Amaurosis fugax	12	13	14	24	13	37	18
All carotid	53	58	51	99	52	157	78
Vertebrobasilar distribution	20	22	10	21	14	40	20
Uncertain location	–	2	–	3	–	5	2

*Age-adjusted to 1980 US white population.
†Age- and sex-adjusted to 1980 US white population.
From Brown RD *et al*. Incidence of transient ischemic attack in Rochester, Minnesota, 1985–1989. *Stroke* 1998; 29: 2109–13, with permission.

Prevalence

Studies of TIA prevalence are more difficult and probably more inaccurate than those of TIA incidence [30]. Estimates of prevalence have varied widely but tend to run between 1% and 6% of different populations. As expected, prevalence has been shown to increase with age. Graphic representation of some estimated prevalence rates by age group can be seen in Fig. 1.1 [27,31–37].

Risk factors

A risk factor for a disease is defined as a characteristic of an individual or a population which indicates that the individual (or population) has an increased risk of disease compared with individuals (or populations) without that characteristic [30]. This implies, but does not establish, that the risk factor plays a causal role in the development of the disease (as the risk factor and disease may both be linked to a separate underlying cause). Knowledge of risk factors can help physicians predict a person's chance of developing disease and lead to risk factor modification.

Risk factors for TIA have been less well defined than those for stroke or ischemic cardiac disease for several reasons. A TIA is less disabling (by definition) than stroke or cardiac events; TIAs are less common than these entities, thereby hindering cohort studies; and TIAs are often elusive and difficult to classify for reasons discussed previously. Finally, it can be argued that risk factors for TIA are only important insofar as TIA itself is a risk factor for ischemic stroke, an important cause of disability and death.

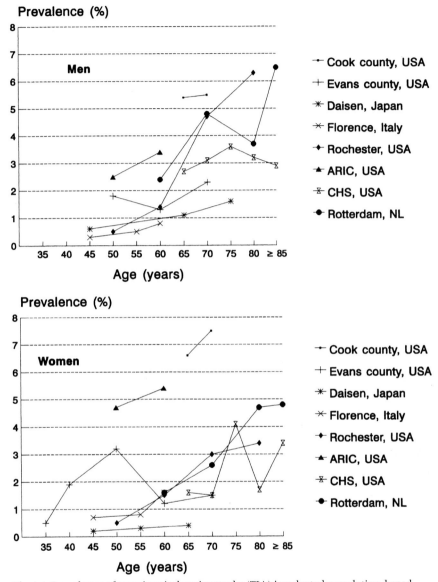

Fig. 1.1 Prevalence of transient ischemic attacks (TIA) in selected population-based studies among (a) men and (b) women. Reprinted with permission, from Bots ML *et al.* Transient neurological attacks in the general population. *Stroke* 1997; 28: 768–73.

However, while it may be true that TIAs alone are of little concern, by studying TIA risk factors one may be able to identify causal mechanisms which are preferentially found in the TIA population but diluted in a larger study of stroke. It is currently unknown whether the mechanisms causing TIA (cardioembolism, large vessel atherosclerosis, small vessel disease, etc.) mirror the mechanisms causing ischemic stroke in type or distribution. If these mechanisms and their associated risk factors differ, treatment and prevention strategies might differ for TIA patients, ischemic stroke patients without TIA, and the general population at risk of stroke.

Studies have not consistently identified differing risk factors between cerebral infarction and TIA. Atrial fibrillation was more common in stroke than TIA patients in some hospital-based studies, but this difference has not been documented in population-based studies and so it is possible that this reflects referral bias [9,38]. A population-based case–control study in Rochester found that the odds ratios for TIA risk factors such as ischemic heart disease, hypertension, atrial fibrillation, diabetes, and cigarette smoking were similar to those produced in an earlier study of ischemic stroke; lipid status, homocysteine levels, and alcohol intake could not be assessed [39,40]. In the Oxfordshire Community Stroke Project (OCSP) the only significant difference in risk factors for TIA and minor ischemic stroke was higher cholesterol levels in the TIA group [9]. Higher cholesterol levels were also found among TIA patients in a hospital-based referral study [41]. The role of cholesterol in stroke and TIA is complex, but one can speculate that higher cholesterol levels predispose patients to carotid atherosclerosis, and that carotid stenosis is a proportionately more common cause of TIA than ischemic stroke. Large vessel atherothrombotic stroke is more commonly preceded by TIA than cardioembolic or lacunar stroke, supporting this contention (see Table 1.4).

Table 1.4 Frequency of transient ischemic attacks prior to various stroke types

Series	Atherothrombotic cerebral infarct (%)	Embolic cerebral infarct (%)	Lacunar cerebral infarct (%)	Intracerebral hemorrhage (%)	Subarachnoid hemorrhage (%)
Harvard Stroke Registry	50	23	11	8	7
Stroke Data Bank	20	13	13	3	1
Lausanne Stroke Registry	29	30	14	6	

Adapted from Feinberg WM *et al.* Guidelines for management of transient ischemic attacks: from the Ad Hoc Committee on Guidelines for the Management of Transient Ischemic Attacks. *Circulation* 1994; 89: 2950–65, with permission.

Given the limited data about risk factors for TIA *per se*, it is reasonable to examine risk factors for ischemic stroke, where much more information is available. Well-established nonmodifiable risk factors for ischemic stroke include increasing age, male sex, positive family history, and race (blacks and Hispanics vs. whites in the USA) [42–44]. The increased incidence of stroke among blacks is due, in part, to a higher stroke burden in younger persons [45]. While some of this difference can be attributed to other risk factors such as hypertension and diabetes, a substantial proportion remains unexplained [46]. The incidence of stroke (particularly intracerebral hemorrhage) is higher in Asians than whites, but this may be more related to environmental and lifestyle factors than race.

Well-established modifiable risk factors for ischemic stroke include diastolic and systolic hypertension, cardiovascular disease, diabetes, cigarette smoking, significant carotid atherosclerosis, and (likely) hyperhomocysteinemia. TIA as a risk factor for stroke will be discussed in the section on prognosis. Within the realm of cardiovascular disease, atrial fibrillation, infective endocarditis, mitral stenosis, congestive heart failure, left ventricular hypertrophy and recent large myocardial infarction are established risks [47,48]. Much recent attention has been paid to less well-defined cardiovascular risks such as patent foramen ovale (PFO), atrial septal aneurysm, spontaneous echocardiographic contrast, valvular strands, mitral valve prolapse, and aortic atherosclerotic debris, but their role in stroke (and TIA) is controversial. For instance, in the case of PFO, case–control studies have shown a higher incidence of PFO in patients with stroke than in controls, and in patients with cryptogenic stroke than in patients with stroke of known cause [49–51]. However, control patients have not been randomly selected and evaluation may not be as aggressive for intracardiac shunts during their studies. Emerging evidence suggests that PFO may not be more common in stroke patients than the general population [52,53]. Other less well-defined stroke risk factors include oral contraceptive use, excessive ethanol consumption, illicit drug use, physical inactivity, obesity, hyperinsulinism, migraine, and hematological abnormalities such as antiphospholipid antibodies, elevated fibrinogen levels, and genetic defects in coagulation cascades [47].

The status of elevated total serum cholesterol as a risk factor for ischemic stroke is not clear. While elevated serum cholesterol plays a definite role in coronary artery disease (CAD), it has not been consistently linked to ischemic stroke in epidemiological studies [54,55]. Meta-analyses of cholesterol reduction with older agents failed to show any benefit upon stroke; conversely, in studies designed primarily for coronary artery disease, the newer 'statin' drugs have reduced rates of ischemic stroke [56–58]. The difference may be due to relative potency in cholesterol reduction [59]. Alternatively, there may be other class-specific causal mechanisms involved, such as stabilization of plaque components or antiplatelet action [48]. As with other preventative measures for stroke, the benefit of statin agents is modest, with an absolute risk reduction of < 1% per year in secondary prevention trials for CAD [59]. Low total serum cholesterol has actually been linked with increased risk of intracerebral hemorrhage [60]. Prospective studies of statins in secondary stroke prevention are underway.

Prognosis following TIA

The prognosis following TIA is an issue of vital importance to patients, their families, and the physicians providing their care. Such information helps determine the rate and scope of diagnostic evaluation for TIA patients, the mode and aggressiveness of their treatment, and the importance of TIA in the realm of public health. The value that patients assign to prognostic information on a personal level, even without treatment implications, should not be underestimated.

Like studies of TIA incidence, studies of prognosis after TIA would ideally be large, prospective, and population based. Such population groups will necessarily include patients receiving a variety of medical and surgical therapies, and thus will not provide true natural history data, which at this time would be impossible and unethical to obtain. Definitions again are important, because patients may be included or excluded from consideration based upon the nature of their symptoms, the methods of their treatment, prior history of TIA, prior history of stroke, or imaging abnormalities [61]. Statistical methods must be sound. In many studies stroke occurrence following TIA is expressed as subsequent strokes divided by the original number of enrolled patients. By ignoring non-stroke deaths (and thus patients no longer at risk of stroke), these studies will underestimate stroke risk. Occurrence of stroke and survival should therefore be determined with actuarial methods [62]. Adequate and reliable follow-up is essential.

A summary of prognosis following TIA is given in Table 1.5.

Community-based studies

Data on prognosis after TIA comes from the OCSP, which has reported on a population-based cohort of 184 patients with incident TIAs who were observed prospectively for a mean of 3.7 years [63]. Only one patient was lost to follow-up. At some point during follow-up, treatment included aspirin in 105 patients, warfarin in 15 patients, and carotid endarterectomy in six patients.

In this study the probabilities of stroke, death, and myocardial infarction were elevated compared with the general population. Risk of death at 5 years was 31.3%, with an annual risk of 6.3% and an overall risk ratio of

Table 1.5 Prognosis following transient ischemic attack (TIA) in selected studies

Study	Patients	Average annual death risk*	Stroke risk at selected time intervals after TIA					Average annual stroke risk*	Average annual MI risk*
			2 days	1 month	3 months	6 months	1 year		
Population-based									
Oxfordshire, UK [63]	184 TIA	6.3%		4.4%		8.8%	11.6%	5.9%	2.4%
Rochester, MN [62]	352 TIA	6.8%		7%		10%	13%	5.6%	
Hospital-based									
Johnston [70]	1707 TIA	2.6% at 3 months	5.3%		10.5%				
Hankey [68]	469 TIA	4.5%						3.4%	2.0%
Treatment trials									
Atrial fibrillation: EAFT Study Group [82]	592 TIA or minor ischemic stroke, NRAF, controls	9–12%						12%	
NASCET [77]	331 TIA or nondisabling ischemic stroke, 70–99% ICA stenosis, controls	3.2%						13.8% (any) 13% (ipsilateral)	

MI, Myocardial infarction; EAFT, European Atrial Fibrillation Trial; NASCET, North American Symptomatic Carotid Endarterectomy Trial; NRAF, nonrheumatic atrial fibrillation; ICA, internal carotid artery.

*Risks documented are arithmetic average annual risks.

1.4. Cardiac disease and sudden death accounted for 35% of fatalities, while stroke accounted for 31%. Stroke was more common than expected in the population, with a 5-year probability of 29.3% and a mean risk of 5.9% per year. Importantly, the danger of stroke was most notable in the first year, with risks of 4.4%, 8.8%, and 11.6% at 1, 6, and 12 months, respectively. The risk ratios for stroke compared with the general population were 13.4 over the first 12 months and 7.0 over 7 years. The risk of myocardial infarction was somewhat lower at 12.1% over 5 years, while the combined annual risk of death, stroke, or myocardial infarction was 8.4%.

In Rochester, outcome data from a large, retrospective, population-based study of incident TIAs [62] demonstrate findings in close agreement with those from Oxfordshire. The risk of death at 5 years was 34%, producing a risk ratio of 1.5. Cardiac deaths were again more common than stroke deaths (41% vs. 31%). Risk of stroke at 5 years (given survival) was 28%, with a mean yearly risk of 5.6%. The probability of stroke at 1, 6, and 12 months in Rochester was 7%, 10%, and 13%, respectively. This resulted in risk ratios of 101, 25, and 16 compared with the general population, again emphasizing the importance of the first months following TIA. The slightly lower early stroke risk in Oxfordshire may be a methodological artifact, as incident TIAs in their study were not necessarily first-ever TIAs, and there was an average 3-day interval between the index TIA and enrollment.

Other population-based studies have published prognostic data which are limited by smaller numbers or short follow-up period [17,22,34,64].

Hospital-based studies

Hospital-based TIA studies necessarily suffer from referral bias and thus are less generalizable than population-based studies. Hospital-referred patients tend to be younger and therefore less likely to suffer from atrial fibrillation and other comorbidities. They are often entered into studies longer after qualifying TIAs, thus selecting out patients who suffer strokes in the interim [65]. In contrast to the population-based studies discussed above, TIAs are not necessarily incident events, and prior stroke may be allowed. However, the information provided by hospital-based studies about selected groups can be quite useful.

Among prospective hospital-based studies with greater than 100 patients, annual risk of death over 5 years has ranged from 3.5% to 4.5% [66–68]. Illustrating the importance of methodology, the study by Heyman *et al.*, which reported a low mortality, did not include TIA patients with symptoms attributable to cardiogenic emboli or 'nonatherosclerotic etiology' or those who had EC-IC bypass. Two studies including patients with RIND found annual mortality rates of 2.2% and 5.9%, with no statistically significant difference between TIA and RIND patients in the former [10,69].

Risk of stroke in the two large prospective TIA studies reporting data was 3.4–4.5% annually (with the caveats previously noted) [66,68]. As in the population-based studies, the greatest risk of stroke came shortly after TIA. In the group reported by Heyman, a good deal of the initial risk was iatrogenic secondary to invasive diagnostic and treatment modalities. Annual stroke risks in the studies combining TIA and RIND discussed above have been calculated at 2.2% and 5.6% [61].

A large, retrospective, emergency department (ED)-based cohort study of TIA by Johnston and colleagues has evaluated risk of stroke and other adverse events following TIA, and potential predictors of stroke [70]. Among 1707 patients with TIA diagnosed in an ED of one of 16 California hospitals in a single health maintenance organization (HMO), crude (non-actuarial) stroke risk over 90 days was 10.5%, with half of strokes occurring in the first 2 days. Two hundred and sixteen patients (12.7%) experienced recurrent TIA, 44 (2.6%) were hospitalized for cardiovascular events (congestive heart failure most commonly) and 45 patients (2.6%) died. More deaths were due to stroke ($n = 20$) than cardiovascular events ($n = 9$). Adverse events, including stroke, recurrent TIA, cardiovascular hospitalization, or death, occurred in 25.1% of patients, with more than half of adverse events occurring in the first 4 days. Review of cases with questionable diagnoses identified 96 patients felt not to have had TIA but rather syncope, migraine, neuropathy, etc. Three had a stroke in the subsequent 90 days. Their exclusion from the larger group did not produce a different overall stroke risk. Among 182 patients lacking documentation of symptom resolution within 24 h of presentation, 19 (10.4%) suffered a stroke during follow-up. The number of iatrogenic strokes was not disclosed, although follow-up was terminated if endarterectomy was performed. Factors noted at the occurrence of TIA which predicted an increased risk of subsequent stroke included: age > 60 years [odds ratio (OR) 1.8], diabetes mellitus (OR 2.0), symptom duration > 10 min (OR 2.3), and weakness (OR 1.9), or speech impairment (OR 1.5) as a symptom of the TIA.

These stroke risk data do not markedly differ from those noted in large population-based studies. In Rochester the 1- and 6-month stroke risks after TIA were 7% and 10%, given survival. The figures were somewhat lower in Oxfordshire for reasons described. While the use of HMO ED patients presents some selection bias, it is probably less than for hospital referrals. The fact that prior stroke was not an exclusion criterion might reduce direct comparison with population-based studies, but is useful in its own right. Most importantly, this study has shown that the early risk of stroke following TIA is considerable. The conclusion that TIA patients often have cardiac conditions is also well known, but easily overlooked by neurologists and internists focusing upon the patient's presenting neurological symptoms. TIA is not a benign condition even in comparison with significant cardiovascular disease. In a case–control study comparing

280 TIA patients with 399 cardiac patients undergoing catheterization, the TIA patients were more likely to suffer from stroke or myocardial infarction within 3 years. The hazard ratio for death for TIA patients was 1.3 after adjustment for age, race, sex, and 'major cardiovascular risk factors'. Only the difference in all-cause mortality failed to reach statistical significance [71].

Whether this enhanced knowledge about timing of stroke risk and cardiovascular comorbidity in TIA patients can be translated into improved outcome through expedited medical or surgical management or screening is unknown. Future prospective clinical trials would be helpful in this regard.

Treatment trials

The exclusion criteria in TIA treatment trials are usually more strict than hospital referral studies, and necessarily more strict than population-based studies. In addition to restrictions set upon age and medical comorbidities, time lag is again important, with many patients passing through the window of highest risk before enrollment and randomization. The goal of treatment trials is comparison of treatment groups rather than general prognosis. Data are thus often presented as odds ratios and not actuarial survival or stroke rates. All of this limits the range of TIA patients to whom the resultant natural history data can be applied. However, the prospective, blinded, meticulous methodology of most treatment trials provides high quality information of great value to clinicians managing TIA patients of similar etiology.

Antiplatelet trials

Among antiplatelet studies, two of the largest trials using placebo were conducted in Europe. Each included patients with TIA or minor ischemic stroke.

In the United Kingdom transient ischaemic attack (UK-TIA) aspirin trial, 2435 patients were randomized to aspirin 300 mg once daily, aspirin 600 mg twice daily, or placebo [72,73]. Patients were over 40, had suffered their stroke or TIA within 3 months of randomization, had not previously experienced a disabling stroke, had not suffered a myocardial infarction within 3 months, and were not 'likely to experience adverse effects from aspirin'. Patients with cardioembolic mechanisms were included if they were not anticoagulated. Patients who 'might have difficulty with follow up, might comply poorly, or had severe intercurrent nonvascular disease' were excluded. In the European Stroke Prevention Study (ESPS) (I), 2500 patients were treated with aspirin plus dipyridamole or placebo and followed for 2 years [74,75]. Inclusion and exclusion criteria were similar to the UK-TIA aspirin trial but less explicit. Dropout rates in both trials were substantial. Among placebo patients, average annual rates of nonfatal stroke following TIA have been calculated at 4.3% (UK-TIA) and 6.1% (ESPS) [61]. In the UK-TIA trial, 25.9% of placebo patients suffered a major stroke, myocardial infarction, or death within 7 years. For placebo patients in the ESPS, the incidence of stroke or death over 2 years was 22.6%.

An overview of randomized trials has been published by the Antiplatelet Trialists' Collaboration [76]. Among patients with prior stroke or TIA who were followed for an average of 3 years, recurrent nonfatal stroke occurred in 600 of 5870 (10.2%) controls vs. 479 of 5837 (8.2%) patients treated with antiplatelets (nonactuarial). Using data from the Antiplatelet Trialists Collaboration consisting of placebo-treated patients in 12 trials, average annual rates of nonfatal stroke, nonfatal myocardial infarction, and stroke, myocardial infarction or vascular death have been calculated at 5.4%, 2.1%, and 8.7%, respectively [61].

Carotid stenosis

The risk of stroke following TIA ipsilateral to carotid stenosis has been investigated by the North American Symptomatic Carotid Endarterectomy Trial (NASCET). In the NASCET patients who had suffered a hemispheric (cerebral) or retinal TIA or nondisabling stroke within 120 days and had 30–99% stenosis of the ipsilateral carotid artery were randomized to antiplatelet treatment (usually 1300 mg/day of aspirin) or antiplatelet therapy plus carotid endarterectomy [77]. Among 331 medically treated patients with stenoses of 70–99%, the 24-month risks of ipsilateral stroke, any stroke, and any stroke or death were 26.0%, 27.6%, and 32.3%, respectively, all considerably higher than among surgically treated patients. Increasing severity of stenosis also correlated with increasing risk until the point of 'near occlusion', at which risk declined somewhat [78]. Medically treated patients with moderate stenoses (50–69%) enrolled within 180 days of their index event had 5-year rates of ipsilateral stroke and any stroke or death of 22.2% and 43.3%. Those with stenosis of < 50% had corresponding rates of 18.7% and 37.0%. Surgery provided a modest benefit for 50–69% stenosis but no benefit for < 50% stenosis [79].

A corresponding European trial of carotid endarterectomy has confirmed a benefit for surgery in patients with symptomatic high-grade carotid stenosis [80]. There was a lower stroke risk in the medically treated group than in NASCET (21.9% risk of any stroke over 3 years), but direct comparisons between studies are limited by methodological differences, including the measurement of stenosis.

The benefit from carotid endarterectomy for high-grade stenosis in the NASCET has proven durable. However, while untreated carotid stenosis continues to pose a risk to patients over time, especially compared with the general population, its effect becomes much less dramatic after 2–3 years [81].

Atrial fibrillation

The rate of adverse events following TIA or minor stroke in patients with nonrheumatic atrial fibrillation has been assessed in the European Atrial Fibrillation Trial (EAFT) [82]. In this study, patients with atrial fibrillation and TIA or minor stroke in the previous 3 months were randomized to open-label anticoagulation or double-blind treatment with aspirin or placebo. Patients with paroxysmal atrial fibrillation documented up to 24 months previously were included, while patients with other potential sources of cardiac emboli were excluded. Patients considered ineligible for anticoagulation due to uncontrolled hypertension, alcoholism, expected poor compliance, or other factors were randomized to aspirin or placebo and tracked as a separate group.

Among all placebo patients, the annual incidence of stroke during a mean follow-up of 2.3 years was 12% (vs. 10% in the aspirin group and 4% in the anticoagulated patients), considerably higher than for controls in primary prevention studies of atrial fibrillation [83,84]. The risk is also greater than that for undifferentiated TIA patients in population-based studies, although results are not directly comparable due to treatment effects in the latter group. Annual incidence of death in the EAFT did not differ between groups. Importantly, benefit in the prevention of primary events (primarily stroke) in the anticoagulant group persisted throughout the study and was not limited to the first few months.

Prognostic indicators

Amaurosis fugax compared with hemispheric TIA

Amaurosis fugax or TMB has traditionally been considered a more benign form of TIA than hemispheric TIA (cerebral ischemia). There is little population-based evidence on the topic. In the OCSP, the risk of death and/or subsequent stroke was lower in TIA patients than in those with minor ischemic strokes, but when amaurosis fugax patients were removed (32 of 184 TIAs), the difference became nonsignificant, suggesting a better prognosis for retinal symptoms [9]. Most referral-based studies have found stroke risk (often including retinal infarct) following amaurosis fugax to be lower than that following hemispheric TIA, with rates ranging from 2 to 4% annually in different populations [85–88]. Amaurosis fugax patients with high-grade (> 70%) ipsilateral carotid stenosis fare better than patients with hemispheric TIAs, although the outcome in this setting is still not benign. Among patients with > 70% carotid stenosis and first-ever TIA in the NASCET, 2-year ipsilateral stroke risks in medically treated amaurosis fugax and hemispheric TIA patients were 16.5% and 43.5%, respectively. In both groups over half of the risk came in the first 2 months. As seen in the larger NASCET analysis, stroke risk increased with increasing degree of carotid stenosis [89,90].

Among those with > 50% ipsilateral carotid stenosis managed medically, the 3-year risk of ipsilateral stroke was 10% in those presenting with amaurosis fugax compared with 20.3% in those with hemispheric TIA. With < 50% carotid stenosis, comparable 3-year risks were 4.1% in those with amaurosis fugax, and 10.3% in hemispheric TIA [90]. Patients who present with transient or permanent visual loss and have retinal emboli on fundoscopic examination appear to be at higher risk of stroke and death than the general amaurosis fugax population [91].

Embolic vs. thrombotic mechanism

TIA has been found to be one of several risk factors which increase the chance of stroke in patients with atrial fibrillation [92,93]. Patients with atrial fibrillation and a recent TIA or minor stroke have a relatively high long-term rate of subsequent stroke. How this applies to other potential cardioembolic sources of TIA is less clear. A study of patients with 'lacunar TIA syndromes' producing isolated motor or sensory symptoms involving two of three body divisions (arm/face/leg) concluded outcomes are better than for 'nonlacunar' TIAs [94]. Population-based, retrospective data comparing ischemic stroke subtypes have shown that a large vessel atherosclerotic mechanism predicts highest short (but not long) term stroke risk, while cardioembolic cerebral infarction is associated with the highest long-term death rates [95]. Similar data for TIA subtypes are sparse.

Anterior vs. posterior circulation

The probability of stroke following anterior vs. posterior circulation TIA did not differ in a population-based series from Rochester [62,96]. Other referral-based studies suggesting lower risk following vertebrobasilar TIAs are not comparable [62,96].

Imaging abnormalities

Several studies have considered whether evidence of infarction on a CT scan obtained during the evaluation of TIA holds any prognostic significance. Between 10 and 30% of such scans have been found to have an area of ischemia appropriate for the TIA symptoms [97]. While a hospital-based study has found shorter survival in TIA patients with infarct on CT (after controlling for stroke history and other covariates), other studies, including the OCSP, found no significant differences in recurrent stroke rate or mortality [97–99]. In the NASCET, patients with 70–99% carotid stenosis and CT evidence of cerebral infarction ipsilateral to their TIA were more likely to have higher degrees of stenosis, plaque ulceration, longer duration of symptoms, and hypertension than patients without infarction. After controlling for patient characteristics, ischemic lesions on CT were not associated with increased ipsilateral stroke risk [100]. An investigation of TIA patients using MRI showed that nearly half had abnormalities on diffusion imaging. Of those with diffusion abnormalities and follow-up imaging, half of those failed to show a corresponding infarct, suggesting a component of reversibility [4]. Another study utilizing MRI found that TIA patients with acute infarcts on MRI have a higher frequency of identifiable vascular or cardiac causes for their symptoms [5]. Whether MRI evidence of acute stroke in clinically defined TIA patients translates into higher risk of recurrent stroke is unknown.

Other prognostic factors after TIA

Other characteristics of TIA patients which have potential prognostic significance have been evaluated. Among large population-based studies, only hypertension and age have been found to be predictive of future stroke among TIA patients (OCSP investigators used univariate regression after controlling for age). Age and 'cardiac disease' predicted shorter survival in Rochester, while age alone was significant in the OCSP [61,62, 101]. Another Rochester population-based study of 330 patients with TIA during 1955–1979 evaluated several potential clinical and demographic factors predicting survival, and an increased risk of future stroke. Several interactions were noted to be significant predictors of survival after TIA, including: (i) age at TIA and gender (with younger women having the best survival), (ii) systolic blood pressure and congestive heart failuare (worst survival in those with low systolic BP and congestive heart failure), and (iii) calendar year of onset and diabetes mellitus (worse survival in those with diabetes, early in the period of study). Age was the only significant predictor of stroke after TIA [102].

The results of multiple regression analyses in hospital-based studies and treatment trials have been summarized [61]. The populations, goals and methods of these various studies are heterogeneous but age, vascular disease (particularly heart disease), and hypertension are frequently found to be modest predictors of stroke or death. Diabetes and male sex are less consistently prognostic. In the study of TIA by Johnston and colleagues, age, diabetes, long duration of symptoms, weakness with TIA, and speech impairment (dysarthria or aphasia) with TIA were independent risk factors for stroke [70]. Several prediction models have been reported, but these have not found widespread clinical use [61,103–105].

Trends in prognosis

Data from both a community and a hospital-based source suggest that the risk of death following TIA declined from the 1950s and 1960s to the 1970s and 1980s [101,106]. What accounted for this improvement (improved prevention, improved cardiac care, improved stroke care, socioeconomic changes among the elderly, etc.) and whether the trend continues is unknown. A thorough discussion of the methodological issues complicating predicting outcome following TIA is also available [107].

Epidemiology of cerebral infarction

Because TIA is so closely intertwined with ischemic stroke, a short discussion of the epidemiology of cerebral infarction is merited.

Incidence and prevalence

The annual incidence of first-ever ischemic stroke in the USA ranges from 127 per 100 000 whites to 246 per 100 000 blacks [42,45]. Ischemic stroke incidence rates among 45–84-year-olds in a variety of Western populations have been tabulated. With the exception of outliers in France and Russia, the rates are comparable, ranging from 262 to 349 per 100 000 [108]. Stroke incidence is substantially higher than TIA incidence. Some data suggest ischemic stroke incidence declined from the 1940s to around 1980 (unlike TIA incidence), after which time it increased slightly [42]. Other studies have not confirmed this finding [109]. Ischemic stroke incidence increases with age and is higher in men than in women.

The prevalence of stroke has varied significantly in different studies [110]. The most recently calculated prevalence rates of ischemic stroke in Rochester were 759 and 917 per 100 000 men and women, respectively [42]. It has been conservatively estimated that approximately 730 000 first-ever and recurrent strokes occur in the USA annually [45].

Ischemic stroke subtypes can be more easily defined than TIA subtypes. In the Rochester population-based studies, incident ischemic strokes from 1985 to 1989 were broken down by mechanism: large vessel cervical or intracranial atherosclerosis with > 50% stenosis, 16%; cardioembolic, 29%; lacunar, 16%; uncertain cause, 36%; and other, 3% [111]. In the black population large vessel stenosis may be a less important cause of stroke, although it has been suggested that blacks are at a higher risk of intracranial stenosis [112].

Only about 10% of strokes are preceded by TIA, although higher values are often seen in hospital-based settings with the potential for referral bias

[101,113,114]. The relationship between ischemic stroke subtype and TIAs is not uniform, with TIA more likely to proceed atherothrombotic infarcts than cardioembolic or lacunar infarcts [115] (Table 1.5).

Mortality and recurrence following cerebral infarction

In Rochester, risk of recurrent stroke following first ischemic stroke was 2%, 4%, 12%, and 29% at 1 week, 1 month, 1 year and 5 years, respectively [116]. The initial risk is somewhat lower than found after TIA, but comparable by 1 year. The 1- and 5-year recurrence rates were very similar in Oxfordshire [117]. Risk of stroke recurrence following first ischemic stroke did not change in Rochester from 1950 through 1979 [101]. The reason why very short-term stroke risk appears to be higher following TIA than cerebral infarction is uncertain.

Survival is slightly worse following first ischemic stroke than following incident TIA. Mortality rates at 1 week, 1 month, 1 year, and 5 years were 7%, 14%, 27%, and 53% in Rochester. In Oxfordshire, death rates were 10%, 23% and 52% at 1 month, 1 year and 5 years [118]. Survival following ischemic stroke improved over most of the twentieth century, but this trend may have ended [48,109,116,119].

Conclusions

Although transient ischemic attacks precede only 10% of ischemic strokes, they are an important indicator of risk for stroke, cardiovascular disease, and death. The current clinical definition of TIA is the basis of extensive epidemiological and clinical investigation and is still useful, although the boundaries between TIA and minor ischemic stroke have blurred with modern neuroimaging. Such distinctions can often be set aside in practical and research settings.

Methodological issues make the study of TIA epidemiology challenging, but its incidence appears to have remained constant through recent decades and falls between 31 and 68 per 100 000 persons. TIA incidence is markedly dependent on age. It is roughly equivalent between sexes, although age at occurrence is somewhat younger in men. The incidence of amaurosis fugax is approximately 13 per 100 000. TIA is quite common, as suggested by TIA prevalence of 1–6%.

Risk factors for TIA have not been as well defined as those for stroke. It is unknown whether the mechanisms causing TIAs mirror those causing ischemic strokes in subtype or distribution, but TIAs are more likely to occur before large-vessel atherosclerotic cerebral infarcts than lacunar or cardioembolic infarcts. In population-based studies, risk factors for TIA and stroke have been similar, with the exception of higher serum cholesterol in TIAs.

The prognosis following TIA is best determined from population-based studies. Among all incident TIA patients (receiving a variety of diagnostic and therapeutic regimens), average annual risk of death is 6–7%, with more deaths caused by cardiac disease than by stroke. Average annual rate of stroke is 5–6% over 5 years. Importantly, the risk is not uniform over time, with the greatest threat coming in the first days to months following TIA. Among TIA mechanisms, untreated atrial fibrillation and symptomatic high-grade carotid stenosis produce high risk of stroke. Fortunately, these conditions are often treatable. Amaurosis fugax has a better prognosis than hemispheric TIA, but when caused by high-grade carotid stenosis the prognosis is still far from benign. There is no apparent difference in prognosis between anterior and posterior circulation TIAs. CT evidence of ischemic infarction found during evaluation of TIA does not clearly change prognosis. This and other evidence suggest TIA and minor ischemic stroke are similar prognostically, especially if cases of amaurosis fugax are excluded. Prediction models to help stratify risk following minor stroke or TIA may be useful in clarifying those at highest risk of subsequent stroke.

The determination of easy and reliable methods to discriminate low- and high-risk TIA patients and the clarification of emerging TIA risk factors are important future goals in cerebrovascular epidemiology.

References

1 Stedman T. *Stedman's Medical Dictionary* (modified from) 27th edn. Philadelphia: Lipincott Williams & Wilkins, 2000.
2 Hankey GJ, Warlow CP. The evolution of the concept of transient ischaemic attacks of the brain and eye. In: *Transient Ischaemic Attacks of the Brain and Eye*. London: W.B. Saunders, 1994: 1–9.
3 Whisnant JP, Basford JR, Bernstein EF *et al*. Classification of cerebrovascular disorders III. Special report from the National Institute of Neurological Disorders and Stroke. *Stroke* 1990; 21: 637–76.
4 Kidwell CS, Alger JR, Di Salle F *et al*. DIffusion MRI in patients with transient ischemic attacks. *Stroke* 1999; 30: 1174–80.
5 Fazekas F, Fazekas G, Schmidt R *et al*. Magnetic resonance imaging correlates of transient cerebral ischemic attacks. *Stroke* 1996; 27: 607–11.
6 Bogousslavsky J, Regli F. Cerebral infarct in apparent transient ischemic attack. *Neurology* 1985; 35: 1501–3.
7 Koudstaal PJ, van Gijn J, Lodder J *et al*. Transient ischemic attacks with and without a relevant infarct on computed tomographic scans cannot be distinguished clinically. Dutch Transient Ischemic Attack Study Group. *Arch Neurol* 1991; 48: 916–20.
8 Wiebers DO, Whisnant JP, O'Fallon WM. Reversible ischemic neurological deficit (RIND) in a community: Rochester, Minnesota, 1955–1974. *Neurology* 1982; 32: 459–65.

9 Dennis MS, Bamford JM, Sandercock PA *et al.* A comparison of risk factors and prognosis for transient ishemic attacks and minor ischemic strokes. The Oxfordshire Community Stroke Project. *Stroke* 1989; 20: 1494–9.

10 Carolei A, Candelize L, Fiorelli M *et al.* Long-term prognosis of transient ischemic attacks and reversible ischemic neurological deficits: a hospital-based study. *Cerebrovasc Dis* 1992; 2: 266–72.

11 Dennis MS, Bamford JM, Sandercock PA *et al.* Incidence of transient ischemic attacks in Oxfordshire, England. *Stroke* 1989; 20: 333–9.

12 Leibson CL, Naessens JM, Brown RD *et al.* Accuracy of hospital discharge abstracts for identifying stroke. *Stroke* 1994; 25: 2348–55.

13 Kraaijeveld CL, van Gijn J, Schouten HJA *et al.* Interobserver agreement for the diagnosis of transient ischemic attacks. *Stroke* 1984; 15: 723–5.

14 Koudstaal PJ, Gerritsma JGM, van Gijn J *et al.* Clinical disagreement on the diagnosis of transient ischemic attack: is the patient or the doctor to blame? *Stroke* 1989; 20: 300–1.

15 Brown RDJ, Petty GW, O'Fallon WM *et al.* Incidence of transient ischemic attack in Rochester, Minnesota, 1985–1989. *Stroke* 1998; 29: 2109–13.

16 Sempere AP, Duarte J, Cabezas C *et al.* Incidence of transient ischemic attacks and minor ischemic strokes in Segovia, Spain. *Stroke* 1996; 27: 667–71.

17 Ricci S, Celani MG, La Rosa F *et al.* A community-based study of incidence, risk factors and outcome of transient ischaemic attacks in Umbria, Italy: the SEPIVAC study. *J Neurol* 1991; 238: 87–90.

18 Whisnant JP, Matsumoto N, Elveback LR. Transient cerebral ischemic attacks in a community. *Mayo Clin Proc* 1973; 48: 194–8.

19 Cartlidge NEF, Whisnant JP, Elveback LR. Carotid and vertebral-basilar transient cerebral ishcemic attacks. *Mayo Clin Proc* 1977; 52: 117–20.

20 Whisnant JP, Melton LJ, Davis PF *et al.* Comparison of case ascertainment by medical record linkage and cohort follow-up to determine incidence rates for transient ischemic attacks and stroke. *J Clin Epidemiol* 1990; 43: 791–7.

21 Terent A. A prospective epidemiological survey of cerebrovascular disease in a Swedish community. *Upsala J Med Sci* 1979; 84: 235–46.

22 Ueda K, Kiyohara Y, Hasuo Y *et al.* Transient cerebral ischemic attacks in a Japanese community, Hisayama, Japan. *Stroke* 1987; 18: 844–8.

23 Zupping R, Roose M. Epidemiology of cerebrovascular disease in Tartu, Estonia, USSR, 1970 through 1973. *Stroke* 1976; 7: 187–90.

24 Lemesle M, Madinier G, Menassa M *et al.* Incidence of transient ischemic attacks in Dijon, France. A 5 year community-based study. *Neuroepidemiology* 1998; 17: 74–9.

25 Feigin VL, Shishkin SV, Tzirkin GM *et al.* A population-based study of transient ischemic attack incidence in Novosibirsk, Russia, 1987–1988 and 1996–1997. *Stroke* 2000; 31: 9–13.

26 Anderson CU, Marquardsen J, Mikkelsen B *et al.* Amaurosis fugax in a Danish community: a prospective study. *Stroke* 1988; 19: 196–9.

27 Bots ML, van der Wilk EC, Koudstaal PJ *et al.* Transient neurological attacks in the general population. *Stroke* 1997; 28: 768–73.

28 Koudstaal PJ, Algra A, Pop GAM *et al.* Risk of cardiac events in atypical transient ischaemic attack or minor stroke. *Lancet* 1992; 340: 630–3.

29 Lemesle M, Milan C, Faivre J *et al.* Incidence trends of ischemic stroke and transient ischemic attacks in a well-defined French population from 1985 through 1994. *Stroke* 1999; 30: 371–7.

30 Hankey GJ, Warlow CP. Incidence, prevalence, and risk factors. In: *Transient Ischaemic Attacks of the Brain and Eye.* London: W.B. Saunders, 1994: 197–250.

31 Ostfeld AM, Shelleke RB, Klawans HL. Transient ischemic attacks and risk of stroke in an elderly poor population. *Stroke* 1973; 4: 980–6.

32 Karp HR, Heyman A, Heyden S *et al.* Transient cerebral ischemia: prevalence and prognosis in a biracial rural community. *JAMA* 1973; 225: 125–8.

33 Urakami K, Igo M, Takahashi K. An epidemiologic study of cerebrovascular disease in western Japan with special reference to transient ischemic attacks. *Stroke* 1987; 18: 396–401.

34 Fratiglioni L, Arfaioli C, Nencini P *et al.* Transient ischemic attacks in a community: occurrence and clinical characteristics. *Neuroepidemiology* 1989; 8: 87–96.

35 Phillips SJ, Whisnant JP, O'Fallon WM *et al.* Prevalence of cardiovascular disease and diabetes mellitus in residents of Rochester, Minnesota. *Mayo Clin Proc* 1990; 655: 344–59.

36 Toole JF, Chambless LE, Heiss G *et al.* Prevalence of stroke and transient ischemic attacks in the Atherosclerosis Risk in Communities (ARIC) Study. *Ann Epidemiol* 1993; 3: 500–3.

37 Mittelmark MB, Psaty BM, Rautaharju P *et al.* Prevalence of cardiovascular diseases among older adults: the Cardiovascular Health Study. *Am J Epidemiol* 1993; 127: 311–7.

38 Harrison MJG, Marshall J. Atrial fibrillation, TIAs and completed strokes. *Stroke* 1984; 15: 441–2.

39 Whisnant JP, Brown RD, Petty GW *et al.* Comparison of population-based models of risk factors for TIA and ischemic stroke. *Neurology* 1999; 53: 532–6.

40 Whisnant JP, Wiebers DO, O'Fallon WM *et al.* A population based model of risk factors for ischemic stroke: Rochester, Minnesota. *Neurology* 1996; 47: 1420–8.

41 Ueda K, Howard G, Toole JF. Transient ischemic attacks (TIAs) and cerebral infarction (CI): a comparison of predisposing factors. *J Chronic Dis* 1980; 33: 13–9.

42 Brown RDJ, Whisnant JP, Sicks JD *et al.* Stroke incidence, prevalence, and survival: secular trends in Rochester, Minnesota, through 1989. *Stroke* 1996; 27: 373–80.

43 Kiely DK, Wolf PA, Cupples LA *et al.* Familial aggregation of stroke: the Framingham Study. *Stroke* 1993; 24: 1366–71.

44 Boden-Ablala B, Gu Q, Kargman DE *et al.* Increased stroke incidence in blacks and Hispanics: the Northern Manhatten Stroke Study. *Neurology* 1995; 45 (Suppl. 4): A300.

45 Broderick J, Brott T, Kothari R *et al.* The Greater Cincinnati/Northern Kentucky Stroke Study: preliminary first-ever and total incidence rates of stroke among blacks. *Stroke* 1997; 29: 415–21.

46 Giles WH, Kittner SJ, Hebel JR *et al.* Determinants of black–white differences in the risk of cerebral infarction. *Arch Intern Med* 1995; 155: 1319–24.

47 Sacco RL, Benjamin EJ, Broderick JP *et al.* Risk factors. *Stroke* 1997; 28: 1507–17.

48 Wolf PA, Kannel WB, D'Agostino RB. Epidemiology of stroke. In: Ginsberg BJ, ed. *Cerebrovascular Disease: Pathophysiology, Diagnosis, and Management.* Malden, MA: Blackwell Science, 1998.

49 Overell JR, Bone I, Lees KR. Interatrial septal abnormalities and stroke: a meta-analysis of case–control studies. *Neurology* 2000; 55: 1172–9.

50 Di Tullio M, Sacco RL, Gopal A. Patent foramen ovale as a risk factor for cryptogenic stroke. *Ann Intern Med* 1993; 117: 461–5.

51 Lechat P, Mas JL, Lascault G. Prevalence of patent foramen ovale in patients with stroke. *N Engl J Med* 1988; 318: 1148–52.

52 Jones EF, Calafiore P, Donnan GA. Evidence that patent foramen ovale is not a risk factor for cerebral ischemia in the elderly. *Am J Cardiol* 1994; 74: 596–9.

53 George W, Petty GW. Personal communication.

54 Prospective Studies Collaboration. Cholesterol, diastolic blood pressure and stroke: 13,000 strokes in 450,000 people in 45 prospective cohorts. *Lancet* 1995; 346: 1647–53.

55 Iso H, Jacobs DRJ, Wentworth D *et al.* Serum cholesterol levels and six-year mortality from stroke in 350,977 men screened for the multiple risk factor intervention trial. *N Engl J Med* 1989; 320: 904–10.

56 Atkins D, Psaty BM, Koepsell TD *et al.* Cholesterol reduction and the risk for stroke in men: a meta-analysis of randomized, controlled trials. *Ann Intern Med* 1993; 119: 136–45.

57 Randomised trial of cholesterol lowering in 4444 patients with coronary heart disease: the Scandanavian Simvastatin Survivial Study (4S). *Lancet* 1994; 344: 1383–9.

58 Byington RP, Jukema JW, Salonen JT *et al.* Reduction in cardiovascular events during pravastatin therapy: pooled analysis of clinical events of the Pravastatin Atherosclerosis Intervention Program. *Circulation* 1995; 92: 2419–25.

59 Di Mascio R, Marchioli R, Tognoni G. Cholesterol reduction and stroke occurrence: an overview of randomized clinical trials. *Cerebrovasc Dis* 2000; 10: 85–92.

60 Yano K, Reed DM, MacLean CJ. Serum cholesterol and hemorrhagic stroke in the Honolulu Heart Program. *Stroke* 1989; 20: 1460–5.

61 Hankey GJ, Warlow CP. Prognosis, prognostic factors and prediction models of outcome. In: *Transient Ischaemic Attacks of the Brain and Eye*. London: W.B. Saunders, 1994: 251–300.

62 Whisnant JP, Wiebers DO. Clinical epidemiology of transient ichemic attacks in the anterior and posterior cerebral circulation. In: Meyer FB, ed. *Sundt's Occlusive Cerebrovascular Disease*, 2nd edn. Philadelphia: W.B. Saunders, 1994: 71–7.

63 Dennis M, Bamford J, Sandercock P *et al*. Prognosis of transient ischemic attacks in the Oxfordshire Community Stroke Project. *Stroke* 1990; 21: 848–53.

64 Terent A. Survival after stroke and transient ischaemic attacks during the 1970s and 1980s. *Stroke* 1989; 20: 1320–6.

65 Hankey GJ, Dennis MS, Slattery JM *et al*. Why is the outcome of individual patients with transient ischaemic attacks different in different groups of patients? *Br Med J* 1993; 306: 1107–11.

66 Heyman AWI, Ikinson WE, Hurwitz BJ. Risk of ishcemic heart disease in patients with TIA. *Neurology* 1984; 34: 626–30.

67 Howard G, Toole JF, Frye-Pierson J *et al*. Factors influencing the survival of 451 transient ischemic attack patients. *Stroke* 1987; 18: 552–7.

68 Hankey GJ, Slattery JM, Warlow CP. The prognosis of hospital-referred transient ischaemic attacks. *J Neurol Neurosurg Psychiatry* 1991; 54: 793–802.

69 Soelberg Sorensen P, Marquardsen J, Pedersen H *et al*. Long-term prognosis and quality of life after reversible cerebral ischemic attacks. *Acta Neurol Scand* 1989; 79: 204–13.

70 Johnston SC, Gress DR, Browner WS *et al*. Short-term prognosis after emergency department diagnosis of TIA. *JAMA* 2000; 284: 2901–6.

71 Howard G, Evans GW, Crouse JR *et al*. A prospective reevaluation of transient ischemic attacks as a risk factor for death and fatal or nonfatal cardiovasular events. *Stroke* 1994; 25: 342–5.

72 UK-TIA Study Group. The United Kingdom transient ischaemic attack (UK-TIA) aspirin trial: final results. *J Neurol Neurosurg Psychiatry* 1991; 54: 1044–54.

73 UK-TIA Study Group. United Kingdom transient ischaemic attack (UK-TIA) aspirin trial: interim results. *Br Med J* 1988; 296: 316–20.

74 ESPS Group. The European stroke prevention study (ESPS). Principle end-points. *Lancet* 1987; 2: 1351–4.

75 ESPS Group. European Stroke Prevention Study. *Stroke* 1990; 21: 1122–30.

76 Antiplatelet Trialists' Collaboration. Collaborative overview of randomised trials of antiplatelet therapy—I. Prevention of death, myocardial infarction, and stroke by prolonged antiplatelet therapy in various categories of patients. *Br Med J* 1994; 308: 81–106.

77 North American Symptomatic Carotid Endarterectomy Trial Collaborators. Beneficial effect of carotid endarterectomy in symptomatic patients with high-grade carotid stenosis. *N Engl J Med* 1991; 325: 445–53.

78 Morgenstern LB, Fox AJ, Sharpe BL *et al.* The risks and benefits of carotid endarterectomy in patients with near occlusion of the carotid artery. North American Symptomatic Carotid Endarterectomy Trial (NASCET) Group. *Neurology* 1997; 48: 911–5.

79 Barnett HJM, Taylor DW, Eliasziw M *et al.* Benefit of carotid endarterectomy in patients with symptomatic moderate or severe stenosis. *N Engl J Med* 1998; 339: 1415–25.

80 European Carotid Surgery Trialists' Collaborative Group. MRC European Carotid Surgery Trial: interim results for symptomatic patients with severe (70–99%) or with mild (0–29%) carotid stenosis. *Lancet* 1991; 337: 1235–43.

81 Paciaroni M, Eliasziw M, Sharpe BL *et al.* Long-term clinical and angiographic outcomes in symptomatic patients with 70% to 99% carotid artery stenosis. *Stroke* 2000; 31: 2037–42.

82 European Atrial Fibrillation Trial Study Group. Secondary prevention in non-rheumatic atrial fibrillation after transient ischemic attack or minor stroke. *Lancet* 1993; 342: 1255–62.

83 The Stroke Prevention in Atrial Fibrillation Investigators. Stroke prevention in atrial fibrillation. Final results. *Circulation* 1991; 84: 527–39.

84 The Boston Area Anticoagulation Trial for Atrial Fibrillation Investigators. The effect of low-dose warfarin on the risk of stroke in patients with non-rheumatic atrial fibrillation. *N Engl J Med* 1990; 323: 1505–11.

85 Poole CJ, Ross Russell RW. Mortality and stroke after amaurosis fugax. *J Neurol Neurosurg Psychiatry* 1985; 48: 902–5.

86 Hurwitz BJ, Heyman A, Wilkinson WE *et al.* Comparison of amaurosis fugax and transient cerebral ischemia: a prospective clinical and ateriographic study. *Ann Neurol* 1985; 18: 698–704.

87 Torem S, Rossman ME, Schneider PA *et al.* The natural history of amaurosis fugax with minor degrees of internal carotid artery stenosis. *Ann Vasc Surg* 1990; 4: 46–51.

88 Nguyen TU, Gans MS, Cote R. The prognosis of amaurosis fugax and hemispheric transient ischemic attacks. *Can J Ophthalmol* 1999; 34: 210–6.

89 Streifler JY, Eliasziw M, Benavente OR *et al.* The risk of stroke in patients with first-ever retinal vs hemispheric transient ischemic attacks and high grade carotid stenosis. *Arch Neurol* 1995; 52: 246–9.

90 Benavente OR, Eliasziw M, Streifler JY *et al.* Prognosis after transient monocular blindness associated with carotid artery stenosis. *New Engl J Med* 2001; 345: 1084–90.

91 Howard RS, Ross Russell RW. Prognosis of patients with retinal embolism. *J Neurol Neurosurg Psychiatry* 1987; 50: 1142–7.

92 Hart RG, Pearce LA, McBride R *et al.* Factors associated with ischemic stroke during aspirin therapy in atrial fibrillation: analysis of 2012 participants in the SPAF I–III clinical trials. The Stroke Prevention in Atrial Fibrillation (SPAF) Investigators. *Stroke* 1999; 30: 1223–9.

93 Gage BF, Waterman AD, Shannon W *et al.* Validation of clinical classification schemes for predicting stroke: results from the National Registry of Atrial Fibrillation. *JAMA* 2001; 285: 2864–70.

94 Landi G, Motto C, Cella E. Pathogenetic and prognostic features of lacunar transient ischaemic attack syndromes. *J Neurol Neurosurg Psychiatry* 1993; 56: 1256–70.

95 Petty GW, Brown RDJ, Whisnant JP *et al.* Ischemic stroke subtypes: a population-based study of functional outcome, survival, and recurrence. *Stroke* 2000; 31: 1062–8.

96 Hornig CR, Lammers C, Buttner T *et al.* Long-term prognosis of infratentorial transient ischaemic attacks and minor strokes. *Stroke* 1992; 23: 199–204.

97 Dennis M, Bamford J, Sandercock P *et al.* Computed tomography in patients with transient ischaemic attacks: when is a transient ischaemic attack not a transient ischaemic attack but a stroke? *J Neurol* 1990; 237: 257–61.

98 Evans GW, Howard G, Murros KE *et al.* Cerebral infarction verified by cranial computed tomography and prognosis for survival following transient ischemic attack. *Stroke* 1991; 22: 431–6.

99 Davalos A, Matias-Guiu J, Torrent O *et al.* Computed tomography in reversible ischaemic attacks: clinical and prognostic correlations in a prospective study. *J Neurol* 1988; 235: 155–8.

100 Eliasziw M, Streifler JY, Spence JD *et al.* Prognosis for patients following a transient ischemic attack with and without a cerebral infarction on brain CT. North American Symptomatic Carotid Endarterectomy Trial (NASCET) Group. *Neurology* 1995; 45: 428–31.

101 Whisnant JP. Natural history of transient ischemic attack and ischemic stroke. In: Whisnant JP, ed. *Stroke: Populations, Cohorts, and Clinical Trials.* Oxford: Butterworth-Heinemann, 1993.

102 Evans BA, Sicks JD, Whisnant JP. Factors affecting survival and occurrence of stroke in patients with transient ischemic attacks. *Mayo Clin Proc* 1994; 69: 416–21.

103 Hankey GJ, Slattery JM, Warlow CP. Transient ischaemic attacks: which patients are at high (and low) risk of serious vascular events? *J Neurol Neurosurg Psychiatry* 1992; 55: 640–52.

104 Dippel DWJ, Koudstaal PJ. We need stronger predictors of major vascular events in patients with a recent transient ischemic attack or nondisabling stroke. *Stroke* 1997; 28: 774–6.

105 Kernan WN, Viscoli CM, Brass LM *et al.* The stroke prognosis instrument II (SPI-II): a clinical prediction instrument for patients with transient ischemia and nondisabling ischemic stroke. *Stroke* 2000; 31: 456–62.

106 Howard G, Brockschmidt JK, Rose LA *et al.* Changes in survival after transient ischemic attacks: observations comparing the 1970s and 1980s. *Neurology* 1989; 39: 982–5.

107 Hankey GJ, Warlow CP. *Transient Ischaemic Attacks of the Brain and Eye.* London: W.B. Saunders, 1994.

108 Sudlow CLM, Warlow CP. Comparable studies of the incidence of stroke and its pathological types: results from an international collaboration. *Stroke* 1997; 28: 491–9.

109 Wolf PA, D'Agostino RB, O'Neal MA *et al.* Secular trends in stroke incidence and mortality. The Framingham Study. *Stroke* 1992; 23: 1551–5.

110 Terent A. Stroke morbidity. In: Whisnant JP, ed. *Stroke. Populations, Cohorts, and Clinical Trials.* Oxford: Butterworth-Heinemann Ltd, 1993: 37–58.

111 Petty GW, Brown RDJ, Whisnant JP. Ischemic stroke subtypes. a population-based study of incidence and risk factors. *Stroke* 1999; 30: 2513–6.

112 Woo D, Gebel J, Miller R. Incidence rates of first-ever ischemic stroke subtypes among blacks: a population-based study. *Stroke* 1999; 30: 2517–22.

113 Matsumoto N, Whisnant JP, Kurland LT *et al.* Natural history of stroke in Rochester, Minnesota, 1955 through 1969: an extension of a previous study, 1945 through 1954. *Stroke* 1973; 4: 20–9.

114 Sandercock PAG, Warlow CP, Jones LN *et al.* Predisposing factors for cerebral infarction: the Oxfordshire Community Stroke Project. *Br Med J* 1989; 298: 75–80.

115 Feinberg WM, Albers GW, Barnett HJM *et al.* Guidelines for the management of transient ischemic attacks: from the Ad Hoc Committee on Guidelines for the Management of Transient Ischemic Attacks of the Stroke Council of the American Heart Association. *Circulation* 1994; 89: 2950–65.

116 Petty GW, Brown RDJ, Whisnant JP *et al.* Survival and recurrence after first cerebral infarction: a population-based study in Rochester, Minnesota, 1975 Through 1989. *Neurology* 1998; 50: 208–16.

117 Burn J, Dennis M, Bamford J *et al.* Long-term risk of recurrent stroke after a first-ever stroke. The Oxfordshire Community Stroke Project. *Stroke* 1994; 25: 333–7.

118 Dennis MS, Burn JPS, Sandercock PAG *et al.* Long-term survival after first-ever stroke. The Oxfordshire Community Stroke Project. *Stroke* 1993; 24: 796–800.

119 Kodama K. Stroke trends in Japan. *Ann Epidemiol* 1993; 3: 524–8.

CHAPTER 2

Pathophysiology of Brain Ischemia

Jin-Moo Lee, Abdullah M. Nassief, Chung Y. Hsu

Introduction

The human brain is exquisitely susceptible to ischemia. Despite its relatively small size (less than 3% of total body weight) the brain receives up to 25% of cardiac output in order to meet its enormous metabolic demands. The brain has little energy reserves, and relies heavily on an uninterrupted supply of oxygen and glucose [1]. If blood flow to the brain is interrupted or critically reduced, compensatory mechanisms of limited capacity are available to preserve homeostasis and viability of brain tissue [2,3]. The assumption that neurological deficits manifest during an ischemic event are synonymous with irreversible brain damage fostered a generally passive and nihilistic attitude towards the management of cerebral ischemia [4]. Neurons and their supportive structures can remain viable under ischemic conditions for longer than had been historically believed [5,6]. Research over the past three decades has resulted in an unprecedented expansion of our knowledge of molecular and cellular processes that accompany or facilitate ischemic brain injury and has paved the way for the identification of biochemical cascades that advance ischemic neurons from dysfunction to death [7,8].

This chapter will begin with a discussion of hemodynamic changes in relation to the pathophysiological consequences in the ischemic brain, then examine our current knowledge of the cellular and biochemical mechanisms that underlie ischemia-induced neuronal dysfunction and brain injury following transient ischemic attack (TIA).

Pathophysiological thresholds of ischemia

Regulation of cerebral blood flow

Brain ischemia has been classically defined as cerebral blood flow (CBF) reduction of sufficient degree to result in symptomatic disruption of normal function [1–3]. Under physiological conditions, cerebral arterioles dilatate or constrict to maintain stable CBF despite variations in cerebral perfusion pressures (CPP, the pressure gradient between mean systemic arterial blood pressure and the intracranial pressure). This autoregulatory mechanism maintains an average basal CBF of approximately 50 mL/min per 100 g brain tissue in healthy subjects within a certain range of mean arterial pressure (approximately 60–150 mmHg) [9]. CBF can also be influenced by a number of factors such as systemic arterial oxygen content, blood carbon dioxide tension, pH, and hematocrit [10,11]. Regional CBF fluctuates in response to changing metabolic demands dictated by local neuronal activity. The coupling of regional CBF and oxygen metabolism is the principle underlying the application of positron emission tomography (PET) and functional magnetic resonance imaging (MRI) for mapping brain activity [12]. Factors that may regulate regional CBF in response to neuronal activity include nitric oxide (NO), prostaglandins, adenosine, vasoactive peptides, neurotransmitters [13–16], and energy metabolites [10].

Compensatory mechanisms in response to reduced CBF

In the face of reduced CBF due to thrombotic or embolic events, or systemic hypotension, autoregulatory vasodilatation is the first-line defense mechanism to restore and maintain optimal CBF. Compensatory vasodilatation may also occur in adjacent vascular beds, contributing to increased collateral blood flow to the ischemic region. Once maximal vasodilatation is reached and fails to meet metabolic demand, a second line of defense is recruited: the efficiency in extracting oxygen from blood is increased. Under physiological conditions, the fraction of arterial blood oxygen extracted by the brain tissue (oxygen extraction fraction, OEF) is relatively low (in the range of 30–40%); however, beyond maximal vasodilatation, OEF may reach as high as 90% before metabolic derangement ensues [17–19]. Thus, vascular response to abrupt reductions in CBF can be depicted to evolve at three levels of perfusion decrement (Fig. 2.1). The first level (normal range) is maintained by autoregulation and may be sufficient to meet the metabolic demands of a functioning brain if the CBF reduction is mild and transient. In the second level (oligemia), metabolic demand is met by increasing OEF beyond maximal compensatory vasodilatation, a more precarious condition at the brink of decompensation if CBF is not restored. The third level (ischemia) is metabolic derangement beyond maximal increase in OEF, leading to neuronal dysfunctional and possibly irreversible ischemic injury (see below). Based on a somewhat simplistic scheme of these three levels of perfusion decrement, it can be predicted that a transient and mild reduction in CBF may not necessarily result in cerebral infarction, but rather in temporary loss of neuronal function, as seen in patients with TIAs.

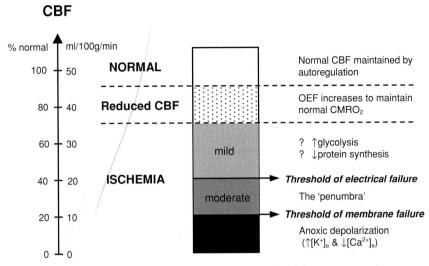

CBF

Fig. 2.1 Brain tissue response to reductions in cerebral blood flow (CBF) can be depicted to evolve at three levels of perfusion decrement. The normal range of CBF (approximately 50–55 ml/100 g per min) is maintained by autoregulation. With further decreases in CBF, oxygen extraction fraction (OEF) increases to maintain normal cerebral metabolic rate of oxygen consumption ($CMRO_2$) (oligemia), which may be sufficient to meet the metabolic demands of a functioning brain. In this range of declining CBF, energy requirements are increasingly dependent on gylcolysis, and protein synthesis decreases. Ischemia, the third level, is defined by CBF below which neurological deficits arise (approximately 20 ml/100 g per min), and coincides with the threshold of 'electrical failure', where the electroencephalogram flattens, evoked potentials are attenuated, and intracellular energy stores are depleted. Neurons experiencing this range of CBF may remain viable for a short period of time (penumbra), as long as they remain above the second ischemic threshold defined by 'ionic failure'. This CBF threshold at approximately 10 ml/100 g per min occurs at the point when normal ion gradients are reversed (anoxic depolarization), as reflected by increases in $[K^+]_e$ and movement of Ca^{2+} into cells, and defines the ischemic core. (Adapted with permission, from Astrup J, Symon L, Branston NM, Lassen NA. Cortical evoked potential and extracellular K^+ and H^+ at critical levels of brain ischemia. *Stroke* 1977; 8: 51–57.) 'Flow gradients' within a hypothetical ischemic stroke are shown on the left panel, depicting normal flow, oligemia, ischemic penumbra and core, corresponding to the shades of gray shown on the right.

Penumbra

Distal to the occlusion of a cerebral artery, the ischemic region does not sustain the same magnitude of flow reduction uniformly. The heterogeneity in blood flow within the affected vascular territory is due to variable degrees of regional neuronal activity, vascular reactivity, collateral flow and OEF increase. Based on neurophysiological and pathological conse-quences of ischemic insults, two ischemic thresholds have been proposed to define the boundaries of the 'ischemic penumbra' [4,20]. The first threshold (electrical failure) refers to a level of ischemia resulting in the loss of the ability of neurons to maintain normal neurophysiological activ-ity. The second and more severe ischemic threshold (membrane failure) entails the loss of neuronal ion homeostasis (Fig. 2.1). Neurons in the penumbra are thought to 'suffer functional but not structural injury' [20], but remain viable for only hours or days. This is in contrast to the 'ischemic core' which sustains a more severe degree of perfusion deficit, resulting in both electrical and membrane failure, and irreversible neuronal death within minutes to hours of ischemic insults. Timely restoration of blood flow in the ischemic zone may salvage tissue in the penumbra. The avail-ability of advanced neuroimaging methods promises to provide noninva-sive methods to delineate the penumbra [21–23], and are discussed in detail in other chapters in this volume (computed tomography and MRI, Chapter 5; PET/SPECT, Chapter 6). In patients experiencing TIA, the entire ischemic region may be considered penumbra; full recovery without residual brain injury may occur if reperfusion takes place within minutes to hours.

In the subsequent sections, ischemia-induced cellular events leading to functional changes in neuronal activity and cell death will be reviewed with attention towards ischemic thresholds.

Cellular events following vascular decompensation

Brain injury caused by cerebral ischemia is accompanied by a multitude of cellular events that may underlie the fundamental mechanisms of neu-ronal death. While neuronal death can occur in the setting of transient ischemia, many of the cellular events that have been linked to neuronal death have also been proposed to enhance brain tolerance against subse-quent lethal ischemia. The cellular events leading to ischemic neuronal death are therefore reviewed in detail here because of their relevance to the possible development of ischemic tolerance after transient ischemic attacks [24,25].

Metabolic derangement

The human brain, under normal conditions, extracts and metabolizes five times more oxygen (165 mmol/100 g per min) than glucose (30 mmol/100 g per min), indicating that the vast majority of the energy required for the brain's work is derived from oxidative metabolism [1,17]. This oxygen to glucose consumption ratio of approximately 5.5 indicates a relat-ively low basal production of lactate via anaerobic glycolysis. When OEF reaches maximum under ischemic conditions, cerebral metabolic rate of oxygen consumption (CMRO$_2$) falls [18]. If ischemia is mild, cerebral electrical function may be maintained despite elevation in brain lactate and hydrogen ion concentrations due to increases in anaerobic glycolysis [1,4,20,26]. At this stage, despite the capacity of tissue to temporarily maintain normal or near normal adenosine triphosphate (ATP) levels, energy production is compromised as reflected by declining tissue phosphocreatinine and elevated inorganic phosphate levels [27]. Indeed, metabolic acidosis, reflected by an early reduction in intracellular and interstitial pH, starts at a time when ATP levels are still relatively high [28]. The interstitial pH begins to decrease within 15 s after the onset of ischemia, with the intracellular pH declining to 6.5–6.8 [29,30]. Protein translation in general may be suppressed, but the products of specific gene families appear in abundance (especially the 'immediate-early genes'; see section on Post-ischemic gene expression, p. 50) [31,32]. When OEF reaches its maximum, brain tissue has little energy reserve to maintain neuronal function and is destined to develop electrical and membrane failure. Furthermore, these tissues are vulnerable to the secondary cellular events including massive release of excitatory neurotransmitters and electrical spreading depression (see below) (Fig. 2.2).

Electrical and membrane failure

Electrical failure
Cerebral blood flow reductions to 18–25 ml/100 g per min, below 40% of normal resting hemispheral CBF, result in slowing of the electroencephalogram, attenuation of the evoked potentials [33,34], and decline of the generation of synaptic potentials by individual cortical neurons [35]. The emergence of neurological deficit corresponds to this stage [36]. It is crucial to emphasize that tissue ATP levels may be normal or only slightly depressed at this stage of functional failure [27]. The exact mechanism(s) of this potentially reversible phemomenon is unknown but may reflect the susceptibility of certain neurotransmitter systems to even moderate hypoxia-ischemia and reductions in tissue pH [37]. The common occurrence of reversible neurological deficit in TIA emphasizes the paramount importance of duration as well as degree of ischemia in producing permanent tissue damage.

Membrane failure

Release of excitatory neurotransmitters and glial swelling
CBF levels needed to produce electrical failure, < 20 ml/100 g per min, parallel the experimentally determined CBF levels needed to produce massive release of excitatory amino acids (EAAs), glutamate and aspartate,

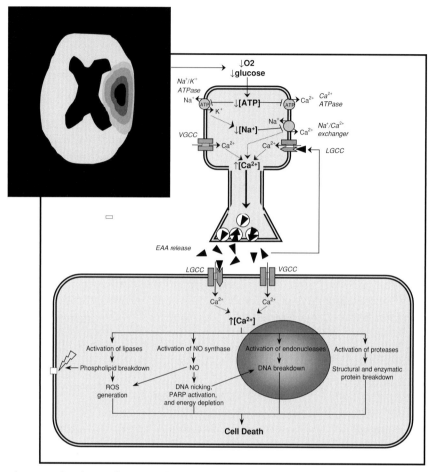

Fig. 2.2 Molecular mechanisms of ischemic neuronal injury. Decreases in cerebral blood flow (CBF) result in depletion of intracellular adenosine triphosphate (ATP), pump failure, activation of voltage-gated Ca^{2+} channels (VGCCs), with resultant increases in $[Na^+]_i$ and $[Ca^{2+}]_i$ (hypoxic depolarization). Large quantities of excitatory amino acids (EAAs) are released, activating ligand-gated Ca^{2+} channels (LGCCs) in postsynaptic neurons, and allowing influx of Ca^{2+} through both LGCCs and VGCCs. Elevated $[Ca^{2+}]_i$ is accompanied by activation of lipases, endonucleases, proteases, and formation of reactive oxygen species (ROS), resulting in the demise of the cell.

into the extracellular fluid (ECF) [38]. The CBF flow threshold for EAA release overlaps with the CBF threshold for early tissue edema formation (approximately = 20 ml/100 g per min). If reduction of CBF is maintained below these levels for approximately 30 min or more, astrocytes will swell, due to their uptake of osmotically active lactate and EAAs from the

ECF [39–41]. There is emerging realization that EAA release, and early edema (associated with moderate ischemia) can occur in tissue in which neither severe energy failure, gross disturbance of cellular ion homeostasis, nor sustained disruption of blood–brain barrier integrity have developed [3,39,40,42].

Calcium influx

The intracellular free Ca2+ concentration [Ca2+]i in neurons is much lower than the extracellular concentration. There are many factors that control the net [Ca2+]i., including Ca2+ influx through voltage-gated Ca2+ channels (VGCCs) and ligand-gated Ca2+ channels (LGCCs), sequestration in storage organelles such as mitochondria and endoplasmic reticulum, buffering by Ca2+-binding proteins, and active Ca2+ extrusion [43]. The expulsion of Ca2+ occurs via a high-affinity Ca2+-activated ATPase and a low-affinity Na+/Ca2+ exchanger, driven by the plasma membrane Na+ gradient. Ca2+ influx and the disturbance of Ca2+ homeostasis are important steps in initiating ischemic cell death. During moderate ischemia, neurons exposed to supraphysiological concentrations of EAAs admit Ca2+, probably through the LGCCs. There is strong indirect *in vitro* evidence suggesting that Ca2+ entry through the N-methyl-D-aspartate (NMDA) receptor-associated channels occurs at a magnitude of membrane depolarization substantially less than that required for Ca2+ entry through VGCCs. This supports the contention that there is a rank order for different routes of Ca2+ entry in the pathogenesis of ischemic injury.

Sodium influx

Following a mild elevation of [Ca2+]i, the Na+—Ca2+ exchanger uses the electrochemical gradient for Na+ to exchange extracellular Na+ for intracellular Ca2+. If cellular energy reserves are sufficient to extrude Ca2+, [Ca2+]i will remain stable and there may be no dire consequences of LGCC-mediated Ca2+ entry. However, excessive entry of Ca2+ through LGCCs can be devastating if neurons lack the energy reserves necessary to contain elevated [Ca2+]i [44] and remedy ionic derangement (see next section). It is likely that an increase in conductance through ligand-operated sodium (Na+) channels by EAAs contributes to excitotoxicity [43,45]. Events associated with increased sodium influx in membrane failure and severe disturbance of ionic homeostasis are detailed below.

Potassium efflux

As CBF reaches levels < 10–12 ml/100 g per min (approximately 20–30% of normal), deterioration of transmembrane ionic gradients ensues, defining the stage of ionic failure. If this level of blood flow is sustained for longer than 1 h, tissue death will occur [12]. ATP is completely degraded as a result of severe substrate depletion and the negative feedback of hydrogen ions at the phosphofructokinase step of glycolysis [19]. Electrophysiological recording from the ECF space detects striking elevations in the concentration of potassium ions (K+), marked declines in Ca2+, indicating Ca2+ entry into cells, and 'anoxic depolarization' [42,46]. Severe ischemia result in anoxic depolarization or rapid depolarization (−20 mV) of all neurons. The process of this anoxic depolarization is poorly understood; it may be the result of reduced intracellular ATP, with consequential inhibition of Na+/K+ ATPase activity and subsequent K+ efflux. These ionic shifts represent multifactorial changes in membrane permeability and the progressive failure of multiple energy-dependent membrane pumps and transport systems (e.g. Na+-K+-ATPase, Ca2+ ATPase, and the Na+-Ca2+ antiporter) that normally preserve the large electrochemical gradients crucial for membrane polarization [47] (see Fig. 2.2).

Maintaining the cell's resting membrane potential in a hyperpolarized state requires functional K^+ channels. The initial increase in extracellular K^+ ($[K^+]_e$) following ischemia is due to the activation of ATP-sensitive K^+ channels. In an attempt to compensate, astrocytes buffer this increase in $[K^+]_e$ by converting to anaerobic glycolysis and swelling, but the attempt by astrocytes to compensate is usually doomed to failure. Increase in $[K^+]_e$ in severely ischemic brain regions may aggravate ischemic injury through several mechanisms. First, high $[K^+]_e$ creates an electrophysiological change that results in the depolarization of neighboring neurons and may provide an important trigger for electrical spreading depression. This spreading wave of depression has been implicated in the extension of tissue injury beyond the region of severe ischemia, due to its ability to promote Ca^{2+} entry into vulnerable ischemic neuronal populations [48]. An ancillary action of rising $[K^+]_e$ is further release of neurotransmitters, especially EAAs. Second, increased $[K^+]_e$ may diffuse toward the cerebral microvasculature and stimulate the activity of Na+-K+-ATPase along the abluminal surface of endothelial cells, resulting in movement of intravascular Na+ and water into the ECF space. This may occur at a level of tissue oxygenation that alters parenchymal Na+-K+-ATPase activity, resulting in a net transfer of Na+ and water from the vasculature into neurons and glia in order to maintain intracellular osmolarity. To promote electrical neutrality, passive entry of Cl− and water occurs, resulting in 'cytotoxic' swelling [49]. Additionally, during ischemia gamma-aminobutyric acid (GABA) release occurs, further increasing Cl−influx [50]. Finally, extremely elevated $[K^+]_e$ may promote vasoconstriction, compromising residual blood flow to already severely ischemic regions [51].

There is evidence that Ca^{2+} entry into neurons via VGCC begins abruptly and massively when $[K^+]_e$ rises to approximately 10–15 mmol [42]. Other mechanisms to increase $[Ca^{2+}]_i$ include second messenger-mediated mobilization of Ca^{2+} from many high-capacity intracellular sites (e.g. phosphatidyl inositol activation), reversal of Na+−Ca2+ exchanger under conditions of cellular Na$^+$ overload, and passage of ions through non-specific 'leak' conductances that may develop across severely damaged cellular membranes. The resting membrane permeability is very low, and transient physiological elevations in [Ca^{2+}]$_i$ are usually rapidly reversed at the expense of metabolic energy by a number of regulating mechanisms and intracellular buffers. However, at the point where massive Ca^{2+} entry through VGCC occurs, the ability of cells to normalize [Ca^{2+}]$_i$ may be severely compromised, and true Ca^{2+} overload is established [50]. Elevations in [Ca^{2+}]$_i$ accompany and probably mediate major pathological processes described below [43].

Molecular mechanisms of ischemic cell injury

Energy depletion is one of the hallmarks of ischemic insults [52]. However, under certain conditions reversible neuronal dysfunction without permanent tissue injury can occur despite significant energy failure. The degree of ATP depletion may correlate better with initial neurological deficits [52] than the final outcome [47]. Protein synthesis, vital for cell survival, may be abnormal at degrees of CBF reduction well above the level needed to produce energy failure [32]. Moreover, brief periods of sufficiently severe ischemia can activate cell death signaling processes, leading to delayed apoptosis of susceptible neuronal populations long after restoration of energy stores [53,54]. In contrast, there is evidence that suggests the presence of many neuronal populations capable of withstanding periods of complete energy failure for as long as 1 h [55]. Finally, neuronal susceptibility to ischemia is determined by a wide variation in cellular expression of receptors and their interaction with certain neurotransmitters [56]. This susceptibility is also determined by other dynamic aspects of neuronal connectivity [57]. Thus, additional factors, independent of energy failure and disruption of ion homeostasis, must come into play to explain these experimental observations. The factors contributing to ischemic neuronal injury are reviewed below (see Fig. 2.2).

Excitotoxicity

EAAs, particularly glutamate, play a crucial role in both the initiation and elaboration of ischemic brain injury. Glutamate is believed to mediate anoxic and hypoglycemic hippocampal and cortical neuronal injury [58,59]. Exposure of neuronal cell cultures to high concentrations of EAAs produces a consistent pattern of structural damage: rapid swelling in cortical neurons—a reflection of increased permeability to Na$^+$ ions and passive influx of chloride and water—and later intracellular accumulation of Ca^{2+} as a result of massive entry through both LGCCs and VGCCs [60,61]. Excitotoxicity, a term first coined by Olney, represents the balanced effects of rapid osmotic disturbance and delayed Ca^{2+} loading [62]. It is now well recognized, however, that glutamate toxicity is far more complex than the simple induction of cation flux. Furthermore, the toxic potential of glutamate analogs may not correlate well with their excitatory potential *per se* [63]. Other mechanisms are believed to be crucial for glutamate and other EAA toxicity. These mechanisms include the production of the potentially toxic compound such as NO, generation of free radicals, and induction of changes in gene structure and expression [64–66] (see below).

The relationship between excitotoxicity and ischemic brain injury is appreciated at several distinct or overlapping levels. First, glutamate is released in supraphysiological quantities into the ECF space. Glutamate then gains access to a broad spectrum of cellular receptors. These glutamate receptors appear to occur temporally 'upstream' from insults leading to disruption of ion homeostasis, cellular membranes, and enzyme systems (Table 2.1). Techniques utilizing brain microdialysis indicate that massive release of glutamate into the ECF space begins when regional CBF is reduced to < 20 ml/100 g per min (40% of normal, CBF above the threshold for ATP depletion, membrane failure, and tissue autocatalysis) [38,67]. Declining cellular energy reserves, K^+ efflux and disturbed Na^+ gradients are thought to result in glutamate release into the ECF. This is compounded by derangements of metabolic function of glial cells leading to impairment of glutamate uptake and further increases in the extracellular

Table 2.1 Genes expressed after cerebral ischemia

Gene group	Representative gene products	Putative roles
Immediate early genes	Fos, Jun	Transactivate genes downstream of AP-1
Neurotrophic genes	TNF, BDNF	Neuroprotective Restore function
Cell death genes	Caspases	Execute apoptosis
Cell survival genes	Bcl-2	Cytoprotective
Receptor genes	Glutamate receptors	Modulate glutamate receptor function
Inflammatory genes	Cytokines	Enhance tolerance to subsequent ischemic attacks
	NOX2, iNOS	Mediate cell death
	Adhesive molecules	Facilitate leukocyte infiltration
Stress genes	Heat shock proteins	Neuroprotective Enhance tolerance
Angiogenic genes	VEGF, FGF	Promote growth of new vessels

level of glutamate [68]. Thus EAAs could be viewed as initiators of ischemic injury. Second, glutamate may be responsible for remote effects, the harmful waves of spreading depression in cortical tissues, from the site of its release [48,69]. The delicate balance of energy supply and demand may be compromised by enhanced neuronal activity caused by EAAs, depleting residual energy reserves under ischemic conditions.

Antagonism of many glutamate receptor subtypes can significantly reduce neuronal necrosis and/or infarct volume in animal models of focal stroke [70,71]. The NMDA receptor, one of three major subtypes of neuronal glutamate receptors, has been widely accepted to play an important role in excitotoxicity. This particular receptor subtype is thought to induce the influx of Ca^{2+} via a LGCC, triggering a host of Ca^{2+}-mediated or accelerated injuries [43] (see Table 2.1). Agonists of the NMDA receptor induce rapid entry of Ca^{2+} into neurons. In contrast, isolated application of specific agonists of the alpha-amino-3-hydroxy-5-methyl-4-isoxazole propionic acid (AMPA) and kainate receptors leads to delayed and less massive Ca^{2+} loading [72]. Moreover, strong evidence indicates that specific antagonists of the NMDA receptor protect cultured neuronal populations, with great efficiency, from lethal oxygen and glucose deprivation [58,72]. However, *in vivo* data suggest a limited role for NMDA antagonists in severe ischemia; this is in part due to down-regulation of these receptors as a result of a change in the local milieu, i.e. reductions in pH and energy charge [73]. It is quite plausible that these and other factors may account for the unmistakable fact that clinical trials of several NMDA receptor antagonists have thus far been disappointing [74]. NMDA antagonists have several serious side-effects, such as psychotic PCP-like reactions, myocardial depression, and formation of neuronal vacuoles and neuronal necrosis [75]. Thus, administration to humans of comparable doses of NMDA antagonists that were shown effective in animal models may not be safe. One approach to address this issue has been to focus on NMDA receptor subtype antagonists that promise to have fewer undesirable side-effects. For example GV150526, a selective inhibitor of the glycine site of the NMDA receptor, is free of circulatory and central nervous system adverse effects and has been put through extensive clinical trials [76,77]. Disappointingly, results from two Phase III trials of GV150526 showed no benefit for stroke patients, although the side-effect profile was favorable. The NR2B subtype selective antagonist, ifenprodil, represents a particularly promising agent, because of its use-dependent inhibition of NR2B receptors, increasing drug effect at overactivated synapses relative to normal synapses [78].

While much attention in the past has focused on NMDA receptor antagonists, more recently AMPA antagonists have been re-examined due to their ability to protect white matter. Classically, white matter was considered resistant to ischemic injury. Mounting *in vivo* data, however, seem to suggest that functional deficit after ischemic insults may be largely due to white matter injury in both the spinal cord [79] and the brain [80]. While the role of glutamate in gray matter injury is well established, its role in white matter ischemia is less clear. However, the role of the AMPA/ kainate glutamate receptor subtype in white matter injury has been recently described. *In vitro* and *in vivo*, activation of the AMPA/kainate receptor causes oligodendrocyte death [81,82]. Moreover, antagonism of this receptor subtype has been shown to selectively salvage white, but not gray, following ischemia in the rat spinal cord [83]. Clinical trials have begun with AMPA/kainate subtype receptor antagonists. These antagonists, through both Ca^{2+}-dependent and Ca^{2+}-independent mechanisms, are believed to exert neuroprotective effects in regions of severe focal or global ischemia [84,85].

Metabolic acidosis

Under ischemic conditions, tissues shift energy metabolism relying on glycolysis rather than oxidative phosphorylation, with detrimental consequences [26,42,86]. Administration of glucose to animals subjected to both global and focal ischemia tends to aggravate brain injury [87,88]. In ischemic brain regions, there is a direct relationship between lactate and hydrogen ion concentrations and glucose and glycogen stores [89], though it is not clear if acidosis *per se* or other aspects of glycolysis and lactate production are responsible for the observed exacerbation of injury. The complexity of tissue acidosis in ischemia is only beginning to emerge; not only does it denature enzymes and structural proteins, low pH produces cellular swelling. In order to cope with the sudden increase of osmoles in the brain ECF, glia absorbs large quantities of these osmoles and increase in volume. Enlarged glial end-feet encroach on their associated capillary walls resulting in impeded blood flow at the microvascular level [90]. Moreover, lactic acidosis results in the consumption of tissue bicarbonate, which in turn enhances iron-catalyzed free radical production and may add to secondary tissue injury [91].

Accumulating *in vitro* evidence seems to support a neuroprotective effect for low pH [92], thought to result from limiting Ca^{2+} entry via the NMDA receptor [93]. These observations may not necessarily be at odds. While supraphysiological acid production may contribute to the physical destruction of glia and endothelial cells in areas of severe ischemia, it may halt events that could lead to selective neuronal death in less severely ischemic brain regions. Under ischemic conditions the interactions between glucose concentration, brain energy metabolism, and tissue acidosis are remarkably complex and preclude universal recommendations. The current consensus, however, favors achieving euglycemia when managing acute ischemic events.

Activation of kinases and proteases

Sustained intracellular Ca^{2+} elevation triggers activation of catalytic enzymes, namely protein kinases, proteases, phospholipases, endonucleases, and others. Kinases are a large family of signaling enzymes that are involved in cell proliferation, differentiation and death. Their physiological role, however, is altered after both focal and global ischemia. The protein tyrosine and serine/threonine kinases, protein kinase A (PKA), the Ca^{2+}/phospholipid-dependent kinase C (PKC) and the Ca^{2+}/calmodulin-dependent kinase II (CaMKII) are rapidly activated during ischemia and may have mixed roles in the pathogenesis of ischemic brain injury. For instance, conflicting results implicating both neuroprotective and deleterious roles for PKC have been reported [94,95]. A recent focal cerebral ischemia study, however, using mice with genetic deletion of PKC γ isoforms, demonstrated increased infarct volumes compared with wild-type controls, suggesting a neuroprotective role for the γPKC [96]. Thus, subtypes of PKC may subserve different roles under ischemia.

Protein kinase B (PKB) (recently renamed Akt), a serine-threonine kinase, is activated by cell survival signals such as trophic factors. Akt is activated after phosphorylation to exert antiapoptotic action by inactivating a number of death signaling processes. Akt activation has been reported after cerebral ischemia and may contribute to the development of ischemic tolerance or reduce ischemic brain injury [97–99]. Another plausible mechanism of the antiapoptotic action of Akt is its negative regulation of mitogen-activated protein (MAP) kinases. Some members of the MAP kinase family have been implicated in mediating ischemic neuronal death. MAP kinase family members, including extracellular signal-regulated kinases (ERK1,2), p38 MAPK, and c-Jun N-terminal kinase (JNK), have all been shown to be activated following cerebral ischemia [100–104]. A number of recent studies have suggested the contributions of MAP kinase activation to ischemic brain injury [105–109]. The exact role of MAP kinase remains to be defined fully, as conflicting results have also appeared [110].

Another cardinal event following ischemia-induced increases in $[Ca^{2+}]_i$ is the activation of proteolytic enzymes, including calpains. Calpains, ubiquitously present in resting brain cells, play a crucial role in the degradation of various structural proteins, including microtubules and probably mitochondrial proteins [111,112]. Leupeptin and other inhibitors of calpain activity [113–115] have been shown to exert neuroprotective effects in both global and focal ischemia models. The blockade of downstream mediators of ischemic injury has the potential advantage of a longer therapeutic window. For example, the calpain inhibitor, MDL 28170, significantly reduced infarct volume even if administered 6 h after ischemia onset [115]. Activation of calpain is also thought to play a role in apoptotic cell death, a process involving the activation of another class of cysteine proteases, namely caspases (see below).

Activation of phospholipid metabolism

Phospholipids, which comprise a significant proportion of the cell membrane, play a crucial role in maintaining normal cell function. Degradation of membrane phospholipids constitutes an important mechanism in ischemic brain injury. When normal energy sources are reduced, the usual balance between anabolic and catabolic processes in cell membranes is reversed: ATP-dependent glycerophospholipid synthetic pathways are shut down, leading to accumulation of diglycerides and increase in Ca^{2+}-dependent membrane lipid catabolism [116–118]. Hydrolysis of diglycerides results in a 10- to 20-fold increase in tissue concentrations of free fatty acid (FFA), which leads to the disruption of cell membranes, affecting permeability to various ions, and decreasing local pH [119]. Arachidonic acid (AA), a particularly important mediator of injury amongst the FFAs, contributes to ischemic brain damage in several ways. During tissue reperfusion, AA metabolism results in the production of eicosanoids, catalyzed through cyclooxygenase and the oxygen-sensitive lipooxygenase pathway, which have complex effects on vascular reactivity, platelet aggregation, leukocyte adhesion, and blood–brain barrier permeability [116]. In addition, the lipooxygenase pathway of AA metabolism results in the increased production of leukotrienes, especially after ischemia reperfusion, affecting broad changes in the permeability of microvascular endothelium and facilitating edema formation [116,117].

There are two types of cyclooxygenases that catalyze prostaglandin formation from AA. The inducible form, COX-2, is of particular relevance to ischemic brain injury. In focal ischemia, transient COX-2 expression occurs in cortical neurons that are at high risk of dying after focal brain ischemia [120]. COX-2 activation leads to increased formation of not only prostaglandin synthesis but also oxygen free radicals [121], and has been directly linked to the pathogenesis of NMDA receptor-mediated neurotoxicity in mixed cortical cell culture [122]. COX-2 activation is thought to occur secondary to post-ischemic activation of proinflammatory transcription factor, NF-κB and its downstream including cytokines and inducible nitric oxide synthase (iNOS) expression [123,124]. (See also section on Post-ischemic inflammatory reaction below, p. 51.)

Reactive oxygen species

The role of reactive oxygen species (ROS) in the pathogenesis of ischemic brain injury has been known for many years. However, it is becoming increasingly clear that ROS tend to populate the perimeter of ischemic brain regions and following reperfusion [125]. ROS, byproducts of AA metabolism and polymorphonuclear leukocyte invasion, accumulate in tissues where Ca^{2+} overload is established, lipolysis is advanced, and secondary vascular injury is underway. Theoretically, ROS may appear at early stages of tissue injury through several pathways. First, under conditions of moderate ischemia, ROS may accumulate when the efficiency of aerobic glycolysis is compromised by the limited availability of molecular oxygen as a final acceptor of electrons within the mitochondria [125]. Second, the formation of ROS is enhanced by the breakdown of metabolites of ATP through the xanthine oxidase pathway. This process is markedly enhanced by the Ca^{2+}-dependent activation of proteolytic enzymes, which, in turn, catalyze the conversion of xanthine dehydrogenase to xanthine oxidase. The breakdown of adenine nucleotides via xanthine oxidase yields superoxide and hydrogen peroxide as byproducts, and the quantity of these ROS will be greatest in tissues with some capacity for ATP regeneration and turnover [125].

Another source of ROS in the ischemic brain is via NOS, an enzyme generating the weak ROS NO, which exists in three different isoforms. Neuronal NOS (nNOS or Type I NOS), a Ca^{2+} calmodulin-dependent enzyme, is likely to be activated immediately downstream of NMDA receptor activation; iNOS (or Type II NOS) is expressed in macrophages, neutrophils, and microglia, and is activated upon immune activation or in inflammation and is thought to contribute to delayed injury following ischemia. Excessive NO can directly inhibit important enzymes needed for vital cellular functions such as energy metabolism and DNA synthesis. The detrimental effects of NO are believed to be due to its affinity for iron and thiol groups [126,127]. NO may also result in ROS generation by forming the powerful oxidant, peroxynitrite ($ONOO^-$), which is capable of generating cytotoxic hydroxyl radicals [65]. Recent data from mutant mice with deletions of the gene encoding the three isoforms of NOS suggest that NO generated by nNOS and iNOS under ischemic conditions may be neurotoxic, whereas that synthesized by the third isoform, endothelial NOS (eNOS or Type III NOS) may protect brain tissue by improving blood flow and exerting antithrombotic actions [65,66,128–130]. Not all effects of NO are cytotoxic. Some of the salutary effects could be related to the interaction of NO with glutathione to form S-nitrosoglutathione (GSNO), a highly potent antioxidant that may protect neurons against oxidative stress [131]. GSNO is probably generated in the endothelial and astroglial cells during oxidative stress and is transferred to neurons, where it neutralizes free radicals via its c-GMP-independent nitrosylation actions [132].

ROS generated under ischemic conditions assail a wide variety of macromolecules, including enzymes and nucleic acids [66,125], and are involved in the demise of multiple cell types. ROS formation may be the final pathway of numerous damaging processes that seem to induce many aspects of ischemic microvascular injury. ROS may destroy naturally occurring antioxidant activities, and affect ATP-dependent DNA repair, resulting in further reductions in already scarce energy reserves [66].

A unique link between the microenvironment of focal ischemia and the generation of ROS comes from the observation that both the reduction of ferric to ferrous iron under acidic conditions and the release of iron from organic stores—delocalization—greatly enhance ROS production [125]. Delocalized iron catalyzes the Haber–Weiss reaction, which in turn converts short-lived and weakly reactive superoxide anions and hydrogen peroxide to highly toxic hydroxyl radicals. The accumulation of lactate, hydrogen ions, and free iron under conditions of ischemia greatly facilitates ROS-induced injury and may promote severe vasogenic edema that can accompany reperfusion [125].

Ischemic neuronal death

Necrosis or apoptosis?

It seems intuitive that brain cells dying after hypoxic-ischemic insult would undergo necrosis, a 'violent' form of cell death associated with swelling of the cell and internal organelles, plasma membrane failure, and ultimately release of genetic material and other proinflammatory cellular contents [133]. Indeed, the implication of excitotoxicity as an important mechanism of ischemic cell injury is consistent with that notion. As discussed above, overstimulation of glutamate receptors resulting in influx of Na^+, Ca^{2+} through ligand- and voltage-gated calcium channels with attendant Cl^- and water entry leads to cell swelling. Furthermore, Ca^{2+} overload induces a diverse array of lethal metabolic derangements and activation of proteases resulting in cell membrane disruption and death, consistent with necrosis. Despite this intuitive link between ischemia and necrosis, growing evidence indicates that after ischemic insult at least some cells may die by an alternative form of cell death, apoptosis, especially if ischemia is mild and transient.

Apoptosis

Apoptosis is the end-result of a more 'altruistic' form of cell death, associated with activation of a specific genetic program resulting in the orderly dismantling of the cell. First described based on morphological criteria, apoptosis was characterized by chromatin condensation and margination in the nucleus, cell and internal organelle shrinkage, and cellular fragmentation resulting in membrane-bound vesicles (apoptotic bodies)

[134]. Intense investigation over the past decade has yielded important insights into the molecular mechanisms underlying apoptosis, providing unique molecular signatures and tools to evaluate cell death in physiological and pathophysiological conditions.

The importance of mitochondria in regulating apoptotic cell death is becoming increasingly recognized [135]. It is the outer mitochondrial membrane that provides the critical regulatory checkpoint, mediated by a group of proteins encoded by the *bcl-2* family of genes, so named by association with human B-cell lymphoma [136]. Members of this family can be classified into antiapoptotic genes (including *bcl-2* and *bcl-xl*) and proapoptotic genes (including *bax, bak, bik,* and *bid*) [137]. The protein products of these opposing groups of genes interact on the outer mitochondrial membrane, through a process that is currently poorly understood, to regulate release of the electron carrier cytochrome c from the intramembranous compartment [138]. Once in the cytoplasm, cytochrome c interacts with another apoptosis regulator, Apaf-1, and dATP to form the 'apoptosome' complex, which activates the effector arm of the apoptotic cascade carried out by a class of cysteine proteases termed caspases [139]. In some cells, caspases can also be activated through an alternate route, independent of mitochondrial regulation, via cell surface death receptors comprising the tumour necrosis factor (TNF) superfamily. These receptors, stimulated by various ligands including fas ligand (fasL, or CD95-L or APO-1-L) and TNF-related apoptosis-inducing ligand (TRAIL), directly lead to the activation of the caspase cascade [140]. Additionally, there is evidence that another caspase-independent pathway for apoptosis may exist through mitochondrial release of apoptosis-inducing factor (AIF) [141].

The caspase family includes over a dozen proteases with sequence homology, but each caspase targets unique amino acid sequences for enzymatic cleavage. Most of the caspases (e.g. caspases-2, -3, -6, -7, -8, -9, -10) appear to be exclusively involved in apoptosis, while others (caspase-1 and -11) play a role in the inflammatory cascade. Under conditions that do not promote apoptosis (or inflammation), this family of enzymes exists in a procaspase form [142]. Upon activation via the apoptosome complex [139] or directly through the receptor-mediated pathway [140], apical procaspases (including caspase-8 or -9) are autocatalytically cleaved, initiating a cascade of proteolytic activation of downstream effector caspases including caspase-3, -6, and -7 [143,144]. These effector caspases, in turn, proteolytically activate other enzymes which mediate cleavage of proteins vital to the survival of the cell. For example, caspase-3 proteolytically inactivates the inhibitory subunit of caspase-activated DNase (CAD) [145], resulting in internucleosomal DNA cleavage; proteolysis of nuclear laminins results in nuclear shrinkage [146]; and cleavage of cytoskeletal proteins results in loss of cell structure [147], resulting in cell morphologies characteristic of apoptosis.

Evidence for apoptosis in brain ischemia

Classic cell morphologies associated with apoptosis are not prominent in ischemic brain cell death; cells dying after ischemia have features of necrosis [148,149]. However, there is a growing consensus fueled by biochemical, pharmacological, and genetic studies that suggest that ischemia can trigger the parallel occurrence of both necrosis and apoptosis. Some of the earliest biochemical evidence supporting a role for apoptosis included the demonstration of internucleosomal DNA fragmentation resulting in a 'DNA-ladder' pattern on agarose gel electrophoresis following global and focal ischemia [150,151], and by TdT-mediated biotinylated dUTP nick end-labeling (TUNEL) of nuclei *in situ* [150,152]. These early biochemical characteristics have since been shown to exist in cells undergoing necrosis as well [153], and thus other criteria for distinguishing apoptosis from necrosis have been used. Several molecular signatures closely associated with apoptosis have been found in the ischemic brain. For example, increased expression of the antiapoptotic genes *bcl-2*, *bcl-x* and *bcl-2* was demonstrated in neurons that survived focal ischemia [154–156], while increased expression of the proapoptotic gene *bax* was found selectively in dying hippocampal CA1 neurons, following transient global ischemia [157]. In addition, translocation of cytochrome c [158] from mitochondria to cytosol, and activation of caspase-3 [159] have been reported following transient focal ischemia in rats.

More convincing evidence that apoptosis participates in ischemic brain cell death comes from experiments that demonstrate neuroprotection after interrupting unique apoptotic pathways. Overexpression of antiapoptotic *bcl-2* by transgenic approaches [160] or by viral vector [161] reduced infarct volume in a mouse model of focal stroke. Likewise, transgenic overexpression of $bcl-x_L$ reduced infarct volume after permanent focal ischemia in mice. Inhibition of caspase-3 activity, by intracerebroventricular (icv) injection of the relatively nonselective caspase-3 inhibitor, *N*-benzyloxycarbonyl-Asp(OMe)-Glu(OMe)-Val-Asp(OMe)-fluoromethylketone (z-DEVD.FMK), also reduced infarct size following transient focal ischemia in rats [162]. The pan-caspase inhibitor, boc-aspartyl(OMe)-fluoromethylketone (BAF), given icv or systemically, dramatically reduced infarction in a neonatal rat model of hypoxia-ischemia [163], raising the possibility that broad-spectrum inhibition of all caspases may be more effective than selective inhibitors. Another approach to blocking caspase activity was demonstrated by virally mediated overexpression of the X chromosome-linked inhibitor of apoptosis protein (XIAP) which markedly reduced the death of CA1 hippocampal neurons following transient global ischemia in rats [164].

More recently, accumulating evidence indicates that apoptosis triggered through the death receptors pathway may play a prominent role in ischemic brain injury. It has been known for some time that the death receptors and their ligands were up-regulated after cerebral ischemia [165–168]. Transient focal ischemia in *lpr* mice, with dysfunctional fasL receptors (fas), results in smaller infarcts than their wild-type counterparts [169]. Moreover, individual gene deletions of the ligands, FasL (*gld* mice) and TNF (TNF knockout mice), resulted in smaller infarcts following transient focal ischemia; combined gene deletions virtually eliminated injury [170]. It is likely that the neuroprotective effects reflected antiapoptotic as well as anti-inflammatory mechanisms. However, the effects of TNF following ischemia remain somewhat puzzling, as rather surprisingly, mice lacking TNF receptors developed larger infarcts than wild-type controls [171]. Dual roles in injury and recovery have been proposed [172].

Apoptosis following TIA?

Apoptosis following ischemia is an intriguing concept, especially as it relates to the phenomenon of delayed cell death after very brief ischemia, and may potentially be relevant to human TIA. Cultured cortical neurons exposed to high concentrations of a variety toxic insults (NMDA, oxidative stress) typically die by necrosis. However, when exposed to relatively short durations or low concentrations, these very same insults induced delayed cell death with prominent features of apoptosis [173]. Likewise *in vivo*, very brief periods of ischemia (15–30 min of middle cerebral artery (MCA) occlusion) in rats, induced small infarcts developing over a period of weeks; progressively longer periods of ischemia resulted in faster evolution of larger infarcts [174]. The very delayed infarction of brain tissue demonstrated features of apoptosis, including DNA fragmentation, TUNEL staining, sensitivity to inhibitors of apoptosis such as cycloheximide [54] or z-DEVD.FMK [164,175]. One may speculate that although neurological deficits may not be detectable after TIA, brain injury may occur through a predominantly apoptotic mechanism. In a similar fashion, many have speculated that necrosis may predominate in the ischemic core, but that apoptosis may find a greater contribution at the periphery, in the ischemic penumbra [8].

Secondary ischemic events

Because of the frequent reversal of arterial occlusion (e.g. spontaneous recanalization of the occluded vessel or compensatory mechanisms described above, especially an increase in collateral flow), ischemia may be followed by partial or even full restoration of blood flow to the ischemic region. Reperfusion of ischemic tissue in a timely manner may prevent irreversible tissue injury; however, delayed reperfusion may contribute to secondary ischemic injury. Key events that have been noted upon reperfusion are briefly reviewed below.

Reperfusion hyperemia

After prolonged ischemia, prompt reconstitution of blood flow may lead to hyperemia, in part due to accumulation of vasodilatating substances such as K^+, hydrogen ions, CO_2, adenosine, and prostacyclin during ischemia. As a result, large increases in CBF frequently follow reperfusion [94,176]. Blood flow to reperfused brain often greatly exceeds the substrate demands of the tissue, resulting in so-called luxury perfusion [14], and may be beneficial. Re-established flow may bring substrates to marginal tissues and remove damaging metabolites produced during ischemia. However, the return of blood flow can paradoxically produce progressive destruction of brain tissues through delivery of large quantities of oxygen to a biochemical environment primed to produce large quantities of potentially harmful AA metabolites and ROS leading to further tissue damage and swelling [57,177–179]. AA metabolites and ROS increase endothelial leukocyte adhesion and permeability, and promote vasogenic edema [178]. Later events involving post-ischemic inflamation and angiogenesis may also affect the restoration of blood flow to the ischemic regions (see below).

Post-ischemic gene expression

Ischemia is a potent modulator of gene expression [180–182]. The first groups of genes, expressed within minutes of cerebral ischemia (immediate early genes) [183], largely code for transcription factors. Massive increases in transcription activity have been noted after cerebral ischemia and a large number of major transcription factors have shown to be activated. Included among these factors are activated protein-1 (AP-1) [183], nuclear factor kappa-beta (NF-κB) [184], hypoxia-inducible factor (HIF) [185], cyclic AMP response element binding protein (CREB) [186], antioxidant/electrophilic response element (ARE) [187], aryl hydro-carbon receptor nuclear translocator 2 (ARNT2) [188], Stat1 [189], Stat3 [190], and SP-1 [191]. The exact role of transcription factors in the ischemic brain remains to be defined. Using NF-κB as an example, both beneficial [192] and detrimental [193] effects have been demonstrated under ischemic conditions. Indeed, it is likely that these factors have multiple roles. Activation of AP-1 and NF-κB also contributes to the post-ischemic inflammatory reaction (see below).

Transcription factors are capable of transactivating multiple down-stream genes that may play major roles in determining the ultimate fate of neurons in the ischemic brain. To implicate specific gene candidates in neuronal injury or recovery from ischemic insults has proven difficult. Varying genetic heterogeneity among animals used for stroke research and the robust changes in gene expression in different cell types over time have confounded interpretation of published results. Recent application of differential display and DNA microarray techniques has led to preliminary studies to assess global gene expression profiles [194]. Completion of human and mouse genome projects and the refinement of DNA microarray and proteomics technology, allowing a large number of genes or proteins to be screened at the same time, may offer a powerful tool in obtaining a comprehensive picture of post-ischemic gene expression in the future to facilitate the delineation of the specific role each gene may play in ischemia [182]. At the present, genes that are transactivated after cerebral ischemia can be grossly categorized into five classes (Table 2.1). Some of these genes have been implicated in the pathogenesis of ischemic neuronal cell death (e.g. caspase genes) or alteration of neurotransmitter receptor responsiveness [195]. Others are expressed as an endogenous defense mechanism to maintain cell viability (e.g. nerve growth factor, Bcl-2, heat shock proteins). There are a large number of genes that may be involved in the development of brain tolerance to sublethal ischemia in preconditioning paradigms (see Brain tolerance to ischemia, p. 53).

Post-ischemic inflammatory reaction

Tissue injury following cerebral ischemia-reperfusion may be exacerbated by post-ischemic inflammatory responses. Most of these inflammatory responses appear to be mediated by various cytokines produced by endothelial cells, microglia, astrocytes, leukocytes, and even neurons. Cerebral ischemia induces many proinflammatory genes by activating transcription factors, such as NF-κB [193], AP-1 [196,197], hypoxia inducible factor-1 [198] and interferon regulatory factor-1 [199]. Induced by these transcription factors, interleukin-1β (IL-1β) and tumor necrosis factor-α (TNF-α) are expressed very early in cerebral ischemia and may contribute to initiating and perpetuating tissue inflammation. IL-1β mRNA levels are dramatically increased after ischemia [124], starting at 3–6 h, peak at 12 h and decline at 5 days after ischemia [200]. It is likely that processing of IL-1β by IL-1β converting enzyme (ICE or caspase-1) contributes to ischemic neuronal death. Transgenic mice that overexpress an ICE inhibitor, resulting in a deficiency in the production of mature IL-1β, had smaller infarctions and better neurological outcomes following permanent MCA occlusion [201]. Along with IL-1β, the level of IL-1 receptor antagonist (IL-1ra), an inhibitor of IL-1 activity, also increases at about the same time point. It is therefore the balance between the levels of IL-1β and IL-1ra expressed after ischemia that may be more critical for the degree of tissue injury. TNF-α expression has also been demonstrated following cerebral ischemia, starting at 1 h, peaking at 12 h and declining at 5 days [193]. TNF-α acts as a local regulator of inflammatory reaction and stimulates the expression of adhesion molecules, and chemokines, and activates NF-κB. However, the roles of TNF-α in ischemic injury are complex and evidence suggesting both deleterious as well as beneficial roles has been shown in different animal models [193]. Other experimental findings relevant to the role of TNF-α in ischemic cell death have been reviewed previously under Ischemic neuronal death.

Tissue injury typically results in increased blood flow and an influx of leukocytes to initiate wound repair. Within the first few hours after ischemia, the CD18 antigen on the surface of activated leukocytes binds to intercellular adhesion molecule-1 (ICAM-1) receptor on endothelial cells. As a result, leukocytes interact with vascular endothelium and induce blood–brain barrier breakdown, plugging of capillaries resulting in a 'no reflow' phenomenon and release deleterious factors including proteases and oxygen free radicals. Additional injury beyond that of ischemia may result from activation of leukocytes, primarily neutrophils. Neutrophils have been detected at the site of ischemia as early as 30 min after arterial occlusion, and peak at 24–48 h, followed by other cells such as macrophages [202]. Therefore, even if reperfusion occurs, secondary tissue destruction may continue.

Intravascular thrombosis has been suggested to occur as a byproduct of the proinflammatory state. Evidence from cell culture experiments suggests that under the influence of proinflammatory mediators (IL-1β and TNF-α) the vascular endothelium adopts a prothrombotic posture. This is evidenced through the expression of platelet-activating factor, inhibition of the thrombomodulin–protein C–protein S system, and inhibition of fibrinolysis [203,204]. There is a large body of evidence that suggests a beneficial effect to inhibiting neutrophil infiltration. However, recent animal studies have suggested that neutrophils are not always detrimental in the settings of acute cerebral ischemia [205,206].

Recent clinical experience with anti-inflammatory strategies has been disappointing: in a Phase III trial, enlimomab (a murine monoclonal anti-human ICAM-1 antibody) increased mortality in a multicentre acute stroke trial [207]. Another trial with humanized monoclonal antibody to CD18 was discontinued after an interim analysis showed no benefit. These clinical failures of anti-inflammatory approaches do not necessarily contradict the possibility that inflammation plays a role in secondary brain injury after ischemia [208].

Post-ischemic inflammatory reactions may not develop fully after a TIA; however, the signaling processes leading to inflammation can occur even with brief ischemic insults, potentially setting the stage for exacerbation of injury [209].

Post-ischemic angiogenesis

The regulation of angiogenesis after cerebral ischemia is an exciting new field of stroke research. Low oxygen tension and glucose deprivation in ischemia lead to compensatory neovascularization, through vascular endothelial growth factor (VEGF) induction, in the affected regions [32–34]. Other data demonstrate that ischemia also regulates the expression of angiogenic genes encoding for VEGF, basic fibroblast growth factor (bFGF) angiopoietin-1 (Angpo-1), angiopoietin-2 (Angpo-2), and receptor tyrosine kinases (Tie-1 and Tie-2) and others [39]. The angiopoietin/Tie receptor system may contribute to angiogenesis and vascular remodeling by mediating interactions of endothelial cells with smooth muscle cells and pericytes. The temporal profile of the angiogenesis factors suggests that Angpo-2 interacts with VEGF in regulating vessel sprouting, whereas Angpo-1 may play a role in stabilizing the vasculature [39]. Transcriptional regulation of angiogenic genes may be driven by HIF [187]. Angiogenesis may be one of the underlying mechanisms of the brain tolerance to recurrent ischemia [210].

Brain tolerance to ischemia

Interest in endogenous mechanisms that limit brain injury after ischemia has led to a large body of literature investigating ischemic tolerance, or preconditioning. Ischemic tolerance, activated by sublethal ischemic attacks, confers resistance to subsequent more severe ischemic insults. A broad spectrum of stressors can induce ischemic tolerance in the brain. It is interesting to note that sublethal cerebral ischemia in animals or in cell cultures (analogous to TIA in clinical situations) can induce the same cellular events that accompany neuronal death under more severe ischemic conditions (see Cellular events following vascular decompensation, above). Some of these post-ischemic events have been proposed to be the underlying mechanism for the development of ischemic tolerance, and include spreading depression [211–216], generation of ROS [217–219], reversible oxidative DNA damage [220–223], activation of glutamate receptor mechanism [222,224–230] or protein kinases [98,231–233], perturbation of adenosine receptor mechanism [234–236], disruption of energy metabolism [237–242], alteration of ion homeostasis [234,243–245], activation of proinflammatory [246–249] or neuroprotective [250,251] transcription factors, the expression of cytokines [223,252–256], other inflammatory gene products or thrombotic mediators [257–260], anti-apoptotic [261], stress proteins [262–265] (see Fig. 2.3), glial activation [266]. A number of transcription factors, especially HIF, and relevant downstream genes such as VEGF, bFGF, and other angiogenic genes may also be activated by sublethal ischemic insults. Angiogenesis may also be a possible mechanism in increasing brain tolerance to ischemia [210]. This is an exciting area that has yet to be explored. The notion that endogenous [224,267] or exogenous [268–272] neurotoxic substances cause neuronal death via mechanisms similar to those involved in ischemic tolerance

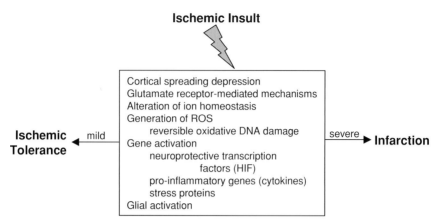

Ischemic Insult

Cortical spreading depression
Glutamate receptor-mediated mechanisms
Alteration of ion homeostasis
Generation of ROS
　　　reversible oxidative DNA damage
Gene activation
　　　neuroprotective transcription
　　　　　　　factors (HIF)
　　　pro-inflammatory genes (cytokines)
　　　stress proteins
Glial activation

Ischemic Tolerance ← mild

severe → **Infarction**

Fig. 2.3 Similar mechanisms lead to either cell death or cell protection via ischemic tolerance depending on the severity of the initial ischemic insult.

suggests that ischemia-induced cellular events are a double-edged sword. Dependent upon the degree of ischemia, these ischemia-triggered processes may either cause irreversible brain damage or build tolerance to protect the brain against subsequent ischemic insults.

Recent experimental studies have begun to shed light on the chronology of ischemic tolerance in the brain. It is believed that two temporally and mechanistically distinct forms of preconditioning, acute and delayed, exist in both the heart and the nervous system. For instance, acute preconditioning, short lived, may be independent of protein synthesis, and is mediated through post-translational protein modification. In contrast, delayed preconditioning, as seen in *in vivo* and *in vitro* models, may be mediated largely through the activation of NMDA receptors resulting in the increase of intracellular calcium and new protein synthesis [273,274].

It is controversial whether sustained modest reductions in CBF, above the CBF threshold for cerebral electrical failure, can ultimately produce clinically significant changes in brain function. However, evidence from models of incomplete global ischemia and graded hypoxia suggest that energy metabolism may deteriorate in a gradual fashion, even in the presence of stable CBF [26]. The measured CBF threshold for energy failure can actually increase over time in marginally perfused tissue [27]. This is the fundamental concept that has driven research in preconditioning. Better understanding of the signaling pathways that are ultimately responsible for preconditioning could potentially provide fertile ground for the development of novel therapeutic interventions, exploiting mechanisms involved in transient ischemia to prevent subsequent more serious ischemic injury.

Conclusions

Transient ischemic attacks and strokes are manifestations of disrupted brain perfusion. Understanding derangements of blood flow and metabolism is an essential starting platform for appreciating the pathophysiology of ischemic injury. In the setting of decreased cerebral perfusion, adaptive mechanisms such as changes in cerebrovascular tone, resistance, and oxygen extraction may sustain sufficient rates of aerobic energy production and therefore survival. However, during critically low levels of perfusion pressure, blood flow decreases, aerobic energy production fails, and a cascade of ionic and biochemical derangements ensue, leading to loss of brain electrical activity and then loss of cellular viability. In an otherwise similar disruption of cerebral perfusion, heterogeneity in ischemia severity is explained mainly by nonuniform collateral circulation and local neuronal activity.

Classic hemodynamic and metabolic considerations are inadequate to explain fully many of the phenomena that occur during or after ischemia. For example, it has been assumed that the deterioration of the ischemic penumbra reflects further reductions in CBF due to mechanical factors such as tissue swelling. Experimental evidence suggests, however, that CBF can be stable for many hours in steadily hypoperfused brain [42,76,96]. Therefore, the determinant of deterioration of the penumbra may not be the restrictions of marginal blood flow but the geographic proximity of susceptible tissues to certain toxic substances or secondary events. Severely ischemic tissue can be seen as a source of mediators of cellular injury that diffuse into adjacent brain tissues. For instance, non-physiological K^+ and glutamate release may trigger harmful waves of spreading depression that induce complex changes in Ca^{2+} homeostasis [47,50]. Moreover, regions of severe ischemia with disrupted blood–brain barrier can serve as a source of edema that, moving down pressure gradients, exposes surrounding tissue to toxic materials from the plasma [87]. Realizing the importance of factors independent of blood flow reduction to the evolution of ischemic injury does not imply that the severity of ischemia in penumbral regions has no bearing on tissue outcome. The impact of excitotoxins and spreading depression in particular may be determined to a large extent by the tissue's ability to compensate for derangements of ion homeostasis [50]. Thus, successful therapeutic interventions aimed at halting the deterioration of the ischemic penumbra will probably be needed to embrace combined strategies integrating reestablishment of CBF and minimizing toxic threats.

Presently, intravenous tissue-type plasminogen activator (t-PA) is the only therapeutic agent with proven benefit in the treatment of acute ischemic stroke, if given within 3 h from symptom onset. Other intravenous agents such as Ancrod, which lower plasma fibrinogen levels and improve reperfusion, have been shown to improve functional outcome [275]. Strategies of local thrombolytic delivery have also proven successful. For instance, intra-arterial pro-urokinase has been shown to be of clinical benefit with a wider therapeutic window [276]. Other strategies, aimed at physical clot disruption, are currently under preliminary investigation. It is likely that with the advent of thrombolytic therapies, the ischemic penumbra predominating in transient ischemic attack may be sustained for longer times and eventually rescued. However, reperfusion of the ischemic brain is a complex matter and is of increasing clinical importance. Future progress in designing pharmacological agents and interventional strategies should also take into consideration the post-ischemic events, including hyperperfusion and inflammatory reaction that can be potentially detrimental after a transient ischemic attack.

References

1 Siesjo BK. Cerebral circulation and metabolism. *J Neurosurg* 1984; 60: 883–908.

2 Ahmed SH. Pathophysiology of ischemic injury. In: Fisher M, ed. *Stroke Therapy*. Woburn, MA: Butterworth-Heinemann, 2001: 25–57.

3 Hossmann KA. Pathophysiology of cerebral infarction. In: Viken PJ, ed. *Handbook of Clinical Neurology*. New York: Elsevier, 1988: 107–54.

4 Astrup J, Siesjo BK, Symon L. Thresholds in cerebral ischemia—the ischemic penumbra. *Stroke* 1981; 12: 723–5.

5 Hossmann KA, Kleihues P. Reversibility of ischemic brain damage. *Arch Neurol* 1973; 29: 375–84.

6 Hossmann KA, Schmidt-Kastner R, Grosse Ophoff B. Recovery of integrative central nervous function after one hour global cerebro-circulatory arrest in normothermic cat. *J Neurol Sci* 1987; 77: 305–20.

7 Lee JM, Zipfel GJ, Choi DW. The changing landscape of ischaemic brain injury mechanisms. *Nature* 1999; 399: A7–14.

8 Dirnagl U, Iadecola C, Moskowitz MA. Pathobiology of ischaemic stroke: an integrated view. *Trends Neurosci* 1999; 22: 391–7.

9 Paulson OB, Strandgaard S, Edvinsson L. Cerebral autoregulation. *Cerebrovasc Brain Metab Rev* 1990; 2: 161–92.

10 Kuschinsky W, Wahl M. Local chemical and neurogenic regulation of cerebral vascular resistance. *Physiol Rev* 1978; 58: 656–89.

11 Brown MM, Wade JP, Marshall J. Fundamental importance of arterial oxygen content in the regulation of cerebral blood flow in man. *Brain* 1985; 108: 81–93.

12 Raichle ME. Behind the scenes of functional brain imaging: a historical and physiological perspective. *Proc Natl Acad Sci USA* 1998; 95: 765–72.

13 Phillis JW. Adenosine in the control of the cerebral circulation. *Cerebrovasc Brain Metab Rev* 1989; 1: 26–54.

14 Iadecola C. Regulation of the cerebral microcirculation during neural activity: is nitric oxide the missing link? *Trends Neurosci* 1993; 16: 206–14.

15 Faraci FM, Heistad DD. Regulation of large cerebral arteries and cerebral microvascular pressure. *Circ Res* 1990; 66: 8–17.

16 Brian JE Jr, Faraci FM, Heistad DD. Recent insights into the regulation of cerebral circulation. *Clin Exp Pharmacol Physiol* 1996; 23: 449–57.

17 Powers WJ, Raichle ME. Positron emission tomography and its application to the study of cerebrovascular disease in man. *Stroke* 1985; 16: 361–76.

18 Powers WJ. Cerebral hemodynamics in ischemic cerebrovascular disease. *Ann Neurol* 1991; 29: 231–40.

19 Yonas H, Pindzola RR. Physiological determination of cerebrovascular reserves and its use in clinical management. *Cerebrovasc Brain Metab Rev* 1994; 6: 325–40.

20 Hossmann KA. Viability thresholds and the penumbra of focal ischemia. *Ann Neurol* 1994; 36: 557–65.

21 Albers GW. Expanding the window for thrombolytic therapy in acute stroke. The potential role of acute MRI for patient selection. *Stroke* 1999; 30: 2230–7.

22 Heiss WD. Ischemic penumbra: evidence from functional imaging in man. *J Cereb Blood Flow Metab* 2000; 20: 1276–93.

23 Kidwell CS, Saver JL, Mattiello J *et al*. Thrombolytic reversal of acute human cerebral ischemic injury shown by diffusion/perfusion magnetic resonance imaging. *Ann Neurol* 2000; 47: 462–9.

24 Weih M, Kallenberg K, Bergk A *et al*. Attenuated stroke severity after prodromal TIA: a role for ischemic tolerance in the brain? *Stroke* 1999; 30: 1851–4.

25 Moncayo J, de Freitas GR, Bogousslavsky J *et al*. Do transient ischemic attacks have a neuroprotective effect? *Neurology* 2000; 54: 2089–94.

26 Baron JC, Rougemont D, Soussaline F *et al*. Local interrelationships of cerebral oxygen consumption and glucose utilization in normal subjects and in ischemic stroke patients: a positron tomography study. *J Cereb Blood Flow Metab* 1984; 4: 140–9.

27 Naritomi H, Sasaki M, Kanashiro M *et al*. Flow thresholds for cerebral energy disturbance and Na^+ pump failure as studied by *in vivo* 31p and 23na nuclear magnetic resonance spectroscopy. *J Cereb Blood Flow Metab* 1988; 8: 16–23.

28 Martin RL, Lloyd HG, Cowan AI. The early events of oxygen and glucose deprivation: setting the scene for neuronal death? *Trends Neurosci* 1994; 17: 251–7.

29 Tombaugh GC, Sapolsky RM. Evolving concepts about the role of acidosis in ischemic neuropathology. *J Neurochem* 1993; 61: 793–803.

30 Hansen AJ. Effect of anoxia on ion distribution in the brain. *Physiol Rev* 1985; 65: 101–48.

31 Sharp FR, Lu A, Tang Y *et al*. Multiple molecular penumbras after focal cerebral ischemia. *J Cereb Blood Flow Metab* 2000; 20: 1011–32.

32 Jacewicz M, Kiessling M, Pulsinelli WA. Selective gene expression in focal cerebral ischemia. *J Cereb Blood Flow Metab* 1986; 6: 263–72.

33 Sharbrough FW, Messick JM Jr, Sundt TM Jr. Correlation of continuous elec-troencephalograms with cerebral blood flow measurements during carotid endarterectomy. *Stroke* 1973; 4: 674–83.

34 Trojaborg W, Boysen G. Relation between EEG, regional cerebral blood flow and internal carotid artery pressure during carotid endarterectomy. *Electroencephalogr Clin Neurophysiol* 1973; 34: 61–9.

35 Heiss WD, Hayakawa T, Waltz AG. Cortical neuronal function during ischemia. Effects of occlusion of one middle cerebral artery on single-unit activity in cats. *Arch Neurol* 1976; 33: 813–20.

36 Jones TH, Morawetz RB, Crowell RM *et al.* Thresholds of focal cerebral ischemia in awake monkeys. *J Neurosurg* 1981; 54: 773–82.

37 Gibson GE, Pulsinelli W, Blass JP *et al.* Brain dysfunction in mild to moderate hypoxia. *Am J Med* 1981; 70: 1247–54.

38 Shimada N, Graf R, Rosner G *et al.* Ischemic flow threshold for extracellular glutamate increase in cat cortex. *J Cereb Blood Flow Metab* 1989; 9: 603–6.

39 Bell BA, Symon L, Branston NM. CBF and time thresholds for the formation of ischemic cerebral edema, and effect of reperfusion in baboons. *J Neurosurg* 1985; 62: 31–41.

40 Staub F, Baethmann A, Peters J *et al.* Effects of lactic acidosis on volume and viability of glial cells. *Acta Neurochir Suppl* 1990; 51: 3–6.

41 Chan PH, Chu L. Mechanisms underlying glutamate-induced swelling of astrocytes in primary culture. *Acta Neurochir (Suppl) (Wien)* 1990; 51: 7–10.

42 Astrup J, Symon L, Branston NM *et al.* Cortical evoked potential and extra-cellular K^+ and H^+ at critical levels of brain ischemia. *Stroke* 1977; 8: 51–7.

43 Choi DW. Calcium-mediated neurotoxicity. Relationship to specific channel types and role in ischemic damage. *Trends Neurosci* 1988; 11: 465–9.

44 Siesjo BK, Bengtsson F. Calcium fluxes, calcium antagonists, and calcium-related pathology in brain ischemia, hypoglycemia, and spreading depression: a unifying hypothesis. *J Cereb Blood Flow Metab* 1989; 9: 127–40.

45 Carter AJ. The importance of voltage-dependent sodium channels in cerebral ischaemia. *Amino Acids* 1998; 14: 159–69.

46 Harris RJ, Symon L. Extracellular pH, potassium, and calcium activities in progressive ischaemia of rat cortex. *J Cereb Blood Flow Metab* 1984; 4: 178–86.

47 Yatsu FM, Lee LW, Liao CL. Energy metabolism during brain ischemia. Stability during reversible and irreversible damage. *Stroke* 1975; 6: 678–83.

48 Back T, Kohno K, Hossmann KA. Cortical negative DC deflections following middle cerebral artery occlusion and KCl-induced spreading depression: effect on blood flow, tissue oxygenation, and electroencephalogram. *J Cereb Blood Flow Metab* 1994; 14: 12–9.

49 Betz AL, Keep RF, Beer ME *et al.* Blood–brain barrier permeability and brain concentration of sodium, potassium, and chloride during focal ischemia. *J Cereb Blood Flow Metab* 1994; 14: 29–37.

50 Madden KP. Effect of gamma-aminobutyric acid modulation on neuronal ischemia in rabbits. *Stroke* 1994; 25: 2271–4; discussion 2274–5.

51 Raichle ME. The pathophysiology of brain ischemia. *Ann Neurol* 1983; 13: 2–10.

52 Sato M, Paschen W, Pawlik G *et al.* Neurologic deficit and cerebral ATP depletion after temporary focal ischemia in cats. *J Cereb Blood Flow Metab* 1984; 4: 173–7.

53 Pulsinelli WA. Selective neuronal vulnerability. Morphological and molecular characteristics. *Prog Brain Res* 1985; 63: 29–37.

54 Du C, Hu R, Csernansky CA *et al.* Very delayed infarction after mild focal cerebral ischemia: a role for apoptosis? *J Cereb Blood Flow Metab* 1996; 16: 195–201.

55 Hossmann KA. Post-ischemic resuscitation of the brain: selective vulnerability versus global resistance. *Prog Brain Res* 1985; 63: 3–17.

56 McDonald JW, Johnston MV. Physiological and pathophysiological roles of excitatory amino acids during central nervous system development. *Brain Res Brain Res Rev* 1990; 15: 41–70.

57 Rothman SM. Synaptic activity mediates death of hypoxic neurons. *Science* 1983; 220: 536–7.

58 Choi DW. Glutamate neurotoxicity and diseases of the nervous system. *Neuron* 1988; 1: 623–34.

59 Choi DW. NMDA receptors and AMPA/kainate receptors mediate parallel injury in cerebral cortical cultures subjected to oxygen-glucose deprivation. *Prog Brain Res* 1993; 96: 137–43.

60 Choi DW. Ionic dependence of glutamate neurotoxicity. *J Neurosci* 1987; 7: 369–79.

61 Choi DW, Lobner D, Dugan LL. Glutamate receptor-mediated neuronal death in the ischemic brain. In: Hsu CY, ed. *Ischemic Stroke: from Basic Mechanisms to Drug Development.* Switzerland: Karger, 1998: 2–13.

62 Olney JW. Neurotoxicity of excitatory amino acids. In: McGeer EG, Olney JW, McGeer PL, eds. *Kainic Acid as a Tool in Neurobiology.* New York: Raven, 1978: 37–70.

63 Koh JY, Choi DW. Vulnerability of cultured cortical neurons to damage by excitotoxins: differential susceptibility of neurons containing NADPH-diaphorase. *J Neurosci* 1988; 8: 2153–63.

64 Dawson VL, Dawson TM, London ED *et al.* Nitric oxide mediates glutamate neurotoxicity in primary cortical cultures. *Proc Natl Acad Sci USA* 1991; 88: 6368–71.

65 Beckman JS, Beckman TW, Chen J *et al.* Apparent hydroxyl radical production by peroxynitrite: implications for endothelial injury from nitric oxide and superoxide. *Proc Natl Acad Sci USA* 1990; 87: 1620–4.

66 Zhang J, Dawson VL, Dawson TM *et al.* Nitric oxide activation of poly (adp-ribose) synthetase in neurotoxicity. *Science* 1994; 263: 687–9.

67 Benveniste H, Drejer J, Schousboe A *et al.* Elevation of the extracellular concentrations of glutamate and aspartate in rat hippocampus during transient cerebral ischemia monitored by intracerebral microdialysis. *J Neurochem* 1984; 43: 1369–74.

68 Swanson RA, Farrell K, Simon RP. Acidosis causes failure of astrocyte glutamate uptake during hypoxia. *J Cereb Blood Flow Metab* 1995; 15: 417–24.

69 Marrannes R, Willems R, De Prins E *et al.* Evidence for a role of the N-methyl-D-aspartate (NMDA) receptor in cortical spreading depression in the rat. *Brain Res* 1988; 457: 226–40.

70 Park CK, Nehls DG, Graham DI *et al.* The glutamate antagonist mk-801 reduces focal ischemic brain damage in the rat. *Ann Neurol* 1988; 24: 543–51.

71 Simon RP, Swan JH, Griffiths T *et al.* Blockade of N-methyl-D-aspartate receptors may protect against ischemic damage in the brain. *Science* 1984; 226: 850–2.

72 Goldberg MP, Choi DW. Combined oxygen and glucose deprivation in cortical cell culture: calcium-dependent and calcium-independent mechanisms of neuronal injury. *J Neurosci* 1993; 13: 3510–24.

73 Buchan AM. Do NMDA antagonists protect against cerebral ischemia: are clinical trials warranted? *Cerebrovasc Brain Metab Rev* 1990; 2: 1–26.

74 Goldberg MP. Stroke trials database.

75 Olney JW. Neurotoxicity of NMDA receptor antagonists: an overview. *Psychopharmacol Bull* 1994; 30: 533–40.

76 Dyker AG, Lees KR. Safety and tolerability of gv150526 (a glycine site antagonist at the N-methyl-D-aspartate receptor) in patients with acute stroke. *Stroke* 1999; 30: 986–92.

77 Phase II studies of the glycine antagonist gv150526 in acute stroke: the North American experience. The North American Glycine Antagonist in Neuroprotection (GAIN) investigators. *Stroke* 2000; 31: 358–65.

78 Kew JN, Trube G, Kemp JA. A novel mechanism of activity-dependent NMDA receptor antagonism describes the effect of ifenprodil in rat cultured cortical neurons. *J Physiol* 1996; 497: 761–72.

79 Follis F, Scremin OU, Blisard KS *et al.* Selective vulnerability of white matter during spinal cord ischemia. *J Cereb Blood Flow Metab* 1993; 13: 170–8.

80 Pantoni L, Garcia JH, Gutierrez JA. Cerebral white matter is highly vulnerable to ischemia. *Stroke* 1996; 27: 1641–6; discussion 1647.

81 McDonald JW, Althomsons SP, Hyrc KL *et al.* Oligodendrocytes from forebrain are highly vulnerable to AMPA/kainate receptor-mediated excitotoxicity. *Nat Med* 1998; 4: 291–7.

82 Matute C, Sanchez-Gomez MV, Martinez-Millan L *et al.* Glutamate receptor-mediated toxicity in optic nerve oligodendrocytes. *Proc Natl Acad Sci USA* 1997; 94: 8830–5.

83 Kanellopoulos GK, Xu XM, Hsu CY *et al.* White matter injury in spinal cord ischemia: protection by AMPA/kainate glutamate receptor antagonism. *Stroke* 2000; 31: 1945–52.

84 Xue D, Huang ZG, Barnes K *et al.* Delayed treatment with AMPA, but not NMDA, antagonists reduces neocortical infarction. *J Cereb Blood Flow Metab* 1994; 14: 251–61.

85 Hollmann M, Hartley M, Heinemann S. Ca^{2+} permeability of ka-AMPA-gated glutamate receptor channels depends on subunit composition. *Science* 1991; 252: 851–3.

86 Plum F, Pulsinelli W. Cerebral metabolism and hypoxic-ischemic brain injury. In: Asbury A, McKhann G, McDonald A, eds. *Diseases of the Nervous System*. Philadelphia: Saunders, 1986: 1086–101.

87 de Courten-Myers G, Myers RE, Schoolfield L. Hyperglycemia enlarges infarct size in cerebrovascular occlusion in cats. *Stroke* 1988; 19: 623–30.

88 Yip PK, He YY, Hsu CY *et al*. Effect of plasma glucose on infarct size in focal cerebral ischemia-reperfusion. *Neurology* 1991; 41: 899–905.

89 Ginsberg MD, Mela L, Wrobel-Kuhl K *et al*. Mitochondrial metabolism following bilateral cerebral ischemia in the gerbil. *Ann Neurol* 1977; 1: 519–27.

90 Garcia JH, Liu K-F, Lian J, Xu J. Astrocytic and microvascular responces to the occlusion of a middle cerebral artery. *J Neuropathol Exp Neurol* ; 1193: 288.

91 Rehncrona S, Hauge HN, Siesjo BK. Enhancement of iron-catalyzed free radical formation by acidosis in brain homogenates: differences in effect by lactic acid and CO_2. *J Cereb Blood Flow Metab* 1989; 9: 65–70.

92 Choi DW. Cerebral hypoxia. Some new approaches and unanswered questions. *J Neurosci* 1990; 10: 2493–501.

93 Giffard RG, Monyer H, Christine CW *et al*. Acidosis reduces NMDA receptor activation, glutamate neurotoxicity, and oxygen-glucose deprivation neuronal injury in cortical cultures. *Brain Res* 1990; 506: 339–42.

94 Hara H, Onodera H, Yoshidomi M *et al*. Staurosporine, a novel protein kinase C inhibitor, prevents postischemic neuronal damage in the gerbil and rat. *J Cereb Blood Flow Metab* 1990; 10: 646–53.

95 Madden KP, Clark WM, Kochhar A *et al*. Effect of protein kinase C modulation on outcome of experimental CNS ischemia. *Brain Res* 1991; 547: 193–8.

96 Aronowski J, Grotta JC, Strong R *et al*. Interplay between the gamma isoform of PKC and calcineurin in regulation of vulnerability to focal cerebral ischemia. *J Cereb Blood Flow Metab* 2000; 20: 343–9.

97 Ouyang YB, Tan Y, Comb M *et al*. Survival- and death-promoting events after transient cerebral ischemia: phosphorylation of akt, release of cytochrome c and activation of caspase-like proteases. *J Cereb Blood Flow Metab* 1999; 19: 1126–35.

98 Yano S, Morioka M, Fukunaga K *et al*. Activation of akt/protein kinase B contributes to induction of ischemic tolerance in the ca1 subfield of gerbil hippocampus. *J Cereb Blood Flow Metab* 2001; 21: 351–60.

99 Noshita N, Lewen A, Sugawara T *et al*. Evidence of phosphorylation of akt and neuronal survival after transient focal cerebral ischemia in mice. *J Cereb Blood Flow Metab* 2001; 21: 1442–50.

100 Campos-Gonzalez R, Kindy MS. Tyrosine phosphorylation of microtubule-associated protein kinase after transient ischemia in the gerbil brain. *J Neurochem* 1992; 59: 1955–8.

101 Hu BR, Wieloch T. Tyrosine phosphorylation and activation of mitogen-activated protein kinase in the rat brain following transient cerebral ischemia. *J Neurochem* 1994; 62: 1357–67.

102 Sugino T, Nozaki K, Takagi Y *et al*. Activation of mitogen-activated protein kinases after transient forebrain ischemia in gerbil hippocampus. *J Neurosci* 2000; 20: 4506–14.

103 Hu BR, Liu CL, Park DJ. Alteration of MAP kinase pathways after transient forebrain ischemia. *J Cereb Blood Flow Metab* 2000; 20: 1089–95.

104 Tian D, Litvak V, Lev S. Cerebral ischemia and seizures induce tyrosine phosphorylation of pyk2 in neurons and microglial cells. *J Neurosci* 2000; 20: 6478–87.

105 Runden E, Seglen PO, Haug FM *et al*. Regional selective neuronal degeneration after protein phosphatase inhibition in hippocampal slice cultures: evidence for a MAP kinase-dependent mechanism. *J Neurosci* 1998; 18: 7296–305.

106 Alessandrini A, Namura S, Moskowitz MA *et al*. Mek1 protein kinase inhibition protects against damage resulting from focal cerebral ischemia. *Proc Natl Acad Sci USA* 1999; 96: 12866–9.

107 Simi A, Ingelman-Sundberg M, Tindberg N. Neuroprotective agent chlomethiazole attenuates c-fos, c-jun, and ap-1 activation through inhibition of p38 MAP kinase. *J Cereb Blood Flow Metab* 2000; 20: 1077–88.

108 Namura S, Iihara K, Takami S *et al*. Intravenous administration of mek inhibitor u0126 affords brain protection against forebrain ischemia and focal cerebral ischemia. *Proc Natl Acad Sci USA* 2001; 98: 11569–74.

109 Barone FC, Irving EA, Ray AM *et al*. Sb 239063, a second-generation p38 mitogen-activated protein kinase inhibitor, reduces brain injury and neurological deficits in cerebral focal ischemia. *J Pharmacol Exp Ther* 2001; 296: 312–21.

110 Kawano T, Fukunaga K, Takeuchi Y *et al*. Neuroprotective effect of sodium orthovanadate on delayed neuronal death after transient forebrain ischemia in gerbil hippocampus. *J Cereb Blood Flow Metab* 2001; 21: 1268–80.

111 Yamashima T. Implication of cysteine proteases calpain, cathepsin and caspase in ischemic neuronal death of primates. *Prog Neurobiol* 2000; 62: 273–95.

112 White BC, Sullivan JM, DeGracia DJ *et al*. Brain ischemia and reperfusion: molecular mechanisms of neuronal injury. *J Neurol Sci* 2000; 179: 1–33.

113 Lee KS, Frank S, Vanderklish P *et al*. Inhibition of proteolysis protects hippocampal neurons from ischemia. *Proc Natl Acad Sci USA* 1991; 88: 7233–7.

114 Bartus RT, Baker KL, Heiser AD *et al*. Postischemic administration of ak275, a calpain inhibitor, provides substantial protection against focal ischemic brain damage. *J Cereb Blood Flow Metab* 1994; 14: 537–44.

115 Markgraf CG, Velayo NL, Johnson MP *et al*. Six-hour window of opportunity for calpain inhibition in focal cerebral ischemia in rats. *Stroke* 1998; 29: 152–8.

116 Chen ST, Hsu CY, Hogan EL *et al*. Thromboxane, prostacyclin, and leukotrienes in cerebral ischemia. *Neurology* 1986; 36: 466–70.

117 Hsu CY, Liu TH, Xu J *et al*. Arachidonic acid and its metabolites in cerebral ischemia. *Ann NY Acad Sci* 1989; 559: 282–95.

118 Sun GY, Hsu CY. Poly phosphoinositide-mediated messengers in focal cerebral ischemia and reperfusion. *J Lipid Med Cell Signal* 1996; 14: 137–45.

119 Gardiner M, Nilsson B, Rehncrona S *et al*. Free fatty acids in the rat brain in moderate and severe hypoxia. *J Neurochem* 1981; 36: 1500–5.

120 Miettinen S, Fusco FR, Yrjanheikki J *et al*. Spreading depression and focal brain ischemia induce cyclooxygenase-2 in cortical neurons through N-methyl-D-aspartic acid-receptors and phospholipase a2. *Proc Natl Acad Sci USA* 1997; 94: 6500–5.

121 Crockard HA, Bhakoo KK, Lascelles PT. Regional prostaglandin levels in cerebral ischaemia. *J Neurochem* 1982; 38: 1311–4.

122 Hewett SJ, Uliasz TF, Vidwans AS *et al*. Cyclooxygenase-2 contributes to N-methyl-D-aspartate-mediated neuronal cell death in primary cortical cell culture. *J Pharmacol Exp Ther* 2000; 293: 417–25.

123 Nogawa S, Zhang F, Ross ME *et al*. Cyclo-oxygenase-2 gene expression in neurons contributes to ischemic brain damage. *J Neurosci* 1997; 17: 2746–55.

124 Minami M, Kuraishi Y, Yabuuchi K *et al*. Induction of interleukin-1 beta mRNA in rat brain after transient forebrain ischemia. *J Neurochem* 1992; 58: 390–2.

125 Chan PH. Reactive oxygen radicals in signaling and damage in the ischemic brain. *J Cereb Blood Flow Metab* 2001; 21: 2–14.

126 Iadecola C. Bright and dark sides of nitric oxide in ischemic brain injury. *Trends Neurosci* 1997; 20: 132–9.

127 Dalkara T, Moskowitz MA. Nitric oxide in cerebrovascular regulation and ischemia. In: Hsu CY, ed. *Ischemic Stroke: from Basic Mechanism to New Drug Development*. Switzerland: Karger, 1998: 28–45.

128 Huang Z, Huang PL, Panahian N *et al*. Effects of cerebral ischemia in mice deficient in neuronal nitric oxide synthase. *Science* 1994; 265: 1883–5.

129 Huang Z, Huang PL, Ma J *et al*. Enlarged infarcts in endothelial nitric oxide synthase knockout mice are attenuated by nitro-L-arginine. *J Cereb Blood Flow Metab* 1996; 16: 981–7.

130 Iadecola C, Zhang F, Casey R *et al*. Delayed reduction of ischemic brain injury and neurological deficits in mice lacking the inducible nitric oxide synthase gene. *J Neurosci* 1997; 17: 9157–64.

131 Rauhala P, Lin AM, Chiueh CC. Neuroprotection by s-nitrosoglutathione of brain dopamine neurons from oxidative stress. *FASEB J* 1998; 12: 165–73.

132 Chiueh CC, Rauhala P. The redox pathway of s-nitrosoglutathione, glutathione and nitric oxide in cell to neuron communications. *Free Radic Res* 1999; 31: 641–50.

133 Wyllie AH, Kerr JF, Currie AR. Cell death. The significance of apoptosis. *Int Rev Cytol* 1980; 68: 251–306.

134 Kerr JF, Wyllie AH, Currie AR. Apoptosis: a basic biological phenomenon with wide-ranging implications in tissue kinetics. *Br J Cancer* 1972; 26: 239–57.

135 Green DR, Reed JC. Mitochondria and apoptosis. *Science* 1998; 281: 1309–12.

136 Tsujimoto Y, Finger LR, Yunis J *et al*. Cloning of the chromosome breakpoint of neoplastic B cells with the t(14;18) chromosome translocation. *Science* 1984; 226: 1097–9.

137 Adams JM, Cory S. The Bcl-2 protein family. Arbiters of cell survival. *Science* 1998; 281: 1322–6.

138 Jurgensmeier JM, Xie Z, Deveraux Q *et al*. Bax directly induces release of cytochrome c from isolated mitochondria. *Proc Natl Acad Sci USA* 1998; 95: 4997–5002.

139 Cecconi F. Apaf1 and the apoptotic machinery. *Cell Death Differ* 1999; 6: 1087–98.

140 Ashkenazi A, Dixit VM. Death receptors: signaling and modulation. *Science* 1998; 281: 1305–8.

141 Joza N, Susin SA, Daugas E *et al*. Essential role of the mitochondrial apoptosis-inducing factor in programmed cell death. *Nature* 2001; 410: 549–54.

142 Thornberry NA, Lazebnik Y. Caspases: enemies within. *Science* 1998; 281: 1312–6.

143 Slee EA, Adrain C, Martin SJ. Serial killers: ordering caspase activation events in apoptosis. *Cell Death Differ* 1999; 6: 1067–74.

144 Nunez G, Benedict MA, Hu Y *et al*. Caspases: the proteases of the apoptotic pathway. *Oncogene* 1998; 17: 3237–45.

145 Nagata S. Apoptotic DNA fragmentation. *Exp Cell Res* 2000; 256: 12–8.

146 Buendia B, Santa-Maria A, Courvalin JC. Caspase-dependent proteolysis of integral and peripheral proteins of nuclear membranes and nuclear pore complex proteins during apoptosis. *J Cell Sci* 1999; 112: 1743–53.

147 Kothakota S, Azuma T, Reinhard C *et al*. Caspase-3-generated fragment of gelsolin: effector of morphological change in apoptosis. *Science* 1997; 278: 294–8.

148 Colbourne F, Sutherland GR, Auer RN. Electron microscopic evidence against apoptosis as the mechanism of neuronal death in global ischemia. *J Neurosci* 1999; 19: 4200–10.

149 Martin LJ, Al-Abdulla NA, Brambrink AM *et al*. Neurodegeneration in excitotoxicity, global cerebral ischemia, and target deprivation: a perspective on the contributions of apoptosis and necrosis. *Brain Res Bull* 1998; 46: 281–309.

150 MacManus JP, Buchan AM, Hill IE *et al*. Global ischemia can cause DNA fragmentation indicative of apoptosis in rat brain. *Neurosci Lett* 1993; 164: 89–92.

151 Tominaga T, Kure S, Narisawa K *et al*. Endonuclease activation following focal ischemic injury in the rat brain. *Brain Res* 1993; 608: 21–6.

152 MacManus JP, Hill IE, Huang ZG *et al*. DNA damage consistent with apoptosis in transient focal ischaemic neocortex. *Neuroreport* 1994; 5: 493–6.

153 Charriaut-Marlangue C, Ben-Ari Y. A cautionary note on the use of the TUNEL stain to determine apoptosis. *Neuroreport* 1995; 7: 61–4.

154 Chen J, Graham SH, Chan PH *et al*. Bcl-2 is expressed in neurons that survive focal ischemia in the rat. *Neuroreport* 1995; 6: 394–8.

155 Isenmann S, Stoll G, Schroeter M *et al.* Differential regulation of bax, Bcl-2, and Bcl-x proteins in focal cortical ischemia in the rat. *Brain Pathol* 1998; 8: 49–62; discussion 62–43.

156 Minami M, Jin KL, Li W *et al.* Bcl-w expression is increased in brain regions affected by focal cerebral ischemia in the rat. *Neurosci Lett* 2000; 279: 193–5.

157 Krajewski S, Mai JK, Krajewska M *et al.* Up-regulation of bax protein levels in neurons following cerebral ischemia. *J Neurosci* 1995; 15: 6364–76.

158 Fujimura M, Morita-Fujimura Y, Murakami K *et al.* Cytosolic redistribution of cytochrome c after transient focal cerebral ischemia in rats. *J Cereb Blood Flow Metab* 1998; 18: 1239–47.

159 Namura S, Zhu J, Fink K *et al.* Activation and cleavage of caspase-3 in apoptosis induced by experimental cerebral ischemia. *J Neurosci* 1998; 18: 3659–68.

160 Martinou JC, Dubois-Dauphin M, Staple JK *et al.* Overexpression of bcl-2 in transgenic mice protects neurons from naturally occurring cell death and experimental ischemia. *Neuron* 1994; 13: 1017–30.

161 Linnik MD, Zahos P, Geschwind MD *et al.* Expression of bcl-2 from a defective herpes simplex virus-1 vector limits neuronal death in focal cerebral ischemia. *Stroke* 1995; 26: 1670–4; discussion 1675.

162 Hara H, Friedlander RM, Gagliardini V *et al.* Inhibition of interleukin 1beta converting enzyme family proteases reduces ischemic and excitotoxic neuronal damage. *Proc Natl Acad Sci USA* 1997; 94: 2007–12.

163 Cheng Y, Deshmukh M, D'Costa A *et al.* Caspase inhibitor affords neuroprotection with delayed administration in a rat model of neonatal hypoxic-ischemic brain injury. *J Clin Invest* 1998; 101: 1992–9.

164 Xu D, Bureau Y, McIntyre DC *et al.* Attenuation of ischemia-induced cellular and behavioral deficits by X chromosome-linked inhibitor of apoptosis protein overexpression in the rat hippocampus. *J Neurosci* 1999; 19: 5026–33.

165 Liu T, Clark RK, McDonnell PC *et al.* Tumor necrosis factor-alpha expression in ischemic neurons. *Stroke* 1994; 25: 1481–8.

166 Matsuyama T, Hata R, Yamamoto Y *et al.* Localization of Fas antigen mRNA induced in postischemic murine forebrain by *in situ* hybridization. *Brain Res Mol Brain Res* 1995; 34: 166–72.

167 Buttini M, Appel K, Sauter A *et al.* Expression of tumor necrosis factor alpha after focal cerebral ischaemia in the rat. *Neuroscience* 1996; 71: 1–16.

168 Saito K, Suyama K, Nishida K *et al.* Early increases in TNF-alpha, IL-6 and IL-1 beta levels following transient cerebral ischemia in gerbil brain. *Neurosci Lett* 1996; 206: 149–52.

169 Martin-Villalba A, Herr I, Jeremias I *et al.* Cd95 ligand (fas-l/apo-1l) and tumor necrosis factor-related apoptosis-inducing ligand mediate ischemia-induced apoptosis in neurons. *J Neurosci* 1999; 19: 3809–17.

170 Martin-Villalba A, Hahne M, Kleber S *et al.* Therapeutic neutralization of CD95-ligand and TNF attenuates brain damage in stroke. *Cell Death Differ* 2001; 8: 679–86.

171 Bruce AJ, Boling W, Kindy MS *et al.* Altered neuronal and microglial responses to excitotoxic and ischemic brain injury in mice lacking TNF receptors. *Nat Med* 1996; 2: 788–94.

172 Shohami E, Ginis I, Hallenbeck JM. Dual role of tumor necrosis factor alpha in brain injury. *Cytokine Growth Factor Rev* 1999; 10: 119–30.

173 Bonfoco E, Krainc D, Ankarcrona M *et al.* Apoptosis and necrosis: two distinct events induced, respectively, by mild and intense insults with N-methyl-D-aspartate or nitric oxide/superoxide in cortical cell cultures. *Proc Natl Acad Sci USA* 1995; 92: 7162–6.

174 Nakano S, Kogure K, Fujikura H. Ischemia-induced slowly progressive neuronal damage in the rat brain. *Neuroscience* 1990; 38: 115–24.

175 Endres M, Namura S, Shimizu-Sasamata M *et al.* Attenuation of delayed neuronal death after mild focal ischemia in mice by inhibition of the caspase family. *J Cereb Blood Flow Metab* 1998; 18: 238–47.

176 Kuroiwa T, Ting P, Martinez H *et al.* The biphasic opening of the blood–brain barrier to proteins following temporary middle cerebral artery occlusion. *Acta Neuropathol (Berl)* 1985; 68: 122–9.

177 Ernster L. Biochemistry of reoxygenation injury. *Crit Care Med* 1988; 16: 947–53.

178 Wei EP, Kontos HA, Dietrich WD *et al.* Inhibition by free radical scavengers and by cyclooxygenase inhibitors of pial arteriolar abnormalities from concussive brain injury in cats. *Circ Res* 1981; 48: 95–103.

179 Kuroiwa T, Shibutani M, Okeda R. Blood–brain barrier disruption and exacerbation of ischemic brain edema after restoration of blood flow in experimental focal cerebral ischemia. *Acta Neuropathol (Berl)* 1988; 76: 62–70.

180 Akins PT, Liu PK, Hsu CY. Immediate early gene expression in response to cerebral ischemia. Friend or foe? *Stroke* 1996; 27: 1682–7.

181 Koistinaho J, Hokfelt T. Altered gene expression in brain ischemia. *Neuroreport* 1997; 8: i–viii.

182 Read SJ, Parsons AA, Harrison DC *et al.* Stroke genomics: approaches to identify, validate, and understand ischemic stroke gene expression. *J Cereb Blood Flow Metab* 2001; 21: 755–78.

183 An G, Lin TN, Liu JS *et al.* Expression of c-fos and c-jun family genes after focal cerebral ischemia. *Ann Neurol* 1993; 33: 457–64.

184 Stephenson D, Yin T, Smalstig EB *et al.* Transcription factor nuclear factor-kappa B is activated in neurons after focal cerebral ischemia. *J Cereb Blood Flow Metab* 2000; 20: 592–603.

185 Semenza GL. Surviving ischemia: adaptive responses mediated by hypoxia-inducible factor 1. *J Clin Invest* 2000; 106: 809–12.

186 Tanaka K. Alteration of second messengers during acute cerebral ischemia —adenylate cyclase, cyclic AMP-dependent protein kinase, and cyclic AMP response element binding protein. *Prog Neurobiol* 2001; 65: 173–207.

187 Campagne MV, Thibodeaux H, van Bruggen N *et al.* Increased binding activity at an antioxidant-responsive element in the metallothionein-1 promoter and

rapid induction of metallothionein-1 and -2 in response to cerebral ischemia and reperfusion. *J Neurosci* 2000; 20: 5200–7.

188 Drutel G, Heron A, Kathmann M *et al*. Arnt2, a transcription factor for brain neuron survival? *Eur J Neurosci* 1999; 11: 1545–53.

189 Planas AM, Justicia C, Ferrer I. Stat1 in developing and adult rat brain. Induction after transient focal ischemia. *Neuroreport* 1997; 8: 1359–62.

190 Planas AM, Soriano MA, Berruezo M *et al*. Induction of stat3, a signal transducer and transcription factor, in reactive microglia following transient focal cerebral ischaemia. *Eur J Neurosci* 1996; 8: 2612–8.

191 Salminen A, Liu PK, Hsu CY. Alteration of transcription factor binding activities in the ischemic rat brain. *Biochem Biophys Res Commun* 1995; 212: 939–44.

192 YuZ, Zhou D, Bruce-Keller AJ *et al*. Lack of the p50 subunit of nuclear factor-kappaB increases the vulnerability of hippocampal neurons to excitotoxic injury. *J Neurosci* 1999; 19: 8856–65.

193 Schneider A, Martin-Villalba A, Weih F *et al*. Nf-kappaB is activated and promotes cell death in focal cerebral ischemia. *Nat Med* 1999; 5: 554–9.

194 Soriano MA, Tessier M, Certa U *et al*. Parallel gene expression monitoring using oligonucleotide probe arrays of multiple transcripts with an animal model of focal ischemia. *J Cereb Blood Flow Metab* 2000; 20: 1045–55.

195 Bennett MV, Pellegrini-Giampietro DE, Gorter JA *et al*. The glur2 hypothesis: Ca(++)-permeable ampa receptors in delayed neurodegeneration. *Cold Spring Harb Symp Quant Biol* 1996; 61: 373–84.

196 Dai WJ, Funk A, Herdegen T *et al*. Blockade of central angiotensin at(1) receptors improves neurological outcome and reduces expression of ap-1 transcription factors after focal brain ischemia in rats. *Stroke* 1999; 30: 2391–8; discussion 2398–9.

197 Domanska-Janik K, Bong P, Bronisz-Kowalczyk A *et al*. Ap1 transcriptional factor activation and its relation to apoptosis of hippocampal ca1 pyramidal neurons after transient ischemia in gerbils. *J Neurosci Res* 1999; 57: 840–6.

198 Bergeron M, Yu AY, Solway KE *et al*. Induction of hypoxia-inducible factor-1 (HIF-1) and its target genes following focal ischaemia in rat brain. *Eur J Neurosci* 1999; 11: 4159–70.

199 Iadecola C, Salkowski CA, Zhang F *et al*. The transcription factor interferon regulatory factor 1 is expressed after cerebral ischemia and contributes to ischemic brain injury. *J Exp Med* 1999; 189: 719–27.

200 Liu T, McDonnell PC, Young PR *et al*. Interleukin-1 beta mRNA expression in ischemic rat cortex. *Stroke* 1993; 24: 1746–50; discussion 1750–41.

201 Friedlander RM, Gagliardini V, Hara H *et al*. Expression of a dominant negative mutant of interleukin-1 beta converting enzyme in transgenic mice prevents neuronal cell death induced by trophic factor withdrawal and ischemic brain injury. *J Exp Med* 1997; 185: 933–40.

202 Kochanek P, Schoettle R, Uhl M *et al*. Platelet-activating factor antagonists do not attenuate delayed post-traumatic cerebral edema in rats. *J Neurotrauma* 1991; 8: 19–25.

203 Plumier JC, Krueger AM, Currie RW *et al*. Transgenic mice expressing the human inducible hsp70 have hippocampal neurons resistant to ischemic injury. *Cell Stress Chaperones* 1997; 2: 162–7.

204 Chen J, Graham SH, Nakayama M *et al*. Apoptosis repressor genes bcl-2 and bcl-x-long are expressed in the rat brain following global ischemia. *J Cereb Blood Flow Metab* 1997; 17: 2–10.

205 Hayward NJ, Elliott PJ, Sawyer SD *et al*. Lack of evidence for neutrophil participation during infarct formation following focal cerebral ischemia in the rat. *Exp Neurol* 1996; 139: 188–202.

206 Ahmed SH, He YY, Nassief A *et al*. Effects of lipopolysaccharide priming on acute ischemic brain injury. *Stroke* 2000; 31: 193–9.

207 Sherman DG. The enlimomab acute stroke trial. Final results (Abstract and Presentation) in 49th Annual Meeting of the American Academy Of Neurology. *Neurology* 1997: A270.

208 del Zoppo GJ, Becker KJ, Hallenbeck JM. Inflammation after stroke: is it harmful? *Arch Neurol* 2001; 58: 669–72.

209 Barone FC, Feuerstein GZ. Inflammatory mediators and stroke: new opportunities for novel therapeutics. *J Cereb Blood Flow Metab* 1999; 19: 819–34.

210 Nariai T, Suzuki R, Matsushima Y *et al*. Surgically induced angiogenesis to compensate for hemodynamic cerebral ischemia. *Stroke* 1994; 25: 1014–21.

211 Kobayashi S, Harris VA, Welsh FA. Spreading depression induces tolerance of cortical neurons to ischemia in rat brain. *J Cereb Blood Flow Metab* 1995; 15: 721–7.

212 Matsushima K, Hogan MJ, Hakim AM. Cortical spreading depression protects against subsequent focal cerebral ischemia in rats. *J Cereb Blood Flow Metab* 1996; 16: 221–6.

213 Kawahara N, Croll SD, Wiegand SJ *et al*. Cortical spreading depression induces long-term alterations of bdnf levels in cortex and hippocampus distinct from lesion effects: implications for ischemic tolerance. *Neurosci Res* 1997; 29: 37–47.

214 Taga K, Patel PM, Drummond JC *et al*. Transient neuronal depolarization induces tolerance to subsequent forebrain ischemia in rats. *Anesthesiology* 1997; 87: 918–25.

215 Matsushima K, Schmidt-Kastner R, Hogan MJ *et al*. Cortical spreading depression activates trophic factor expression in neurons and astrocytes and protects against subsequent focal brain ischemia. *Brain Res* 1998; 807: 47–60.

216 Kawahara N, Ruetzler CA, Mies G *et al*. Cortical spreading depression increases protein synthesis and up-regulates basic fibroblast growth factor. *Exp Neurol* 1999; 158: 27–36.

217 Kato H, Kogure K, Araki T *et al*. Immunohistochemical localization of superoxide dismutase in the hippocampus following ischemia in a gerbil model of ischemic tolerance. *J Cereb Blood Flow Metab* 1995; 15: 60–70.

218 Mori T, Muramatsu H, Matsui T *et al*. Possible role of the superoxide anion in the development of neuronal tolerance following ischaemic preconditioning in rats. *Neuropathol Appl Neurobiol* 2000; 26: 31–40.

219 Bordet R, Deplanque D, Maboudou P *et al.* Increase in endogenous brain superoxide dismutase as a potential mechanism of lipopolysaccharide-induced brain ischemic tolerance. *J Cereb Blood Flow Metab* 2000; 20: 1190–6.

220 Baek SH, Kim JY, Choi JH *et al.* Reduced glutathione oxidation ratio and 8 ohdg accumulation by mild ischemic pretreatment. *Brain Res* 2000; 856: 28–36.

221 Sugawara T, Noshita N, Lewen A *et al.* Neuronal expression of the DNA repair protein ku 70 after ischemic preconditioning corresponds to tolerance to global cerebral ischemia. *Stroke* 2001; 32: 2388–93.

222 Douen AG, Akiyama K, Hogan MJ *et al.* Preconditioning with cortical spreading depression decreases intraischemic cerebral glutamate levels and down-regulates excitatory amino acid transporters eaat1 and eaat2 from rat cerebal cortex plasma membranes. *J Neurochem* 2000; 75: 812–8.

223 Jander S, Schroeter M, Peters O *et al.* Cortical spreading depression induces proinflammatory cytokine gene expression in the rat brain. *J Cereb Blood Flow Metab* 2001; 21: 218–25.

224 Kasischke K, Ludolph AC, Riepe MW. NMDA-antagonists reverse increased hypoxic tolerance by preceding chemical hypoxia. *Neurosci Lett* 1996; 214: 175–8.

225 Grabb MC, Choi DW. Ischemic tolerance in murine cortical cell culture: critical role for NMDA receptors. *J Neurosci* 1999; 19: 1657–62.

226 Yamaguchi K, Yamaguchi F, Miyamoto O *et al.* The reversible change of glur2 RNA editing in gerbil hippocampus in course of ischemic tolerance. *J Cereb Blood Flow Metab* 1999; 19: 370–5.

227 Bond A, Lodge D, Hicks CA *et al.* NMDA receptor antagonism, but not AMPA receptor antagonism attenuates induced ischaemic tolerance in the gerbil hippocampus. *Eur J Pharmacol* 1999; 380: 91–9.

228 Slusher BS, Vornov JJ, Thomas AG *et al.* Selective inhibition of naaladase, which converts naag to glutamate, reduces ischemic brain injury. *Nat Med* 1999; 5: 1396–402.

229 Plamondon H, Blondeau N, Heurteaux C *et al.* Mutually protective actions of kainic acid epileptic preconditioning and sublethal global ischemia on hippocampal neuronal death: involvement of adenosine a1 receptors and k(ATP) channels. *J Cereb Blood Flow Metab* 1999; 19: 1296–308.

230 Aizenman E, Sinor JD, Brimecombe JC *et al.* Alterations of N-methyl-D-aspartate receptor properties after chemical ischemia. *J Pharmacol Exp Ther* 2000; 295: 572–7.

231 Shamloo M, Wieloch T. Changes in protein tyrosine phosphorylation in the rat brain after cerebral ischemia in a model of ischemic tolerance. *J Cereb Blood Flow Metab* 1999; 19: 173–83.

232 Shamloo M, Rytter A, Wieloch T. Activation of the extracellular signal-regulated protein kinase cascade in the hippocampal ca1 region in a rat model of global cerebral ischemic preconditioning. *Neuroscience* 1999; 93: 81–8.

233 Shamloo M, Kamme F, Wieloch T. Subcellular distribution and autophosphorylation of calcium/calmodulin-dependent protein kinase ii-alpha in rat hippocampus in a model of ischemic tolerance. *Neuroscience* 2000; 96: 665–74.

234 Heurteaux C, Lauritzen I, Widmann C *et al.* Essential role of adenosine, adenosine a1 receptors, and ATP-sensitive K+ channels in cerebral ischemic preconditioning. *Proc Natl Acad Sci USA* 1995; 92: 4666–70.

235 Perez-Pinzon MA, Mumford PL, Rosenthal M *et al.* Anoxic preconditioning in hippocampal slices: role of adenosine. *Neuroscience* 1996; 75: 687–94.

236 Kawahara N, Ide T, Saito N *et al.* Propentofylline potentiates induced ischemic tolerance in gerbil hippocampal neurons via adenosine receptor. *J Cereb Blood Flow Metab* 1998; 18: 472–5.

237 Riepe MW, Esclaire F, Kasischke K *et al.* Increased hypoxic tolerance by chemical inhibition of oxidative phosphorylation: "chemical preconditioning". *J Cereb Blood Flow Metab* 1997; 17: 257–64.

238 Bruer U, Weih MK, Isaev NK *et al.* Induction of tolerance in rat cortical neurons: hypoxic preconditioning. *FEBS Lett* 1997; 414: 117–21.

239 Vannucci RC, Towfighi J, Vannucci SJ. Hypoxic preconditioning and hypoxic-ischemic brain damage in the immature rat: pathologic and metabolic correlates. *J Neurochem* 1998; 71: 1215–20.

240 Yu ZF, Mattson MP. Dietary restriction and 2-deoxyglucose administration reduce focal ischemic brain damage and improve behavioral outcome: evidence for a preconditioning mechanism. *J Neurosci Res* 1999; 57: 830–9.

241 Wiegand F, Liao W, Busch C *et al.* Respiratory chain inhibition induces tolerance to focal cerebral ischemia. *J Cereb Blood Flow Metab* 1999; 19: 1229–37.

242 Plaschke K, Weigand MA, Michel A *et al.* Permanent cerebral hypoperfusion: 'preconditioning-like' effects on rat energy metabolism towards acute systemic hypotension. *Brain Res* 2000; 858: 363–70.

243 Ohta S, Furuta S, Matsubara I *et al.* Calcium movement in ischemia-tolerant hippocampal ca1 neurons after transient forebrain ischemia in gerbils. *J Cereb Blood Flow Metab* 1996; 16: 915–22.

244 Reshef A, Sperling O, Zoref-Shani E. Opening of ATP-sensitive potassium channels by cromakalim confers tolerance against chemical ischemia in rat neuronal cultures. *Neurosci Lett* 1998; 250: 111–4.

245 Connor JA, Razani-Boroujerdi S, Greenwood AC *et al.* Reduced voltage-dependent Ca^{2+} signaling in ca1 neurons after brief ischemia in gerbils. *J Neurophysiol* 1999; 81: 299–306.

246 Yoneda Y, Kuramoto N, Azuma Y *et al.* Possible involvement of activator protein-1 DNA binding in mechanisms underlying ischemic tolerance in the ca1 subfield of gerbil hippocampus. *Neuroscience* 1998; 86: 79–97.

247 Domoki F, Perciaccante JV, Veltkamp R *et al.* Mitochondrial potassium channel opener diazoxide preserves neuronal-vascular function after cerebral ischemia in newborn pigs. *Stroke* 1999; 30: 2713–8; discussion 2718–9.

248 Blondeau N, Widmann C, Lazdunski M *et al.* Activation of the nuclear factor-kappaB is a key event in brain tolerance. *J Neurosci* 2001; 21: 4668–77.

249 Kapinya K, Penzel R, Sommer C et al. Temporary changes of the ap-1 transcription factor binding activity in the gerbil hippocampus after transient global ischemia, and ischemic tolerance induction. *Brain Res* 2000; 872: 282–93.

250 Semenza GL. Hypoxia-inducible factor 1. Oxygen homeostasis and disease pathophysiology. *Trends Mol Med* 2001; 7: 345–50.

251 Mabuchi T, Kitagawa K, Kuwabara K et al. Phosphorylation of cAMP response element-binding protein in hippocampal neurons as a protective response after exposure to glutamate *in vitro* and ischemia *in vivo*. *J Neurosci* 2001; 21: 9204–13.

252 Ohtsuki T, Ruetzler CA, Tasaki K et al. Interleukin-1 mediates induction of tolerance to global ischemia in gerbil hippocampal ca1 neurons. *J Cereb Blood Flow Metab* 1996; 16: 1137–42.

253 Tasaki K, Ruetzler CA, Ohtsuki T et al. Lipopolysaccharide pretreatment induces resistance against subsequent focal cerebral ischemic damage in spontaneously hypertensive rats. *Brain Res* 1997; 748: 267–70.

254 Dawson DA, Furuya K, Gotoh J et al. Cerebrovascular hemodynamics and ischemic tolerance: lipopolysaccharide-induced resistance to focal cerebral ischemia is not due to changes in severity of the initial ischemic insult, but is associated with preservation of microvascular perfusion. *J Cereb Blood Flow Metab* 1999; 19: 616–23.

255 Liu J, Ginis I, Spatz M et al. Hypoxic preconditioning protects cultured neurons against hypoxic stress via TNF-alpha and ceramide. *Am J Physiol Cell Physiol* 2000; 278: C144–53.

256 Wang X, Li X, Currie RW et al. Application of real-time polymerase chain reaction to quantitate induced expression of interleukin-1beta mRNA in ischemic brain tolerance. *J Neurosci Res* 2000; 59: 238–46.

257 Barone FC, White RF, Spera PA et al. Ischemic preconditioning and brain tolerance: temporal histological and functional outcomes, protein synthesis requirement, and interleukin-1 receptor antagonist and early gene expression. *Stroke* 1998; 29: 1937–50; discussion 1950–31.

258 Wang X, Yaish-Ohad S, Li X et al. Use of suppression subtractive hybridization strategy for discovery of increased tissue inhibitor of matrix metalloproteinase-1 gene expression in brain ischemic tolerance. *J Cereb Blood Flow Metab* 1998; 18: 1173–7.

259 Gidday JM, Shah AR, Maceren RG et al. Nitric oxide mediates cerebral ischemic tolerance in a neonatal rat model of hypoxic preconditioning. *J Cereb Blood Flow Metab* 1999; 19: 331–40.

260 Striggow F, Riek M, Breder J et al. The protease thrombin is an endogenous mediator of hippocampal neuroprotection against ischemia at low concentrations but causes degeneration at high concentrations. *Proc Natl Acad Sci USA* 2000; 97: 2264–9.

261 Shimizu S, Nagayama T, Jin KL et al. Bcl-2 antisense treatment prevents induction of tolerance to focal ischemia in the rat brain. *J Cereb Blood Flow Metab* 2001; 21: 233–43.

262 Kato H, Araki T, Itoyama Y *et al.* An immunohistochemical study of heat shock protein-27 in the hippocampus in a gerbil model of cerebral ischemia and ischemic tolerance. *Neuroscience* 1995; 68: 65–71.

263 Chen J, Graham SH, Zhu RL *et al.* Stress proteins and tolerance to focal cerebral ischemia. *J Cereb Blood Flow Metab* 1996; 16: 566–77.

264 Tanaka S, Uehara T, Nomura Y. Up-regulation of protein-disulfide isomerase in response to hypoxia/brain ischemia and its protective effect against apoptotic cell death. *J Biol Chem* 2000; 275: 10388–93.

265 Yagita Y, Kitagawa K, Ohtsuki T *et al.* Induction of the hsp110/105 family in the rat hippocampus in cerebral ischemia and ischemic tolerance. *J Cereb Blood Flow Metab* 2001; 21: 811–9.

266 Liu J, Bartels M, Lu A *et al.* Microglia/macrophages proliferate in striatum and neocortex but not in hippocampus after brief global ischemia that produces ischemic tolerance in gerbil brain. *J Cereb Blood Flow Metab* 2001; 21: 361–73.

267 Nawashiro H, Tasaki K, Ruetzler CA *et al.* TNF-alpha pretreatment induces protective effects against focal cerebral ischemia in mice. *J Cereb Blood Flow Metab* 1997; 17: 483–90.

268 Sugino T, Nozaki K, Takagi Y *et al.* 3-nitropropionic acid induces ischemic tolerance in gerbil hippocampus *in vivo*. *Neurosci Lett* 1999; 259: 9–12.

269 Kasischke K, Huber R, Li H *et al.* Primary hypoxic tolerance and chemical preconditioning during estrus cycle in mice. *Stroke* 1999; 30: 1256–62.

270 Weih M, Bergk A, Isaev NK *et al.* Induction of ischemic tolerance in rat cortical neurons by 3-nitropropionic acid: chemical preconditioning. *Neurosci Lett* 1999; 272: 207–10.

271 Kuroiwa T, Yamada I, Endo S *et al.* 3-nitropropionic acid preconditioning ameliorates delayed neurological deterioration and infarction after transient focal cerebral ischemia in gerbils. *Neurosci Lett* 2000; 283: 145–8.

272 Brambrink AM, Schneider A, Noga H *et al.* Tolerance-inducing dose of 3-nitropropionic acid modulates bcl-2 and bax balance in the rat brain: a potential mechanism of chemical preconditioning. *J Cereb Blood Flow Metab* 2000; 20: 1425–36.

273 Gonzalez-Zauluet. Requirement for nitric oxide activation of p21(ras)/extracellular regulated kinase in neuronal ischemic preconditioning. *Proc Natl Acad Sci USA* 2000; : 436–41.

274 Kato H, Liu Y, Araki T *et al.* Mk-801, but not anisomycin, inhibits the induction of tolerance to ischemia in the gerbil hippocampus. *Neurosci Lett* 1992; 139: 118–21.

275 Sherman DG, Atkinson RP, Chippendale T *et al.* Intravenous ancrod for treatment of acute ischemic stroke: the STAT study: a randomized controlled trial. Stroke Treatment with Ancrod Trial. *JAMA* 2000; 283: 2395–403.

276 Furlan A, Higashida R, Wechsler L *et al.* Intra-arterial prourokinase for acute ischemic stroke. The proact II study: a randomized controlled trial. Prolyze in acute cerebral thromboembolism. *JAMA* 1999; 282: 2003–11.

CHAPTER 3

Clinical Syndromes—Brain

Sandeep Kumar, Louis R. Caplan

Transient symptoms resulting from brain ischemia have been recognized for a nearly a century. As early as 1914, Hunt described episodes of 'cerebral intermittent claudication' in patients who had carotid artery stenosis [1]. Forty years later, Denny-Brown referred to hemodynamic crises from 'episodic insufficiency in the Circle of Willis of a temporary nature' [2]. The term 'transient ischemic attacks' (TIA) was initially coined by Fisher to describe short-lived episodes of neurological symptoms in patients with carotid artery disease [3,4]. The term has gained widespread acceptance and has been refined over the years. According to the most cited classification, TIA is defined as a brief episode of focal loss of brain function attributable to ischemia, involving one or more of the vascular symptoms and lasting by convention less than 24 h [5].

The present definitions of TIAs are primarily based on clinical phenomenology and do not consider the underlying pathophysiology or presence or absence of target organ damage. For example, TIA may be caused by a penetrating artery arteriopathy, embolization from a cardiac or a large artery source, hypoperfusion from a low flow state, or arterial spasm to name a few mechanisms. Moreover, the cut-off time period of 24 h is chosen arbitrarily, as prolonged TIAs that resolve well within the 24 h often have evidence of brain infarction on imaging studies [6,7]. Efforts are now underway to change the definition of TIA to reflect the fact that most TIAs are brief (< 1 h) and longer TIAs are indicative of brain infarction. Certain non-ischemic conditions like seizures, multiple sclerosis, subdural hematoma, neoplasms can also mimic TIA.

The diagnosis of TIA largely hinges on clinical history and only occasionally by observation of an episode by a physician. Between attacks, the neurological examination is often normal. One of the root problems in characterizing these episodes accurately lies in the inadequacies of clinical history. Quite often, the spells are frightening or may affect the patient's sensorium, making a detailed recall of symptoms difficult. Patients with an unsophisticated knowledge of the nervous system and no previous episodes may not know how to interpret and describe their experience. Patients with right hemispheric ischemia may be unaware of their deficits, others may have evanescent symptoms or symptoms such as field defects, etc., which may be difficult to recognize. Symptoms may occur during sleep or some may simply be forgotten. Despite these limitations, the patient should be questioned closely and repeatedly. A thorough examination should be performed and appropriate investigations obtained. The questions should be directed at determining the loss of function of different body parts which would convey information about the site and degree of brain ischemia, duration of symptoms, tempo of evolution of deficits, accompanying features, activity at time of onset and history of previous episodes.

Temporal profile

The present definition of TIAs includes all reversible clinical deficits lasting < 24 h. In reality, most TIAs are much briefer, and last between 2 and 30 min [5,8,9–11]. Bogousslavsky et al. [12] found that in attacks lasting more than 45–60 min, the risk of infarction as visible on computed tomography scan was > 80%. Kimura et al. [13] reported a similarly high incidence of infarcts on magnetic resonance imaging scans with TIAs lasting > 60 min. Prolonged TIAs, i.e. those lasting > 1 h, are more common with cardioembolic and large artery disease. Tsuda et al. [14] found that short attacks (< 30 min) tended to correlate with mild internal carotid artery (ICA) stenosis and longer attacks with ICA occlusion. TIAs from lacunar disease or from perfusion failure are much briefer in duration.

The symptoms of TIA are typically abrupt in onset and negative in nature, that is they involve a loss of function. This contrasts with migraine, where there is a 'march' of symptoms over a few minutes and symptoms are positive in nature, such as parasthesias, visual scintillations, etc. Neurological deficits in patients with embolism are characteristically abrupt in onset, whereas a nonsudden onset is more typical of thrombosis. A fluctuating or a nonsudden onset occurs in 5–6% of documented embolic strokes compared with almost 30% in lacunes [15–17]. Presumably emboli, which are loosely attached to a vessel wall, dislodge and migrate distally leading to a fluctuating clinical course. The movement of emboli most often occurs during the first 48 h after symptom onset [18]. Distinguishing between mechanisms of ischemia based on clinical presentation can often be difficult. Suddenness of onset suggests but does not confirm the diagnosis of embolism [19]. A single transitory episode, especially if it lasts more than an hour, or multiple episodes of different patterns suggest embolism. This should be distinguished from brief (2–10 min) attacks of the same pattern, which are more indicative of hypoperfusion or atherothrombosis.

Strokes resulting from large vessel atherosclerosis are much more likely to be preceded by TIAs. In the Harvard Stroke Registry, TIAs occurred in 50% of patients with large artery atherosclerosis vs. 23% in patients with lacunar disease [20]. TIAs from lacunar disease typically are limited to a time span of a few days, whereas those from large artery disease may occur over a period of weeks to months. Occasionally some patients have multiple TIAs occurring over a short period of time, often with increasing duration or severity. These have been called 'crescendo TIAs' [21–23], though their significance continues to be debated. Several authorities believe that it represents a condition of impending brain infarction—presumably the TIAs become more frequent as the artery occludes progressively. In the Harvard Stroke Registry, patients who eventually developed strokes from carotid occlusive disease were more likely to do so within a week of their last TIA. Thus, a recent TIA is more ominous and should be evaluated more urgently than an episode that occurred months ago.

Activity at onset

It is widely believed that most thrombotic strokes occur when the circulation is sluggish such as during sleep, whereas embolism is more likely to occur when the circulation is more active. New data show that most ischemic strokes occur in the morning hours between 10.00 h to noon [24]. It is unusual for a thrombotic stroke or TIA to develop during vigorous physical activity. A particularly common time for embolism to occur is on arising at night to urinate, the so-called matudinal (morning) embolus. A TIA that occurs in the setting of relative hypotension (such as orthostasis or a hot bath) is likely to be hemodynamic in nature. Similarly, hemodynamic mechanisms are suspected for vertebrobasilar attacks related to prolonged head and neck turning [25]. A previous history of neck trauma or manipulation, especially with an associated headache or neck pain, is suspicious for an arterial dissection. Types of trivial trauma reported to antedate dissection include almost all varieties of sports activities, violent coughing, vigorous nose blowing, sexual activity, chiropractic manipulation, anesthetic administration and sudden neck turning [26,27].

Associated symptoms

Headache

Headaches occur often in patients who have TIAs; close to half the patients with TIAs report having unacustomed headache during the time span of their ischemic symptoms [28,29]. The pain is present at onset, is mostly ipsilateral to the site of ischemia and is not severe in nature. Headaches are more likely to occur with cortical ischemia [30]. Vertebrobasilar TIAs are more frequently associated with headaches, probably due to a richer trigeminal innervation of the posterior circulation vessels [28]. Emboli to the top of the carotid and basilar arteries or the origin of middle cerebral artery often have associated pain, whereas emboli affecting distal vessels are usually painless [31].

Headache is also a prominent feature of arterial dissection. In extracranial carotid artery dissection, head and neck pain precedes the onset of ischemic symptoms by several hours to a few weeks. Ischemic events most often develop within a week of onset of local symptoms [32]. The headache is most often nonthrobbing and severe, and ipsilateral scalp tenderness may occur. Radiation of pain to the neck and jaw is characteristic. Almost a third of patients have a Horner's syndrome and one-quarter report pulsatile tinnitus or a subjective bruit [33]. Headache immediately precedes or coexists with the onset of neurological deficits in patients with intracranial carotid dissection and TIAs are uncommon. Dissection of an extracranial vertebral artery produces pain localized to the back of neck, head and the occiput. The onset of ischemic symptoms is more variable. Intracranial vertebral artery dissection may present with subarachnoid hemorrhage or brainstem or cerebellar symptoms. Prodromal headaches are uncommon in patients presenting with subarachnoid hemorrhage.

Dizziness and vertigo

Isolated dizziness, especially of a nonrotatory type, is rarely a symptom of TIA and usually results from diverse causes such as orthostatic hypotension, cardiac arrhythmias or hyperventilation. Occasionally, severe stenosis of multiple arteries in the carotid or vertebrobasilar system may give rise to symptoms of global hypoperfusion such as dimness of vision, dizziness and even syncope. Dizziness is a common symptom of extracranial vertebral artery disease, though it is unlikely to be the only symptom. In some attacks, it is accompanied by other symptoms of brainstem or cerebellar dysfunction such as diplopia, oscillopsia, weakness of both legs, hemiparesis or numbness. Rostral basilar artery syndrome or superior cerebellar artery (SCA) territory ischemia may also cause dizziness but is frequently accompanied by other prominent symptoms such as vomiting, visual field defects, ataxia, dysarthria, motor weakness or clumsiness of limbs [34,35].

Although dizziness is a common symptom, it is rarely the sole presentation of a TIA. Patients with dizziness should be closely questioned about any other accompanying symptoms.

Vertigo, which refers to a sensation of spinning, or a sensation of motion, results from a mismatch between the visual, vestibular and somatosensory systems. Ischemia can result in a number of vestibular syndromes, of which vertigo is only one component. In the lateral medullary syndrome, patients often describe a sensation of being off balance, feeling of tilting, or being pulled towards one side or frank spinning [36]. This occurs in conjunction with other symptoms of lateral medullary ischemia such as dysarthria, dysphagia, numbness and ataxia. Examination during the episode reveals an ocular torsion with ipsilateral eye and ear located in a down position, nystagmus including both horizontal and rotatory components with the rapid component of the rotatory nystagmus moving the upper pole of the iris towards the side of the lesion. Ischemia of the anterior inferior cerebellar artery, which supplies the anterolateral pons, middle cerebellar peduncle and flocculus, as well as the inner ear, can result in a spectrum of symptoms that involves vertigo, unilateral tinnitus and hearing loss along with brainstem and cerebellar signs and symptoms. Rostral pontomesencephalic ischemia can give rise to a head tilt that is contraversive, i.e. the contralateral eye is undermost with an associated skew deviation and ocular tilt reaction. Vertigo is also a common neurological symptom of subclavian steal syndrome and usually has a spinning character. It may be accompanied by diplopia, oscillopsia or staggering and is occasionally brought on by exercise of the ischemic arm. However, recurrent isolated episodes of vertigo without neurological signs and symptoms are an uncommon manifestation of vertebrobasilar disease [37].

Other associated symptoms

Loss of consciousness rarely occurs as a symptom of a TIA [38]. Seizures at stroke onset or a cardiac arrhythmia are more likely to cause impairment of consciousness. However, ischemia of deep diencephalic, mesencephalic structures or widespread bihemispheric ischemia as a result of either bilateral carotid or vertebrobasilar occlusive disease can result in loss of consciousness.

Vomiting is commonly seen with ischemia of the posterior circulation, especially when it involves the caudal brainstem. Vomiting occurs infrequently in ischemic events of the anterior circulation. Hiccups are one of the transient symptoms seen at onset of lateral medullary infarcts. It may also occur in association with pontine or bulbar ischemia [39,40].

Angina or palpitations are rarely reported with TIAs. In one series of 205 patients, their prevalence was 2%, though their occurrence clearly suggested an underlying cardiac source of embolism [9].

Carotid disease and TIA

A strong correlation exists between TIAs and carotid artery disease. Patients who eventually develop strokes from carotid artery stenosis have a known prior TIA incidence of 50–75% [19,41,42]. The pathophysiology can be artery-to-artery embolism, perfusion failure from a tight carotid stenosis, or anterograde propagation of carotid artery thrombus. Embolism is the predominant mechanism and causes different clinical attacks during different spells. Most of the embolic TIAs affect the middle cerebral artery (MCA) territory. The episodes are longer than the typical 5–7-min spells seen with severe carotid stenosis [10].

Transient monocular blindness (TMB) and other ocular symptoms are described in Chapter 4. Transient hemispheric symptoms from transient cerebral ischemia can cause weakness or numbness of the contralateral body parts. The motor symptoms are commonly reported as weakness, heaviness or clumsiness, whereas the sensory symptoms are described as numbness, tingling, novocaine like or a dead sensation. Involvement of the left hemisphere can result in aphasia, reported as difficulty in understanding or producing spoken or written language. At times, it may be difficult to distinguish dysarthria from dysphasia, while at other times they may coexist. Facial and tongue weakness are often underreported and should be suspected in dysarthric patients, especially in the absence of cerebellar or truncal dysfunction. Neglect of the opposite side of the visual space and an attentional hemianopia may occur if the right hemisphere is involved. However, unless the patient is examined during the episode, these symptoms may be difficult to reconstruct retrospectively.

Several studies have attempted to characterize features of hemispheric TIAs from carotid disease. In a study by Pessin *et al.* [10], the most common symptoms were motor and sensory involvement of contralateral limbs, followed by pure motor dysfunction, pure sensory dysfunction and lastly isolated dysphasia. Fractional arm weakness, i.e. hand and distal arm weakness that is greater than proximal weakness, can be quite often found in patients with carotid TIAs and may be the only symptom. Presumably, part of the homunculus representing hand and arm lies in the most distal field of the carotid circulation, making this region vulnerable to either perfusion failure or embolism.

Patients with severe ICA stenosis may have recurrent episodes of involuntary, irregular, shaking, trembling or wavering movements of the contralateral arms or legs. These have been called 'limb shaking TIAs' and probably arise from hemodynamic mechanism in the setting of a tight carotid lesion [43–45]. They typically occur when the patient is standing or active and usually involve the arm [43]. Some patients may have abnormal leg movements [46]. Occasionally, these symptoms may develop in patients with ICA occlusion who are intravascularly volume depleted.

On examination, detection of a cervical bruit ipsilateral to the involved hemisphere is a reliable indicator of carotid disease, in a patient with TIA [9]. A local bruit can be heard in approximately 70–87% of patients with tight ICA stenosis [47,48]. The site of maximal intensity corresponds to the ICA bifurcation. Ocular bruit can occur with siphon stenosis or contralateral ICA occlusion.

Middle cerebral artery

Embolism is the commonest mechanism of TIAs or stroke within the MCA territory [19]. *In situ* thrombosis from an underlying atherosclerotic plaque is much less common. MCA disease is more prevalent in women, blacks, and people of Asian descent [49].

Occlusion of the MCA stem by an embolus produces a large area of ischemia involving the superficial and deep territories of the MCA. This may result in a contralateral hemiplegia equally affecting the face, arm and leg along with hemianesthesia and hemi-inattention. Involvement of the dominant hemisphere produces a global aphasia, while anasognosia results from the involvement of the nondominant hemisphere. Occlusion of the upper division produces similar findings, except that the hemiparesis involves the face and arm more than the leg and the aphasia may be more of an anterior type. Lower division syndromes result in a pure aphasia when the dominant hemisphere is involved and behavioral disturbances with involvement of the nondominant hemisphere. A superior quadrantanopia or a hemianopia may be found if the patient is examined during the attack. Involvement of the lenticulostriate branches leads to a variety of motor deficits with varying severity and distribution, usually unaccompanied by sensory, visual, language or behavioral disturbance.

Occasionally, a transient occlusion of the distal ICA or proximal MCA by an embolus results in a major hemispheric syndrome followed by rapid recovery due to early migration of the embolus. This phenomenon has been named 'spectacular shrinking deficit' [50]. The typical initial presentation is of a full hemispheric syndrome followed by a fading hemiparesis with a persistent posterior type of an aphasia or complete recovery, as the embolus migrates across the MCA stem and lodges into the terminal branches of the inferior division. It is more likely to occur in nondiabetic men, with a potential cardiac source of embolism, who are < 60 years of age [51]. In the series reported by Minematsu, most of the recovery took place within 4 h and almost all patients recovered by 24 h.

TIAs also occur in patients with atheromatous MCA disease. The frequency of TIAs is, however, less than that of ICA disease and they occur over a shorter span of time [49,52]. Symptoms typically have a more gradual onset and progressive course, which can fluctuate with time. In a series of 370 patients (58% Asians, 34% blacks, 18% whites) from the EC/IC Bypass Study, reported by Bogousslavsky *et al.* [53], the frequency of TIAs was much higher, which may have been due to a selection bias. The most common clinical picture was unilateral motor weakness, often with arm and leg involvement and facial sparing, and dysarthria or dysphasia. Sensory TIAs were less frequent and involvement of the arm only (31%), of the arm and leg (24%), or of the face, arm and leg (24%) were most common. In patients with repetitive TIAs, stereotypy of symptoms was very common. The mean duration of symptoms varied between 77 and 138 min. In three series of predominantly white patients with MCA occlusive disease, TIAs were a more frequent presentation than stroke, whereas in blacks the incidence of stroke was higher [54–56].

Anterior cerebral artery syndromes

Intrinsic disease of the anterior cerebral artery (ACA) is uncommon, and most of the ACA territory infarcts are embolic [57]. Leg weakness with a distal gradient, which is greatest in the foot but also involves the thigh, is an important clue of ACA territory ischemia, especially if it spares the deeper territories. On examination during the episode, the patient has some weakness of shoulder shrug but hand and face are typically spared. A grasp reflex is often present in the contralateral hand. Another helpful sign is apraxia of the left arm. Cortical sensory loss may be present in the weak limbs but is usually mild. Patients with unilateral or bifrontal ischemia are usually abulic. They appear apathetic with a decrease in spontaneity, are slow to respond to queries and use terse speech, which is limited in amount. Some patients with medial frontal ischemia have prominent motor neglect.

Ischemia of the left ACA territory and supplementary motor cortex can result in a transcortical motor and sensory aphasia. Involvement of the deeper branches, such as the recurrent artery of Heubner, results in ischemia of the head of caudate and anterior limb of internal capsule. The signs and symptoms are very variable but prominent among them are a transient hemiparesis, dysarthria and occasional choreoathetosis of the contralateral limbs. Not uncommonly, changes in behavior such as abulia, slowness, restlessness or hyperactivity can be seen.

Vertebral artery syndromes

Occlusion or severe narrowing of the subclavian or innominate arteries can produce the subclavian steal syndrome. Obstruction in the proximal subclavian artery produces a low-pressure system in the ipsilateral vertebral artery and blood vessels of the ipsilateral arm, diverting blood flow from the contralateral vertebral and basilar arteries into the ipsilateral vertebral artery and into the arm. Most patients with subclavian steal are asymptomatic. In symptomatic patients, most complaints relate to arm ischemia. Fatigue, aching after exercise, and coolness are described. Neurological symptoms are uncommon and are only occasionally brought on by arm exercise. The most common neurological symptom is dizziness, which usually has a vertiginous character [58]. Diplopia, blurring of vision, oscillopsia and staggering are less common. The attacks are brief and although frequent episodes of posterior circulation ischemia may occur, development of a posterior circulation stroke is rare [59,60]. An important clue on examination is a difference in the pulse or blood pressure between the arms and occasionally a supraclavicular bruit can be heard.

The most common transient symptom of vertebral artery disease is dizziness or vertigo, usually accompanied by other symptoms. Chronic, recurrent spells of isolated vertigo lasting longer than 6 weeks are seldom attributable to vertebral occlusion or other vascular etiologies [61]. Patients with isolated vertigo, who eventually develop an infarct, do so within 3 weeks of symptom onset. The most well-recognized symptoms of vertebral artery disease include components of the lateral medullary syndrome. The most common constellation of signs and symptoms includes dizziness or vertigo, often accompanied by staggering and double vision, nausea and vomiting, dysarthria, dysphagia, ipsilateral Horner's syndrome, gait and limb ataxia, diminished sensation of the ipsilateral face and loss of pain and thermal sensation of contralateral limb and trunk. Gait and trunk ataxia, axial lateropulsion or a combination of these two makes standing or walking difficult.

Bilateral stenosis of the intracranial vertebral arteries usually results in multiple TIAs, which are stereotyped, and position sensitive. In the NEMC Posterior Circulation Registry, most of the patients with bilateral disease had TIAs—43% had TIAs prior to stroke, 38% had TIAs only and only 19% had strokes without TIAs [62]. Vertigo, dizziness, dysarthria, diplopia and headache were the most common symptoms.

Basilar artery syndromes

TIAs are uncommon in patients with basilar artery embolism, which typically produces strokes without any preceding TIAs [59]. In contrast, patients with primary atherosclerosis of the basilar and intracranial vertebral arteries have TIAs followed by strokes.

Widespread occlusive disease involving multiple posterior circulation arteries in addition to the basilar artery produces predominantly TIAs often followed by strokes. TIAs from lacunar disease do occur in the posterior circulation but they are less common than with large vessel disease [20].

The most commonly reported symptoms in patients with basilar artery occlusive disease include diplopia, dizziness often without vertigo, weakness of both legs or weakness alternating between different limbs in different attacks. When examined during the episode, patients may have bilateral weakness of limbs or may have a hemiparesis. Most of the hemiparetic patients show motor or reflex abnormalities on the other side [59]. Occasionally, abnormal spontaneous movements such as shivering, twitching, shaking or jerking may be seen on the relatively spared side [63]. Weakness of cranial musculature causes dysarthria, dysphonia, hoarseness, dysphagia or tongue weakness. Abnormality of eye movements such as internuclear ophthalmoplegia, paresis of conjugate gaze, nystagmus or ocular skewing may be seen. Some patients may have ptosis with small pupils. Somatosensory or special sensory abnormalities are not prominent.

Pontine lacunes and infarcts from atheromatous basilar branch disease are very common in hypertensive and diabetic patients. Some patients with pontine branch disease have frequent, brief, stereotyped TIAs. The term 'capsular warning syndrome' originally used to describe repeated attacks of hemiparesis in patients who eventually developed internal capsular infarcts, also occurs in relation to pontine ischemia [64]. In some patients with repetitive attacks, persistent neurological symptoms do not develop.

Basilar migraine

Basilar migraine often presents with transient ischemic symptoms referable to the vertebrobasilar artery territory. This syndrome is probably more common than is appreciated and occurs in a wide spectrum of ages. Most of the patients have a strong family history of migraine. Sturzenegger and Meinberg et al. [65] reported that 65% of the patients had their first attack in the second or third decade. The most common symptom was bilateral visual impairment occurring in 86% of the patients followed by some impairment of consciousness, parasthesias, vertigo, weakness, ataxia or dysarthria. In the original description by Bickerstaff, the signs and symptoms lasted between 2 to 45 min and were invariably followed by a pulsating headache [66]. Many individuals have other migraine accompaniments during the attack. Strokes are probably more common in patients with basilar artery migraine than in those with just scintillating scotomas.

Posterior cerebral artery

Embolism is the most common cause of posterior cerebral artery (PCA) territory ischemia [59,67]. The embolus may arise from the heart or from a proximal source in the posterior circulation, such as the extracranial or intracranial vertebral arteries. Intrinsic atheromatous disease of the PCA is infrequent and tends to involve the proximal (peduncular and ambient) segments of the artery [11].

TIAs are the most frequent from of presentation in patients with PCA stenosis [11]. The episodes tend to be brief, typically lasting between 2 and 10 min, and are often multiple. In the series reported by Pessin et al. [11], TIAs were more frequent than infarcts, with a predominance of visual and sensory symptoms. Visual symptoms included flashing lights, graying or darkening of vision on one side, and red and white lights. Scintillations, shimmering, brightness, and fortifications did not occur in patients with either PCA stenosis or embolism, and the episodes of photopsias in patients with PCA ischemia were brief, lasting < 30 s, compared with the usual 20 min or more in patients with migraine. All the patients with visual symptoms in the series reported by Pessin *et al.* also had other symptoms, including parasthesias, or clumsiness and involuntary limb movement. Embolism to the PCA usually presents with a sudden-onset neurological deficit. When the donor source of the embolism is the extracranial or intracranial vertebral artery, patients may have TIAs related to local ischemia in proximal intracranial territory (medulla and posteroinferior cerebellum) before their PCA stroke.

Headache occurs frequently in patients with PCA territory ischemia [59]. It may precede TIA symptoms in patients with intrinsic PCA stenosis. It is often located in or just above the eye, in the forehead, or in the frontal or parietal region. A number of cognitive and behavioral abnormalities can occur with PCA territory ischemia. These may be difficult to discern based purely on history. However, some may be detected more easily when the patient is examined during the episode. Ischemia of the left occipital lobe and splenium can result in alexia without agraphia. In this syndrome, there is a loss of previously fluent reading skill, despite the ability to write, speak and comprehend spoken language. Reading is, however, a complex process and involves vision, form perception, attention, and scanning eye movements and can be impaired for a variety of reasons. When the lesion is large and involves the angular gyrus as well, patient can develop alexia with agraphia. In this syndrome, patients can neither read, write nor spell correctly. Some patients with left PCA territory ischemia may have an anomic or transcortical aphasia. Acquisition of new memories can be impaired when both mesial temporal lobes are affected, but may also occur with ischemia limited to the left temporal lobe. Ischemia of the right PCA territory can cause prosopagnosia, when the patient has difficulty recognizing familiar faces. Individuals can only be identified by their voice, hairstyle or clothing, etc. Disorientation to place and reduplicative paramnesia occurs in relation to right PCA territory ischemia. Patients often report being in a different locale that does not bear any relation to their current location. Bilateral PCA territory ischemia, which is almost always caused by embolism to the top of the basilar artery, can result in a triad of abnormalities: (i) bilateral visual field abnormalities sometimes extensive enough to cause cortical blindness; (ii) memory loss, involving both anterograde and retrograde amnesia; (iii) agitated delirium in which patients are hyperactive, loquacious, and often aggressive [59].

Transient global amnesia

Transient global amnesia (TGA) occurs mostly after the age of 50 with an observed incidence of 23.5–32 per 100 000 per year [68–70]. The etiological basis of the syndrome remains unsettled, though transient ischemia of the inferomedial parts of the temporal lobes from vasoconstriction has been put forward as one of the possible mechanisms to explain its pathogenesis [69,71]. Most consider it a benign condition. Reports of poor outcome in literature are probably due to loose application of the term to conditions which may mimic TGA. Strokes, epilepsy, brain tumor or head trauma are all known to cause memory dysfunction. The unqualified diagnosis of TGA should be reserved for those cases without any obvious cause.

The symptoms of TGA are fairly typical and consist of an abrupt impairment in the ability to form new memories as well as an amnesia for past events dating back a variable length of time. Patients appear perplexed and restless. Most patients engage in repetitive questioning frequently concerning the time of day, recent activity, or how they got to their present locale. Working memory, personal identity, and consciousness are well preserved, and patients are able to perform accustomed and even routine complex behavior quite well during the episode. A minority of patients report headaches, which can occur during the episode but most often follow after the event. The duration of the attack varies between 4 and 7 h and is almost always less than 24 h [68,72]. Following the attack there is a permanent memory loss for the period of the attack, and for a few hours preceding it. A number of precipitants have been reported in literature including strenuous physical exercise, sexual intercourse, hot and cold baths, emotional stress, and medical procedures such as angiography, cystoscopy, etc. However, in a number of episodes an established precipitant is missing. Multiple attacks do occur in a minority of patients with a reported recurrence rate between 14.4 and 23.8% [68]. The average time interval between attacks in the series reported by Miller *et al.* [68] was 28.5 months, which was strikingly different from patients with TIAs, who have attacks hours, days, weeks or at most a few months apart.

The senior author has suggested the following criteria for the diagnosis of TGA [72].

(1) The information about the beginning of attack should be available preferably from an articulate observant witness This criterion is designed to guard against missing the diagnosis of post-traumatic amnesia or epilepsy. Patients who live alone may fall or hit their head and post-traumatic retrograde amnesia might erase any personal recollection of the injury. Similarly, it is well known that patients with epileptic attacks, especially complex partial seizures, can experience significant periods of amnesia.

(2) Dysfunction during the attacks should be limited to repetitive queries and amnesia Information about the patient's behavior during the attack can come from an observant witness or by a physician's examination during the attack.

(3) There should be no important accompanying neurological signs PCA or watershed infarcts can cause memory disturbances like TGA, but are always accompanied by other neurological signs and symptoms such as drowsiness, diplopia, ataxia, parasthesias, motor or visual field deficits, visual or color agnosia, prosopagnosia or aphasia [73]. Similarly unilateral thalamic infarcts can cause amnestic strokes, with other associated features, which vary with lesion site. Tuberothalamic lesions can cause variable cognitive deficits including aphasia from a left-sided lesion and neglect or visuospatial impairments from right-sided lesions along with transitory sensorimotor signs and a facial paresis for emotional movements [73]. Paramedian infarcts typically present with somnolence and supranuclear vertical gaze palsies. Neuropsychologial deficits including amnesia appear as the patient improves. Occasionally, anterior choroidal territory ischemia may produce an amnestic syndrome accompanied by hemiparesis, hemiataxia and visual field defects [73]. Minor or trivial abnormalities like visual flickering or minor and transient parasthesias should not disqualify the diagnosis of TGA.

(4) The memory loss should be transient Amnestic strokes usually cause lasting memory loss, which seldom clear in 24 h. Similarly, other structural lesions like tumor, abscesses, encephalitis are more likely to produce longer memory loss.

When the above criteria are not met, the chance of a more sinister pathology as a cause of TGA increases greatly. If all criteria are met, the likelihood of future strokes or other serious disease is similar to age matched population that share similar risk factors [72].

Lacunar TIAs

A lacune refers to a small, deep infarct in the territory of a small, penetrating branch arising from a large cerebral artery. The size of the infarcts at autopsy has been small, varying between 0.2 and 15 mm [3,16]. The majority of patients have hypertension and/or diabetes. A number of clinical syndromes from lacunar disease have been described. These include pure motor stroke, pure sensory stroke, sensorimotor stroke, ataxic hemiparesis, dysarthria clumsy-hand syndrome, various movement disorders, and disorders of speech. It is beyond the scope of this chapter to give a detailed account of each syndrome. However, for present discussion a brief summary of the important syndromes is provided below.

Pure motor stroke or pure motor hemiparesis (PMH) is by far the most common lacunar syndrome, accounting for more than half of the cases [74–76]. Most of the infarcts have involved the internal capsule, pons, corona radiata, and medullary pyramid. The deficits equally affect the face, arm, leg on the same side, and spare sensation, vision, language and cognition. The deficits may affect one region more than the other and include minor abnormalities of sensation. However, pure motor mono-paresis is almost never due to a lacunar infarct [77]. Pure sensory stroke, which is the sensory counterpart of the PMH, occurs less frequently. The sensory disturbance may involve the entire hemicorpus, including the scalp and genitilia or may affect different body parts including lips, tongue and mouth in varying combinations. Syndrome of ataxic hemiparesis has elements of both cerebellar and pyramidal dysfunction and was initially described as homolateral ataxia with crural paresis. It usually presents with weakness of the leg or foot, without any weakness of arm or face, and is accompanied by ataxia of the arm or leg on the same side. In dysarthria clumsy-hand syndrome, dysarthria and ataxia of the upper extremity are most prominent and can include facial weakness, dysphagia, and minor weakness of the hand or leg.

In contrast to lacunar strokes, lacunar TIAs have been less well defined. Some general features of lacunar TIAs have been mentioned in the previous sections. Lacunar TIAs present with more episodes compared with TIAs from large arteries, have a longer duration of neurological deficit in each attack, and a shorter latency between the first and last TIA and definitive infarction [19]. The attacks are usually stereotyped and are often either pure motor or pure sensory. Stepwise or stuttering onset is more common in lacunes than large vessel disease or cardiac embolism. It may be possible to differentiate lacunar TIAs from cortical TIAs using the same clinical criteria as is used for lacunar infarction, i.e. if a right-handed patient has a transient right-sided facial and/or upper motor neuron TIA symptoms and attempts to speak at the same time, dysphasia may occur when the TIA involves the cortical branches of the left MCA (cortical TIA), whereas the speech may be normal or dysarthric if penetrating lenticulos-triate branches are involved (lacunar TIA) [78]. If the speech is normal or the patient remains silent, the syndrome may be distinguished clinically provided that the motor and/or sensory disturbance involves only one body area (face, arm, or leg) or incompletely affects two such areas, since permanent deficits of this type are usually caused by cortical ischemia [79]. In a series of 580 patients with left hemispheric symptoms reported by Hankey *et al.* [78], lacunar and cortical TIA could be reliably distinguished using the above criteria.

Prognosis

Patients with TIAs have an increased risk of stroke and vascular death. The risk of stroke has been reported to be 4.4–8% during the first month [85–87], 11.6–13% during the first year [80,81], and 24–29% during the first 5 years [80–82]. The risk of death has varied between 8 and 37% in different studies, during the first 5 years after a TIA [83–85]. Despite a number of studies on TIAs, numerous methodological differences exist between them limiting their general applicability. These include differences in defining incident cases, differences in study population (community vs. hospital cohorts), differences in duration of follow-up, prospective vs. retrospective case reviews, failure to report treatment details such as antiplatelet therapy or prophylactic carotid surgery, etc. A number of these studies lump all TIAs together, ignoring important differences between the various etiologies and mechanisms. TIAs are a heterogeneous group of disorders with different underlying pathophysiologies, each of which may confer a different prognosis. For example, in the NASCET study, Kaplan–Meier estimates of patients with hemispherical symptoms and high-grade carotid stenosis (> 70%) had a 43.5 ± 6.7% risk of ipsilateral stroke [86], while the yearly risk of stroke in patients with MCA stenosis in the EC/IC Bypass study was 5.8% [53]. However, in even more homogeneous cohorts such as patients with TIA due to atherothromboembolism, lipohyalinosis or cardiogenic embolism, the prognosis was quite variable among individual TIA patients, mainly due to differences in prevalence and level of risk factors [82,87].

Several studies have attempted to identify adverse prognostic factors. These include increasing number of TIAs in 3 months prior to presentation [23,88], increasing age [23,89,90], peripheral vascular disease [88,90], left ventricular hypertrophy [23,91], TIA of the brain (compared with amaurosis fugax only) [23,86], multiple TIAs involving both vertebrobasilar and carotid territories [88], and ischemic heart disease [88,90]. Patients with significant cardiac source of embolism such as atrial fibrillation [91,92], valvular heart disease [93], recent anterior or apical myocardial infarction with or without mural thrombus [94,95], congestive heart failure [95], and significant carotid stenosis [96] (with or without plaque ulceration) are all at higher risk of subsequent strokes.

However, there is clearly a dearth of clinical data and much more research needs to be done to identify those variables, which put a patient at higher risk of stroke. This should include information on clinical details such as number and type of clinical attacks, timing and description of attacks, situations that provoke attacks, stereotypy or heterogeneity of attacks, vascular and cardiac data, and information about other blood parameters. This would ultimately help clinicians diagnose and make a more rational risk assessment of individual patients, order appropriate tests in a cost-effective way and manage their patients more judiciously.

References

1 Hunt JR. The role of the carotid arteries in the causation of vascular lesions of the brain with remarks on certain special features of symptomatology. *Am J Med Sci* 1914; 147: 704–13.

2 Denny-Brown D. The treatment of recurrent cerebrovascular symptoms and the question of vasospasm. *Med Clin N Am* 1951; 35: 1457–74.

3 Fisher CM. Occlusion of the carotid arteries. *Arch Neurol Psychiatry* 1954; 72: 187–204.

4 Fisher CM. Intermittent cerebral ischemia. In: Wright TS, Millikan CH, eds. *Cerebral Vascular Disease*. New York: Grune & Stratton, 1958.

5 Ad Hoc Committee on Cerebrovascular Diseases. Classification of cerebrovascular diseases III. *Stroke* 1990; 21: 637–76.

6 Perrone P, Candelize L, Scotti G *et al*. CT evaluation in patients with transient ischemic attacks; correlation between clinical and angiographic findings. *Eur Neurol* 1979; 18: 217–21.

7 Waxman SG, Toole JF. Temporal profile resembling TIA in the setting of cerebral infarction. *Stroke* 1983; 14: 433–7.

8 Hevy DE. How transient are transient ischemic attacks ? *Neurology* 1988; 38: 674–7.

9 Bogousslavsky J, Hachinski V, Barnette HJM *et al*. Clinical predictors of cardiac and arterial lesions in carotid ischemic attacks. *Arch Neurol* 1986; 43: 229–33.

10 Pessin MS, Mohr JP, Poskanzer DC *et al*. Clinical and angiographic features of carotid transient ischemic attacks. *N Engl J Med* 1977; 296: 358–62.

11 Pessin MS, Kwan E, DeWitt LD *et al*. Posterior cerebral artery stenosis. *Ann Neurol* 1987; 21: 85–9.

12 Bogousslavsky J, Regli F. Cerebral infarct in apparent transient ischemic attack. *Neurology* 1985; 35: 1501–3.

13 Kimura K, Minematsu K, Yamaguchi T *et al*. The duration of symptoms in transient ischemic attack. *Neurology* 1999; 52: 976–80.

14 Tsuda Y, Kimura K, Yoneda S *et al*. CBF and CO_2 reactivity in transient ischemic attacks: comparison between transient ischemic attacks due to internal carotid artery occlusion and internal carotid artery mild stenosis. *Neurol Res* 1983; 5: 17–37.

15 Fisher CM, Pearlman A. The non sudden onset of cerebral embolism. *Neurology (Minneap)* 1967; 17: 1025–32.

16 Fisher CM. Capsular infarcts. *Arch Neurol* 1979; 36: 65–73.

17 Fisher CM. Thalamic pure sensory stroke: a pathological study. *Neurology* 1978; 28: 1141–4.

18 Caplan LR. *Caplan's Stroke: a Clinical Approach*, 3rd edn. Boston: Butterworth Heinemann, 2000.

19 Fieschi C, Sette G, Fiorelli M *et al*. Clinical presentation and potential sources of embolism in acute ischemic stroke patients: the experience of the Rome Acute Stroke Registry. *Cerebrovasc Dis* 1995; 5: 75–8.

20 Mohr J, Caplan LR, Melski J *et al*. The Harvard Cooperative Stroke Registry: a prospective registry. *Neurology* 1978; 28: 754–62.

21 Feinberg WM, Albers GW, Barnett HJM *et al*. Guidelines for management of transient ischemic attacks. *Stroke* 1994; 25: 1320–35.

22 North American Symptomatic Carotid Endarterectomy Trial Collaborators. Beneficial effect of carotid endarterectomy in symptomatic patients with high grade carotid stenosis. *N Engl J Med* 1991; 325: 445–543.

23 Hankey GJ, Slattery JM, Warlow CP. Transient ischemic attacks? Which patients are at high (and low) risk of serious vascular events? *J Neurol Neurosurg Psychiatry* 1992; 55: 640–52.

24 Marler J, Price TR, Clark GL *et al*. Morning increase in onset of ischemic stroke. *Stroke* 1989; 20: 473–6.

25 Berciano J, Coria F. Occipitoatlantal instability. a hemodynamic cause of vertebrobasilar ischemia after neck motion. *Stroke* 1992; 23: 921.

26 Bostrom K, Liliequist B. Primary dissecting aneurysm of the extracranial part of the internal carotid and vertebral arteries. *Neurology* 1967; 17: 179–86.

27 Hart RG, Easton JD. Dissection of cervical and cerebral arteries. *Neurol Clin* 1983; 1: 155–82.

28 Grindal AB, Toole JF. Headache and transient ischemic attack. *Stroke* 1974; 5: 603–6.

29 Portenoy RK, Abissi CJ, Lipton RB *et al*. Headache in cerebrovascular diseases. *Stroke* 1984; 15: 1009–12.

30 Koudstaal PJ, Van Ginj J, Kapelle LJ for the Dutch TIA Study Group. Headache in transient or permanent cerebral ischemia. *Stroke* 1991; 22: 754–9.

31 Estol CJ. Headache. Stroke symptoms and signs. In: Bogousslavsky J, Caplan LR, eds. *Stroke Syndromes*. Cambridge: Cambridge University Press, 2001.

32 Biousse V, D'Anglejean-Chatillon J, Bousser H-G *et al*. Time course of symptoms in extracranial carotid artery dissections. *Stroke* 1995; 26: 235–9.

33 Saver JL, Easton JD. Dissection and trauma of cervicocerebral arteries. In: Barnette HJM, Mohr JP, Yatsu FM, eds. *Stroke: Pathophysiology, Diagnosis and Management*, 3rd edn. New York: Churchill Livingstone, 1998.

34 Amarenco P, Hauw J-J. Cerebellar infarction in the territory of the superior cerebellar artery. A clinicopathological study of 33 cases. *Neurology* 1990; 40: 1383–90.

35 Kase C, Norring B, Levine S *et al*. Cerebellar infarction. Clinical and anatomic observations in 66 cases. *Stroke* 1993; 24: 76–83.

36 Caplan LR. Intracranial vertebral arteries and proximal intracranial territory infarcts. In: *Posterior Circulation Disease: Clinical Findings, Diagnosis and Management*. Cambridge, MA: Blackwell Science, 1996.

37 Estol C, Caplan LR, Pessin MS. Isolated vertigo: an uncommon manifestation of vertebrobasilar ischemia. *Cerebrovasc Dis* 1996; 6 (Suppl. 2): 161.

38 Bousser MG, Dubois B, Castaigne P. Transient loss of consciousness in ischemic cerebral events. A study of 557 ischemic strokes and transient ischemic attacks. *Ann Med Interne (Paris)* 1981; 132: Abstract.

39 Shibaski H, Kakigi R, Masukawa S *et al*. Somatosensory and acoustic brainstem reflex myoclonus. *J Neurol Nsurg Psychiatry* 1988; 51: 572–5.

40 Palmer JP, Tippett DC, Wolf JS. Synchronous positive and negative myoclonus due to pontine hemorrhage. *Muscle Nerve* 1991; 14: 124–32.

41 Russo LS Jr. Carotid system transient ischemic attacks: clinical, racial and angiographic correlations. *Stroke* 1981; 12: 470–3.

42 Pessin MS, Hinton RC, Davis KR *et al*. Mechanisms of acute carotid stroke. *Ann Neurol* 1979; 6: 245–52.

43 Baquis GD, Pessin MS, Scott RM. Limb shaking—a carotid TIA. *Stroke* 1985; 16: 444–8.

44 Tatemichi TK, Young WL, Mohr JP *et al*. Perfusion insufficiency in limb shaking transient ischemic attacks. *Stroke* 1990; 21: 341–7.

45 Yanagihara T, Klass DW. Rhythmic involuntary movement as a manifestation of transient ischemic attacks. *Trans Am Neurol Assoc* 1981; 106: 46–8.

46 Yanagihara T, Sundt TM Jr, Piepgras DG. Weakness of the lower extremity in carotid occlusive disease. *Arch Neurol* 1988; 45: 297–301.

47 Pessin MS, Panis W, Prager RJ *et al*. Auscultation of cervical and ocular bruits in extracranial carotid occlusive disease: a clinical and angiographic study. *Stroke* 1983; 14: 246–9.

48 Gautier JC, Rosa A, Lhermitte F. Carotid auscultation: correlation in 200 patients with 332 angiograms. *Rev Neurol (Paris)* 1975; 131: Abstract.

49 Yoo K-M, Shin HK, Caplan LR *et al*. Middle cerebral artery occlusive disease: the New England Medical Center stroke registry. *J Stroke Cerebrovasc Dis* 1988; 7: 344–51.

50 Mohr JP, Lazar RM, Hier DB *et al*. Middle cerebral artery. In: Barnett HJM, Mohr JP, Stein BM, Yatsu FM, eds. *Stroke: Pathophysiology, Diagnosis and Management*, 3rd edn. New York: Churchill Livingstone, 1988.

51 Minematsu K, Yamaguchi T, Omae T. 'Spectacular shrinking deficit': rapid recovery from a major hemispheric syndrome by migration of an embolus. *Neurology* 1992; 42: 157–62.

52 Caplan LR, Babikian V, Hegalson C *et al*. Occlusive disease of the middle cerebral artery. *Neurology* 1985; 35: 975–82.

53 Bogousslavsky J, Barnett HJM, Taylor W *et al*. Atherosclerotic disease of the middle cerebral artery. *Stroke* 1986; 17: 1112–20.

54 Hinton R, Mohr JP, Ackerman R *et al*. Symptomatic middle cerebral artery stenosis. *Ann Neurol* 1979; 5: 152–7.

55 Corston RN, Kendall BE, Marshall J. Prognosis in middle cerebral artery stenosis. *Stroke* 1984; 15: 237–41.

56 Moulin DE, Lo R, Chiang J *et al*. Prognosis in middle cerebral artery occlusion. *Stroke* 1985; 16: 282–4.

57 Bogousslavsky J, Regli F. Anterior cerebral artery territory infarction in the Lausanne Stroke Registry: clinical and etiological patterns. *Arch Neurol* 1990; 47: 144–50.

58 Caplan LR. Large vessel occlusive disease of the posterior circulation. In: *Caplan's Stroke: a Clinical Approach*, 3rd edn. Boston: Butterworth-Heinemann, 2001.

59 Caplan LR. *Posterior Circulation Disease. Clinical Findings, Diagnosis and Management*. Boston: Blackwell, 1996.

60 Hennerici M, Klemm C, Rautenberg W. The subclavian steal phenomenon: a common vascular disorder with rare neurological deficits. *Neurology* 1988; 38: 669–73.

61 Fisher CM. Vertigo in cerebrovascular disease. *Arch Otolaryngol* 1967; 85: 529–34.

62 Shin H-K, Yoo K-M, Caplan LR *et al*. Bilateral intracranial vertebral artery disease in the New England Medical Center Posterior Circulation Registry. *Arch Neurol* 1999; 56: 1353–8.

63 Ropper AH. 'Convulsions' in the basilar artery occlusion. *Neurology* 1988; 38: 1500–1.

64 Farrar J, Donnan GA. Capsular warning syndrome preceding pontine infarction. *Stroke* 1993; 24: 762.

65 Sturzenegger MH, Meienberg O. Basilar artery migraine: a follow up study of 82 cases. *Headache* 1985; 25: 408–15.

66 Bickerstaff ER. Basilar artery migraine. *Lancet* 1961; 1: 15–7.

67 Yamammoto Y, Georgiadis AL, Caplan LR. Posterior cerebral artery territory infarcts in the New England Medical Center Posterior Circulation Registry. *Arch Neurol* 1999; 56: 824–32.

68 Miller JW, Petersen RC, Yanagihara T *et al*. Transient global amnesia: clinical characteristics and prognosis. *Neurology* 1987; 37: 733–7.

69 Hodges JR, Warlow CP. The etiology of transient global amnesia: a case controlled study of 114 cases with prospective follow up. *Brain* 1990; 113: 639–57.

70 Koski KJ, Martilla RJ. Transient global amnesia: incidence in an urban population. *Acta Neurol Scand* 1990; 81: 358–60.

71 Caplan LR, Chendru F, Mayman C. Transient global amnesia and migraine. *Neurology* 1981; 31: 1167–70.

72 Caplan LR. Transient global amnesia: characteristic features and overview. In: Markowitsch HJ, ed. *Transient Global Amnesia and Related Disorders*. Toronto: Hogrefe and Huber, 1990.

73 Ott BR, Saver J. Unilateral amenstic stroke: six new cases and review of literature. *Stroke* 1993; 24: 1033–42.

74 Arboix A, Marti-Vilalta JL, Garcia JH. Clinical study of 227 patients with lacunar infarcts. *Stroke* 1990; 21: 842–7.

75 Mohr JP, Kase CS, Wolf PA *et al*. Lacunes in the NINCDS Pilot Stroke Data Bank. *Ann Neurol* 1982; 12: 84.

76 Tuszynski MH, Petito CK, Levy DE. Risk factors and clinical manifestations of pathologically verified lacunar infarction. *Stroke* 1989; 20: 990–9.

77 Melo TP, Bogousslavsky J, Van Melle G *et al*. Pure motor stroke: a reappraisal. *Neurology* 1992; 42: 789–95.

78 Hankey GJ, Warlow CP. Lacunar transient ischemic attacks: a clinically useful concept? *Lancet* 1991; 337: 353–38.

79 Kase CS. Middle cerebral artery syndromes. In: Vinkin PJ, Bruyn GW, Toole JF, eds. *Handbook of Clinical Neurology*. Amsterdam: Elsevier, 1988: 353–70.

80 Dennis M, Bamford J, Warlow C *et al.* Prognosis of transient ischemic attacks in the Oxfordshire Community Stroke Project. *Stroke* 1990; 21: 848–53.

81 Whisnant JP, Wiebers DO. Clinical epidemiology of transient ischemic attacks (TIA) in the anterior and posterior circulation. In: Sundt TM Jr, ed. *Occlusive Cerebrovascular Disease: Diagnosis and Surgical Management.* New York: W.B. Saunders Co., 1987: 60–5.

82 Heyman A, Wilkinson WE, Gore TB *et al.* Risk of ischemic heart disease in patients with TIA. *Neurology* 1984; 34: 626–30.

83 Muuronen A, Kaste M. Outcome of 314 patients with transient ischemic attacks. *Stroke* 1982; 13: 24–31.

84 Goldner JC, Whisnant JP, Taylor WF. Long-term prognosis of transient cerebral attacks. *Stroke* 1971; 2: 160–7.

85 Simonsen N, Pederson HE, Sorenson PS *et al.* Long-term prognosis after transient ischemic attacks. *Acta Neurol Scan* 1981; 63: 156–68.

86 Streifler JY, Eliasizw M, Fox AJ *et al.* Angiographic detection of carotid plaque ulceration. Comparison with surgical observations in a multicenter study. North American Symptomatic Carotid Endarterectomy Trial. *Stroke* 1994; 25: 1130.

87 Hankey GJ, Slattery JM, Warlow CP. Prognosis of hospital-referred transient ischemic attacks. *J Neurol Neurosurg Psychiatry* 1991; 54: 793–801.

88 Kernan WN, Horwitz RI, Taylor KJN *et al.* A prognostic system for transient ischemic attacks or minor stroke. *Ann Intern Med* 1991; 114: 552–7.

89 American–Canadian Cooperative Study Group. Persantin and aspirin trial in cerebral ischemia. Part III. Risk factors for stroke. *Stroke* 1986; 17: 12–8.

90 The Dutch TIA Trial Study Group. A comparison of two doses of aspirin (30 mg vs. 283 mg a day) in patients after a transient ischemic attack or minor ischemic stroke. *N Engl J Med* 1991; 325: 1261–6.

91 The Stroke Prevention in Atrial Fibrillation Investigators. Predictors of thromboembolism in atrial fibrillation: 1. Clinical features of patients at risk. *Ann Intern Med* 1992; 116: 1–5.

92 Atrial Fibrillation Investigators. Risk factors for stroke and efficacy of antithrombotic therapy in atrial fibrillation: analysis of pooled data from five randomized controlled trials. *Arch Intern Med* 1994; 154: 1449–57.

93 Cerebral Embolism Task Force. Cardiogenic brain embolism. *Arch Neurol* 1986; 43: 71–84.

94 Loh E, Sutton M, Wun C-C *et al.* Ventricular dysfunction and the risk of stroke after myocardial infarction. *N Engl J Med* 1997; 336: 251–7.

95 Caplan LR. Brain embolism. In: Caplan LR, Hurst JW, Chimowitz M, eds. *Clinical Neurocardiology.* New York: Marcell Dekker, 1999.

96 Barnett HJM, Taylor DW, Eliasziw M *et al.* Benefit of carotid endarterectomy in patients with symptomatic moderate or severe stenosis. North American Symptomatic Carotid Endarterectomy Trial Collaborators. *N Engl J Med* 1998; 339: 1415–25.

CHAPTER 4

Clinical Syndromes—Ocular: Transient Visual Loss

Gregory P. Van Stavern

Introduction

Transient visual loss (TVL) reflects a heterogeneous group of disorders, some relatively benign and others with grave neurological or ophthalmological implications. The task of the clinician is to use the history and examination to localize the problem to a region in the visual pathways, identify potential etiologies, and in some cases perform a focused battery of laboratory tests to confirm or exclude certain causes. The therapeutic and prognostic implications for certain causes of transient visual loss may differ markedly, so it is important to identify the underlying pathological process.

Approach to transient visual loss

The majority of patients with TVL present after the episode has resolved, so the neurological and ophthalmological examination is often normal. The nature of the visual symptoms, associated features, and pertinent medical and family history provide valuable clues to the underlying diagnosis. The examination may reveal residual deficits that localize the lesion (perhaps the visual loss was not actually transient), and suggest possible etiologies.

It is important to establish whether the visual loss was monocular or binocular. Transient monocular visual loss (TMVL) implies a disorder anterior to the optic chiasm, including ocular causes as well as ischemia due to ipsilateral carotid artery disease. Transient binocular visual loss (TBVL) suggests a process posterior to the chiasm, such as migraine, seizure, or vertebrobasilar insufficiency. Since the visual field is slightly larger temporally than nasally, patients with homonymous visual field defects often report monocular visual loss, localizing it to the eye with the temporal field cut. The patient should be asked specifically whether each eye was alternately covered during the attack.

The duration of the event provides helpful information regarding etiology. Transient visual obscurations due to papilledema typically last seconds, and are often provoked by postural change. Thrombo-embolic events generally last 2–10 min, and may be associated with hemispheric symptoms. Migraine aura lasts 20–30 min, and may be followed by a characteristic headache.

The actual visual symptoms should be explored. Positive visual phenomena such as scintillations that march across the visual field suggest migraine as the most likely diagnosis. Visual seizures often involve positive visual symptoms, but are typically maximal at onset, and lack the evolution or build-up characteristic of migraine. A curtain or shade descending over vision is highly suggestive of ipsilateral carotid disease, but is infrequently reported. The patient should be questioned about any precipitating factors. Dimming of vision in one eye after exposure to bright light or after eating has been associated with carotid occlusive disease [1,2]. Loss of vision after exercise or a hot shower (Uhthoff's symptom) is characteristic of demyelinating disease, and reflects transient conduction block due to pre-existing optic nerve demyelination [3].

Pertinent medical and family history may be relevant. A history of diabetes mellitus, hypertension, or hyperlipidemia raises concern about a vascular etiology. TVL in a patient with known cardiac disease might suggest a cardioembolic event. A history of rash and fetal wastage is a feature of the antiphospholipid antibody syndrome, which may cause TVL. A family history of young stroke or unexplained thrombosis in a patient with TVL might prompt evaluation for an underlying hereditary hypercoagulable disorder.

The examination should first focus on the involved organ, and determine whether there are any residual deficits. Although a complete neurological and ophthalmological examination is essential, certain components deserve special mention.

The visual acuity should be measured using either a Snellen card (for near vision) or standardized visual acuity chart at 6 m (for distance vision). When testing near visual acuity, patients over the age of 45 years should wear their reading correction to account for presbyopia. Neurogenic causes of visual loss affect distance and near vision equally; therefore, a patient reporting difficulty only with near vision is unlikely to have a neurogenic etiology. Similarly, a patient with normal near visual acuity but poor distance vision probably has a refractive error rather than a lesion in the visual pathways.

Accurate visual field testing is essential in any patient complaining of visual loss, transient or otherwise. Although formal visual field testing using either static (automated) or kinetic (Goldmann or tangent screen) perimetry is preferred, these resources are not always readily available. Confrontation visual field testing is an acceptable alternative, and is easily performed in clinic or at the bedside. The examiner should pay careful attention to the vertical meridian; defects that respect the vertical midline are highly localizing, and indicate a lesion either at or behind the optic chiasm. Desaturation to red is a sensitive method of detecting lesions in the afferent visual pathways. A small red target is moved in from the periphery, and the patient is asked to identify when the color red is detected. Using this technique, subtle visual field defects may be found which other methods (e.g. finger counting in all four quadrants) would overlook.

The fundus should be carefully evaluated. Although a complete dilated fundoscopic examination is preferred, a great deal of information is obtained by observing the optic disc, macula, and vascular arcades, all of which can be readily seen using a direct ophthalmoscope through an undilatated pupil. Disc swelling in a patient with sudden visual loss suggests an acute event involving the optic nerve, and may represent ischemia or inflammation. Optic atrophy does not develop until approximately 4–6 weeks after an injury, regardless of severity. Therefore, optic disc pallor suggests a subacute or chronic process, rather than an acute event. Retinal whitening often reflects ischemia of the nerve fiber layer, and may be seen after a branch or central retinal artery occlusion. However, retinal edema may not develop for 1–2 h after an acute ischemic event, so it possible for a severely ischemic retina to appear normal hyperacutely. Examination of the arterioles should focus on caliber as well as the presence of embolic plaques. Investigators have attempted to classify plaques in a way that would suggest a possible proximal source, but in practice the distinction is often difficult.

The 'Hollenhorst plaque' (Fig. 4.1) typically appears at vascular bifurcations, and has a highly refractile appearance. It is strongly suggestive of ipsilateral carotid artery disease, but cholesterol emboli may arise from a more proximal source, such as the aortic arch [4]. Platelet-fibrin and calcific emboli are less common. The characteristics of each plaque are summarized in Table 4.1.

Transient monocular visual loss

As a symptom, TMVL has carried a variety of names throughout the years. While amaurosis fugax was a term originally used to describe loss of sight from any cause, it has more recently referred to fleeting visual loss from a vascular etiology. TMVL is preferable, since it is purely descriptive, and carries no connotation regarding etiology.

As previously mentioned, TMVL suggests a disturbance anterior to the optic chiasm and ipsilateral to the visual symptoms. Therefore, this may reflect dysfunction anywhere from the cornea to the posterior optic nerve.

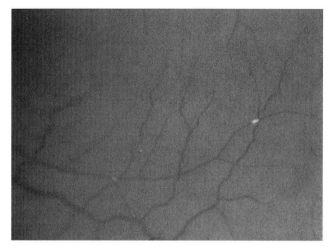

Fig. 4.1 Fundus photograph showing a typical cholesterol embolus, or 'Hollenhorst' plaque. Note the characteristic location at a vascular bifurcation, and the refractile appearance. Note also that the retina served by the involved arteriole is not ischemic. This was an asymptomatic retinal embolus found during routine eye examination. Photograph courtesy of Dean Eliott, MD.

Table 4.1 Retinal emboli

Characteristic	Cholesterol	Platelet-fibrin	Calcium
Appearance	Elongated pulsatile	White, creamy	Gray-white
Number	Multiple	Often multiple	Usually single
Location	Bifurcations	Temporal arcades	On or near disc
Mobility	Can fragment and propagate	Mobile or fixed	Fixed
Retinal ischemia	Rare	Frequent	Frequent
Source	Ipsilateral ICA (most often)	ICA, arch, heart	Hear

Ocular causes of TMVL

Ocular disease may cause TMVL. Although a detailed eye examination may not be possible at the time the patient is evaluated, a directed series of questions may suggest an ocular cause. A dry eye is a common cause of transient visual blurring, particularly in the elderly. The vision loss is mild, brief (several seconds), and is often relieved by blinking or eye rubbing. The patient may also report eye irritation and tearing. Acute angle closure glaucoma is an uncommon cause of TMVL. The episodes are usually painful, and associated with conjunctival injection and a mid-position, dilated pupil. Recurrent hyphema (hemorrhage into the anterior chamber) has been reported as a cause of TMVL, but is uncommon, and readily detected on ophthalmological examination.

Neurogenic causes of TMVL

Neurogenic etiologies of TMVL represent either retinal or optic nerve dysfunction. Uhthoff's symptom is a transient dimming of vision after elevation in body temperature (such as after a hot bath or exercise). The events typically last several seconds to several minutes. Although classically associated with multiple sclerosis, Uhthoff's has been described in other inflammatory optic neuropathies [5].

The transient visual obscurations due to papilledema (i.e. optic disc swelling secondary to elevated intracranial pressure) typically last seconds, and are often provoked by postural change. Patients often have other symptoms of increased intracranial pressure (headache, pulsatile tinnitus), and the examination is notable for bilateral optic disc edema. The mechanism probably involves vascular compression from the swollen optic nerve head, as well as altered cerebral perfusion dynamics due to elevated intracranial pressure.

Congenital optic disc anomalies such as drusen may cause TMVL. The episodes are brief (seconds to minutes), and the anomalous discs are usually evident on fundoscopic examination. The presumed mechanism is transient vascular dysfunction.

Thrombo-embolic causes of TMVL

The most common etiology of TMVL is retinal vascular occlusion, particularly in the elderly. Transient vascular events affecting the optic nerve are less common. The blood supply to the retina and optic nerve originates from the ophthalmic artery (Fig. 4.2). The inner two-thirds of the retina is served by the central retinal artery, which travels within the optic nerve for a short distance behind the disc, then branches out to supply the four quadrants of the retina. The short posterior ciliary arteries (SPCAs) provide the main blood supply to the anterior optic nerve and the outer one-third of the retina. An anastomotic ring of SPCAs wreathes the optic nerve head, and is functionally divided into superior and inferior divisions. Therefore, although all potential mechanisms of ischemia (thrombosis, embolism, hypoperfusion, vasospasm) may cause TMVL, embolic events are far more likely to involve the retina than the optic nerve. Ischemia to the optic nerve is more commonly a result of local or generalized hypoperfusion.

Although concurrent hemispheric symptoms may accompany transient visual loss, the visual symptom is often an isolated manifestation of thrombo-embolism. Several theories have been advanced to explain this

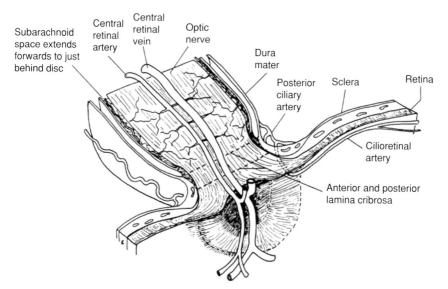

Fig. 4.2 The vascular anatomy of the optic nerve, retina, and choroid.

phenomenon [6]: (i) fleeting visual loss is a symptom more readily detected than fleeting weakness or numbness; (ii) the visual system is topographically organized, with little functional reduplication, so that ischemia of a small area will be clinically expressed; (iii) the retinal circulation is collateralized, and the parieto-occipital cortex is a circulatory watershed area, so both regions are vulnerable to reduced flow; (iv) laminar flow favors the ocular circulation, so that emboli are preferentially directed toward the eye. Vascular events affecting the retina typically cause dramatic fundoscopic changes that develop rapidly, while events that affect the optic nerve will result in either a swollen or normal-appearing optic disc.

The classic symptom of TMVL from a vascular etiology is a curtain or shade descending over vision. This is relatively uncommon; in the North American Symptomatic Carotid Endarterectomy Trial (NASCET), 53.4% of patients with TMVL had sudden, diffuse loss of vision, while 23.8% reported altitudinal visual loss [7]. Donders *et al.* [8] identified several clinical features that increased the probability of high-grade carotid stenosis. These included rapid onset of symptoms, altitudinal visual loss, and duration of 1–10 min. Although examination of the fundus may reveal a plaque, the absence of an embolus does not exclude central retinal artery occlusion as a cause of TMVL, even if the patient is seen during the attack. Emboli located behind the lamina cribosa (Fig. 4.3) are not evident fundoscopically. Further, the presence or absence of an embolus does not help identify those patients with hemodynamically significant carotid artery stenosis [9].

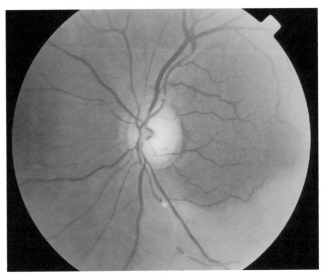

Fig. 4.3 Fundus photograph of a branch retinal artery occlusion in the left eye. Note the Hollenhorst plaque at the vascular bifurcation, as well as the retinal whitening in the distribution of the involved artery. Photograph courtesy of Dean Eliott, MD.

Retinal emboli are often asymptomatic. In a large population study [10], 1.4% of 3654 asymptomatic Australian patients > 49 years of age were found to have retinal emboli. There was significant correlation of asymptomatic emboli with hypertension, smoking, and vascular disease.

Central and branch retinal artery occlusion

Central retinal artery occlusion (CRAO) may be thrombotic, embolic, or hemodynamic. Patients report sudden, painless central visual loss. Visual acuity is profoundly decreased in most cases. A dense relative afferent pupillary defect (RAPD) will be present immediately, reflecting damage to the ganglion cells and the nerve fiber layer. The classic fundoscopic appearance of CRAO is retinal whitening surrounding a cherry-red spot in the macula (Fig. 4.4). This occurs because the retina is thin at the macular region, and the underlying choroidal circulation (which is supplied by the SPCAs) shows distinctly against the white, surrounding retina. A visible embolus is present in 10–20% of patients with CRAO. Acutely, the optic disc will appear normal, since it is not perfused by the central retinal artery. There may be segmentation of the arteriolar blood column, and reduction of the arteriolar lumen. Within 4–6 weeks, the optic nerve becomes pale, reflecting irreversible injury to the ganglion cells and nerve fiber layer. The retinal vessels become narrowed and sheathed over time. Acute management is still debated, and most often involves a variety of

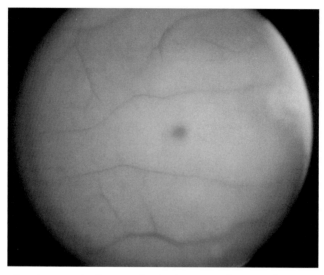

Fig. 4.4 Fundus photograph of a central retinal artery occlusion right eye. The prominent cherry-red spot represents intact choroidal circulation. No embolus is present. Photograph courtesy of Dean Eliott, MD.

maneuvers designed to improve circulation to the retina. These may include ocular massage, anterior chamber paracentesis, and administration of medications to lower intraocular pressure. More recently, thrombolytic therapy, administered by either ophthalmic artery infusion or systemically, has been used. Results have been mixed, with some anecdotal reports of beneficial effect. Although considered the most common cause of CRAO, the prevalence of hemodynamically significant carotid artery stenosis ranges from 11 to 45% with central or branch retinal artery occlusions [11]. Therefore, other, more proximal sources (i.e. cardiac, aortic arch) should be considered as well.

Approximately 15% of patients have a cilio-retinal artery, directly supplying the macula. These patients may have CRAO but retain good visual acuity, since the macular circulation is spared.

In a branch retinal artery occlusion (BRAO), the area of retinal whitening, as well as the visual field defect, are determined by the location and amount of retina subserved by the involved vessel (Fig. 4.3). The mechanism may be thrombotic or embolic, but not (as with CRAO) hemodynamic. Acute treatments are similar to CRAO.

Ocular ischemic syndrome

Ocular ischemic syndrome results from chronic hypoperfusion of the eye, and is associated with severe carotid occlusive disease. Eye pain is often present, and visual acuity is usually decreased. Other features that may be present include iris and retinal neovascularization, mid-peripheral retinal hemorrhages, and cotton-wool spots (reflecting ischemia to the nerve fiber layer). Venous stasis retinopathy may be present, and is characterized by dilatated and tortuous retinal veins and peripheral microaneurysms. Patients may experience episodes of hemodynamic TMVL. These may include visual loss induced by postural change, after exposure to bright light [1], during exercise [12], or after eating [2].

Ocular ischemic syndrome has high morbidity and mortality due to systemic vascular disease. In one series [13], 31% of patients had coronary artery disease, and 38% had a previous hemispheric stroke or transient ischemic attack (TIA). The visual prognosis is likewise poor.

Treatment for ocular ischemia due to carotid occlusive disease remains difficult and controversial. Panretinal photocoagulation is performed to prevent neovascularization of the iris (leading to neovascular glaucoma) and retina. Reducing intraocular pressure to improve ocular perfusion is critical. Carotid endarterectomy would seem to be the treatment of choice, both to revascularize the eye as well as to prevent subsequent stroke. However, the benefits are uncertain, and in some cases the condition worsens after surgery. It has been suggested that reperfusion of an ischemic eye results in generation of oxygen free radicals leading to further damage [14]. In one series [13], seven patients with eight affected eyes underwent carotid endarterectomy. None of the patients improved, but none had further vascular complications.

Evaluation and management of thrombo-embolic TMVL

When a vascular etiology is suspected in patients with TMVL, effort should be directed toward identifying a possible embolic source, as well as modifying vascular risk factors. Duplex color imaging, combining B-mode real-time ultrasound imaging with continuous and/or pulsed Doppler ultrasound techniques, accurately measures the degree of extracranial carotid artery stenosis, and provides important information about vessel wall configuration and morphology. Magnetic resonance angiography (MRA) of the neck is another non-invasive measure of carotid diameter, but had a tendency to overestimate stenosis. There is as yet no consensus whether duplex ultrasound or MRA are adequate tests of the carotid artery prior to endarterectomy, thereby avoiding the risks and cost of conventional angiography. Some preliminary studies suggest that either a high-quality non-invasive test alone or both in combination may be adequate [15]. The ophthalmic artery may be demonstrated on conventional angiography, but the smaller, distal vessels (SPCAs, central retinal artery) are unable to be visualized adequately. Color Doppler of the orbit can evaluate these distal vessels, and may demonstrate ophthalmic artery stenosis, retrolaminar emboli, and reversal of direction of ophthalmic artery flow in ocular ischemic syndrome [16]. Fluorescein retinal angiography is used to evaluate the retinal and choroidal circulation, and may demonstrate occlusive disease, retinal edema, and hypoperfusion.

Evaluation of the heart is accomplished with electrocardiography (ECG), as well as transthoracic or transesophageal echocardiography (TTE or TEE). TEE is clearly the more sensitive test, and has been shown to demonstrate more emboligenic lesions than TTE in patients with retinal vascular occlusions [17]. When a cardiac etiology is suspected, and ECG and TEE are unrevealing, a Holter monitor may be indicated to identify emboligenic arrhythmias, such as paroxysmal atrial fibrillation.

In selected patients (young, no vascular risk factors, family history of unexplained thrombosis), laboratory testing for systemic and hypercoagulable disorders (particularly those associated with arterial thrombosis) may be indicated. In elderly patients with appropriate symptoms, a temporal artery biopsy might be indicated, particularly in the setting of an elevated erythrocyte sedimentation rate (ESR).

The prognosis of TMVL varies depending upon etiology. The NASCET showed that the 2-year risk of stroke in patients with high-grade carotid stenosis (70–99%) was 43.5% if the episode was hemispheric, and 16.6% if the event was a retinal TIA. The risk increased with the degree of stenosis [7].

In patients with high-grade (> 70%) symptomatic internal carotid artery stenosis, endarterectomy is superior to medical therapy alone in preventing stroke. However, the morbidity and mortality of the surgical procedure must be low (< 3–4%) to achieve this benefit. Benavente *et al.* [18] reviewed the subset of NASCET patients experiencing amaurosis fugax. They found that patients with amaurosis had a lower risk of stroke than those with hemispheric events, and that the strokes that occurred were less disabling. There was a trend toward increased efficacy of endarterectomy in those patients with amaurosis and one or more vascular risk factors. Perioperative stroke and death rates are substantially lower in patients presenting with amaurosis, compared with those presenting with hemispheric TIA or minor stroke [19]. In the absence of cardioembolic or high-grade carotid disease, antiplatelet agents are the first-line treatment for patients with ischemic causes of TMVL. Somewhat surprisingly, the risk of permanent visual impairment following a retinal TIA is relatively low, approximately 1%/year [20]. The risk of vascular death in patients with TMVL due to carotid disease is 3.5%/year, and is largely due to cardiac morbidity. However, the risk of stroke-related death is not inconsiderable [21]. Conventional wisdom as well as recent data [22] suggest that the risk of stroke is highest soon after the initial TIA, or when the frequency of the event increases.

Transient binocular visual loss

TBVL implies a process posterior to the optic chiasm, and may include migraine, seizure, and vertebrobasilar ischemia. In rare cases, TBVL may reflect bilateral, simultaneous involvement of the anterior visual pathways.

Migraine

Migraine is a common cause of TBVL in young adults. The presence of positive visual phenomena such as scintillations suggests migraine as the most likely diagnosis, particularly given a history of episodic headaches with migrainous features. Migraine aura typically lasts 20–30 min, in contrast to thromboembolic events, which are shorter (1–10 min). Migraine visual equivalents have a characteristic build-up, or evolution, a feature that is notably lacking in other causes of TBVL (ischemia, seizure). TIAs may rarely cause positive visual phenomena [23], but the duration and lack of build-up help distinguish these episodes from migraine. The mechanism of visual loss in migraine is thought to be neuronal depression after a period of cortical excitation ('spreading depression of Leao') [24].

All patients with TBVL should be questioned about previous headache history. Migraine is often underdiagnosed, or misclassified as 'tension' or 'sinus' headache. A history of recurrent headaches with migrainous features (throbbing, unilateral pain, photophobia, nausea), as well as a childhood history of motion sickness (common in migraineurs) lends support to the diagnosis of migraine equivalent.

Migraine visual aura may occur independently of headache ('ocular migraine'). C. Miller Fisher described 'later life migrainous accompaniments', or migraine aura (often not accompanied by headache) occurring in older patients, some with a previous history of migraine headache [25]. He identified a number of clinical features suggestive of migraine accompaniment, including binocular visual symptoms, build-up of scintillations, and duration of 15–20 min. He also reported a mid-life 'flurry' of identical episodes, and a benign course. In the Framingham cohort [26], the incidence of migrainous visual symptoms was 1.33% for women and 1.08% for men. These episodes may occur after the age of 50, independent of concurrent headaches, and in the absence of a history of recurrent headaches. These episodes did not appear to be associated with an increased incidence of stroke. Therefore, in patients with typical presentations (binocular symptoms, build-up of scintillations, duration < 1 h) and a normal neurological and neuro-ophthalmic examination (including visual field testing), extensive diagnostic testing is not routinely indicated. In patients with atypical presentations (brief duration lack of build-up), non-invasive testing (MR imaging and angiography, echocardiography) is reasonable.

Retinal migraine is a monocular migraine equivalent. The duration, presence of positive visual phenomena, and build-up of symptoms are in all other ways similar to binocular migraine equivalent. The presumed mechanism is localized vasospasm. Indeed, fluorescein angiography performed during an attack has demonstrated retinal vasospasm [27].

There are many prophylactic and abortive treatments available for migraine headache, but their efficacy for migraine aura remains unclear. Many neurologists employ a combination of aspirin and calcium channel blockers to prevent these symptoms.

Visual seizure

Visual seizure is an uncommon cause of TBVL. The visual loss may be ictal or postictal. When postictal, the visual loss is often preceded by a period of positive visual phenomena, which may range from unformed photopsias to complex visual hallucinations, depending upon the cortical area involved. Ictal blindness may be either an isolated epileptic phenomenon, or accompanied by other manifestations, such as tonic eye deviation, altered consciousness, or motor impairment. Postictal blindness typically lasts minutes to hours, but may last days or weeks [28,29]. As with Todd's paralysis (postictal weakness following a motor seizure), the mechanism is presumed to be prolonged enhancement of inhibitory stimuli in response to prolonged excitation (similar in some ways to migraine). Prolonged ictal blindness ('status epilepticus amauroticus') is rare, but has been reported [30].

Benign occipital epilepsy is a childhood seizure disorder with usual age of onset between 15 months and 17 years. The visual events may be positive (hallucination, illusions) or negative (blindness). They may be followed by tonic-clonic seizures or remain isolated. Migraine-like headaches may follow. The neurological and neuro-ophthalmological examination is normal, but the interictal EEG demonstrates occipital spike-wave discharges. Although these episodes are often misdiagnosed as migraine, the visual events are usually briefer (3–5 min), and are maximal at onset, without the gradual evolution of migraine. The seizures are generally well controlled with conventional anticonvulsants, and most cases remit in the early teens.

Adult-onset visual seizures are more commonly associated with a fixed lesion in the posterior visual pathways, and a corresponding visual field defect. Therefore, visual field testing (preferably using static or kinetic perimetry) is important in all patients with TBVL.

Vertebrobasilar ischemia

Ischemia to the visual cortex caused by vertebrobasilar atheroma may result in TBVL. If only one hemisphere is ischemic, the patient will experience homonymous visual field loss contralateral to the lesion, but visual acuity will remain normal. As mentioned previously, the patient may report visual loss only in the eye with the temporal visual field loss. Reduction in visual acuity (cerebral visual loss) can only occur with bilateral involvement of the posterior visual pathways, usually due to bilateral occipital lesions. This is due to bilateral macular representation: a patient with a complete homonymous hemianopia will still be able to read 20/20 in the intact macular hemifield. Visual loss may be an isolated symptom or may be accompanied by symptoms of brainstem ischemia (dysarthria, dysphagia, vertigo, lightheadedness, diplopia). The attacks are generally briefer than those associated with carotid disease, lasting less than 1 min. Positive visual phenomena are rare, but may occur. However, they typically are maximal at onset, and do not progress across the visual field, as with migraine. Episodes of vertebrobasilar insufficiency are not uncommon in elderly patients, and are often precipitated by head-turning or postural change.

As with anterior circulation ischemia, the mechanism may involve thrombosis, embolism, or hypoperfusion. Evaluation of the vertebrobasilar system is accomplished by transcranial Doppler studies, MR or computed tomography angiography, or conventional catheter angiography. For patients with atherosclerotic vertebrobasilar disease, antiplatelet therapy is generally the first-line treatment. In certain circumstances, invasive therapy such as angioplasty and stenting may be warranted, but these procedures are not, at this time, part of standard treatment algorithms.

Ischemic optic neuropathies

Anterior ischemic optic neuropathy (AION) is the most common acute optic neuropathy in patients > 50 years old. The vast majority of cases are non-arteritic in origin; i.e. not associated with systemic vasculitis such as giant cell arteritis (GCA). The annual incidence of non-arteritic anterior ischemic optic neuropathy (NAION) is 2.3–10.2/100 000. It is far more common in the white population than in African-Americans, possibly due to racial differences in optic disc configuration. Arteritic AION occurs more frequently in females, but there is no gender predisposition to NAION.

Non-arteritic AION

Typical presentation of NAION is abrupt onset of painless, unilateral visual loss. Preceding episodes of TMVL are rare, and should raise suspicion of an arteritic etiology. A visual field defect is invariable, and is most commonly altitudinal (Fig. 4.5). However, arcuate defects, cecocentral scotomas, nasal or generalized depression may also be seen. An ipsilateral RAPD is present unless there is concurrent damage to the contralateral optic nerve. The term 'anterior' refers to optic nerve head involvement, so by definition the optic disc is swollen acutely. The swelling is most often diffuse, but

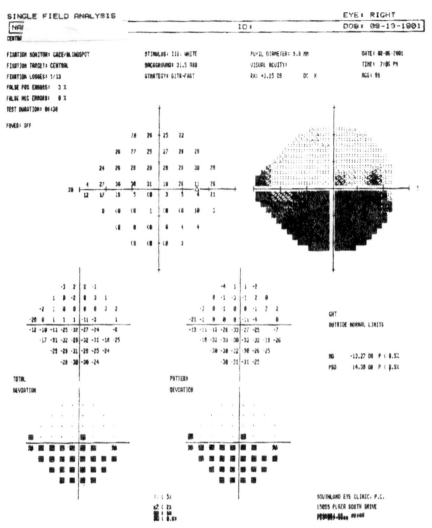

Fig. 4.5 Humphrey automated 24–2 visual field demonstrating inferior altitudinal defect. The patient presented with a 3-day history of painless visual loss in the left eye. He had a swollen left optic disc, and was diagnosed with non-arteritic anterior ischemic optic neuropathy.

may be segmental (Fig. 4.6), correlating with an altitudinal visual field defect. The optic disc in the fellow eye is typically small and crowded, demonstrating a small or absent cup. This configuration has been called the 'disc at risk', referring to structural crowding of axons at the level of the lamina cribosa [31,32]. Visual loss may progress for 7–10 days, and then stabilizes. The swelling resolves over 4–6 weeks, and the optic disc

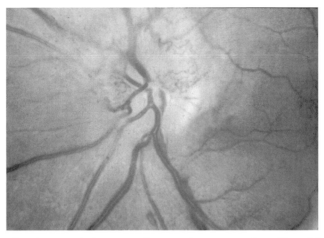

Fig. 4.6 Fundus photograph demonstrating superior segmental swelling of the optic nerve. The patient had a corresponding inferior altitudinal visual field defect.

becomes visibly atrophic. Persistence of swelling beyond this point suggests an alternate diagnosis. The 5-year risk of fellow eye involvement is 12–19%, but recurrence in the same eye is rare [33].

The presumed mechanism of NAION is insufficiency of the optic disc circulation. Localized hypoperfusion, exacerbated by structural crowding of the nerve and its supporting structures at the nerve head, reaches a threshold at which inadequate oxygenation produces ischemia and swelling of the disc. Further axonal swelling may lead to microvascular compression and progressive nerve damage. Hayreh suggested that nocturnal systemic hypotension and the location of the optic disc in a watershed zone between the distributions of the lateral and medial SPCAs may contribute to the development of ischemia [34].

Although the presence of a small crowded disc may be the most important pathogenic risk factor, a substantial number of patients with NAION have conventional vascular risk factors such as hypertension (up to 49%) and diabetes mellitus (up to 25%). Diabetes may predispose patients to developing NAION at a younger age. Other potential risk factors include smoking, hyperlipidemia, migraine, and hyperhomocysteinemia [35–37].

There is no known treatment for NAION. The Ischemic Optic Neuropathy Decompression Trial (IONDT) was a multicentered, randomized study evaluating the role of optic nerve sheath decompression in NAION [38]. The postulated mechanism was that reduction of perineural subarachnoid cerebrospinal fluid pressure would improve local vascular flow or axoplasmic transport within the optic nerve head, thus reducing tissue injury in reversibly damaged axons. The study showed no benefit of optic nerve sheath decompression over careful observation. However, 42.7% of control patients (careful observation) improved by at least three lines of visual acuity at 6 months, suggesting that the visual prognosis may not be as bleak as previously believed. Other treatments such as anticoagulation and hyperbaric oxygen have been used, with no proven results. Johnson *et al.* [39] have suggested a beneficial effect of levodopa on NAION, but the results are controversial.

Neuroimaging is not typically indicated unless the onset of visual loss is uncertain, the disc is pale at presentation, or the fellow disc is not small and crowded. A basic evaluation for modifiable vascular risk factors (hypertension, diabetes mellitus, hyperlipidemia) is reasonable. In selected patients (< 50 years, no obvious vascular risk factors, family history of thrombosis), screening for hypercoagulable disorders associated with arterial thrombosis might be indicated, and might include antinuclear antibody (ANA), prothrombin time (PT), partial thromboplastin time (PTT), anticardiolipin antibodies, lupus anticoagulant, homocysteine, and sickle cell screen. Since most cases of NAION are due to local vascular factors involving a small, crowded optic disc, carotid ultrasound examination is not indicated for patients with typical presentations [40].

However, if a bruit is heard over the carotid, if the patient complains of visual symptoms suggesting hypoperfusion of the eye (i.e. blurred vision with postural change, with bright light, or after exercise), if the event was preceded by episodes of visual loss, or if the visual loss is painful or progressive, then carotid ultrasonography may be warranted.

There is no proven prophylactic agent for a recurrent episode of NAION. Most clinicians recommend daily aspirin, based on its proven effect in reducing the risk of recurrent stroke in patients at risk. However, retrospective studies have not demonstrated a prolonged beneficial effect [41,42].

NAION may occasionally be misdiagnosed as optic neuritis, with all the attendant neurological implications that diagnosis entails. However, in the vast majority of cases, historical and clinical features serve to differentiate the two disorders [43]. The demographics of the two disorders differ, in that NAION affects patients > 50 years, while optic neuritis typically affects women 20–50 years old. Further, pain on eye movements is present in 90–92% of patients with optic neuritis, and occurs rarely in NAION. Finally, the natural history of optic neuritis is spontaneous complete or nearly complete recovery over weeks, while NAION remains relatively stable, with minimal recovery.

Giant cell arteritis and arteritic AION

Arteritic AION most commonly occurs in patients with GCA, although it has been reported in a variety of systemic vasculitides, including Wegener's, Behçet's, and Takayasu's disease. An arteritic etiology occurs in 5–10% of AION cases.

Giant cell arteritis, also known as temporal arteritis, is a T-cell-mediated inflammation of medium and large sized arteries. It is the most common vasculitis in the elderly, with a strong predilection for women and whites, particularly those of Scandinavian and Northern European origin. It affects patients > 50 years, with highest incidence in patients 70 and older.

The clinical manifestations of GCA are diverse, reflecting the heterogeneous nature of the disease. Transient visual loss and transient diplopia may be the presenting symptoms. Indeed, permanent visual loss is more common in patients with preceding episodes of visual loss or diplopia. Headache is the most common symptom, occurring in 90% of patients. It is most commonly temporal, but may be occipital. Jaw claudication is caused by ischemia of the muscles of mastication, and in one study had the highest predictive value for a positive temporal biopsy [44].

The American College of Rheumatology established five clinical criteria for the diagnosis of GCA [45]:

1 age > 50 years
2 new-onset localized headache
3 temporal artery tenderness
4 ESR > 50 mm/h
5 superficial temporal artery biopsy consistent with GCA.

The presence of three out of five criteria yields 93.5% sensitivity and 91.2% specificity. Although these criteria do not necessarily require a temporal artery biopsy for the diagnosis of GCA, most authorities strongly recommend obtaining pathological confirmation in all cases of suspected GCA, even in the setting of classic clinical findings and strong corroborating laboratory results.

Arteritic AION is the most common cause of permanent visual loss in patients with GCA. CRAO occurs less frequently, and BRAO rarely. Visual loss is typically profound. Systemic symptoms of GCA are often present, but 'occult GCA' is not rare. By some reports [46], 21.2% of patients with GCA and visual loss had no systemic symptoms of the disease. Pallid edema of the optic disc is more frequent in arteritic AION than NAION. Cotton-wool spots may be present in arteritic AION, but are exceedingly rare in NAION. They reflect inner retinal ischemia and involvement of the central retinal arterial circulation. The optic disc in the fellow eye may be of any configuration. Table 4.2 summarizes the clinical and historical features differentiating non-arteritic and arteritic forms of AION.

In many cases, the presenting signs and symptoms of GCA (TMVL, AION), may be identical to those caused by other disorders (carotid occlusive disease, NAION). A high index of suspicion as well as a thorough and pertinent review of systems often helps identify patients harbouring GCA. Laboratory testing may be of value. The ESR is elevated in 80–90% of patients with GCA, but is nonspecific. The ESR increases with age, making interpretation difficult in the elderly. A suggested age correction formula is: normal

Table 4.2 Arteritic vs. non-arteritic anterior ischemic optic neuropathy

	Non-arteritic	Arteritic
Age	Mean, 60	Mean, 70
Gender	M = F	F > M
Visual acuity	> 20/200 in > 60%	< 20/200 in > 60%
Disc appearance	Pallid edema or hyperemic; fellow disc small and crowded	Generally pale swelling; fellow disc of any configuration; cotton-wool spots
Natural history	16–42.7% improve; 20% risk in fellow eye at 5 years	Rare improvement; fellow eye involved 54–95%
Treatment	None proven	Systemic corticosteroids

ESR = age/2 for men and (age + 10)/2 for women. A complete blood count should be obtained at the same time as the ESR, as anemia may cause elevation of the ESR. Although it is also nonspecific, the C-reactive protein is not affected by hematological abnormalities. The combination of ESR and C-reactive protein may have the greatest predictive value for GCA [44]. Although a positive temporal artery biopsy is 100% specific for GCA, negative results may occur due to inadequate length of specimen, the presence of skip lesions, the sectioning technique, and the duration of treatment. Biopsy results are not influenced by corticosteroid treatment initiated within the previous 2 weeks [47]. Therefore, treatment should be started as soon as the disease is strongly suspected, and the biopsy arranged in a timely fashion.

Systemic corticosteroids are the mainstay of treatment for GCA. Dosages vary, but are generally in the range of 1 mg/kg per day. Case reports and small case series have demonstrated a beneficial effect of intravenous methylprednisolone as the initial treatment in patients with visual loss, but this remains unproven [48,49]. A typical regimen in such cases would be 500 mg intravenous methylprednisolone every 6 h for 3–5 days. The tapering regimen and duration of treatment are guided by the clinical manifestations and laboratory data. Therapy is usually required for at least 6 months and in most cases for 1–2 years. Alternate day dosing may be associated with a recurrence of symptoms and ischemic complications during the treatment-free days [50]. The steroid-sparing potential of several agents, including methotrexate, azathioprine, and cyclosporine, have been studied with no conclusive recommendations [51].

Summary

Transient visual loss reflects a heterogeneous array of disorders, ranging from the benign to the catastrophic. Table 4.3 summarizes the features of

Table 4.3 Causes of transient visual loss

Etiology	Duration	Pattern of visual loss	Associated findings	Mechanism
Migraine with aura	15–30 min	Binocular, hemianopic, scintillations typical build-up of symptoms	Usually followed by headache with migrainous quality	Spreading cortical depression
Retinal migraine	15–30 min	Monocular; retinal (quadrantic, altitudinal) choroidal (concentric)	Headache, positive family history	Vasospasm
Vertebrobasilar insufficiency	Seconds	Binocular, concentric or blurring	Posture-related, vertigo, diplopia	Orthostastic hypotension, arrythmia, autonomic insufficiency, V-B stenosis
Retinal emboli	2–10 min	Monocular, quadrantic, altitudinal	Hollenhorst plaque, ipsilateral carotid bruit	Emboli form ipsilateral ICA, aortic arch heart, paradoxical
Papilledema	Seconds	Monocular with each occurrence; gray out, blur	Headache, pulsatile tinnitus, diplopia	Venous stasis, poor arterial perfusion
Seizure	3–5 min (ictal) 10–20 min (postictal)	Binocular, may have positive phenomena, no build-up	Altered consciousness, eye deviation	Idiopathic (children); occipital lesion (adults)

common causes of transient visual loss. Recognition of the common etiologies, a high index of suspicion for the uncommon but vision-threatening etiologies, and a general understanding of the neuroanatomy of the primary visual pathways serve in most cases to establish a diagnosis. The judicious use of laboratory testing and neuroimaging helps confirm or exclude the possible etiologies generated by the history and examination.

References

1 Kaiboriboon K, Piriyawat P, Selhorst JB. Light-induced amaurosis fugax. *Am J Ophthalmol* 2001; 131: 674–6.

2 Levin LA, Mootha V. Postprandial visual loss. A symptom of critical carotid stenosis. *Ophthalmology* 1997; 104: 397–401.

3 Smith KJ, McDonald WI. The pathophysiology of multiple sclerosis: the mechanisms underlying the production of symptoms and the natural history of the disease. *Phil Trans R Soc Lond* 1999; 354: 1649–73.

4 Miller NR. Embolic causes of transient monocular visual loss. Appearance, source and assessment. *Ophthalmol Clin N Am* 1996; 9: 359–80.

5 Shults WT. Compressive optic neuropathies. In: Miller NR, Newman NJ, ed. *Clinical Neuro-Ophthalmology*, 5th edn. Detroit, MI: Williams & Wilkins, 1998: 649–662.

6 Burde RM, Savino PJ, Trobe JD. *Clinical Decisions in Neuro-Ophthalmology*. Boston: Mosby, 1992.

7 Streifler JY, Eliasziw M, Benavente OR *et al*. The risk of stroke in patients with first-ever retinal vs hemispheric transient ischemic attacks and high-grade carotid stenosis. North American Symptomatic Carotid Enderaterectomy Trial. *Arch Neurol* 1995; 52: 246–9.

8 Donders RCJM, for the Dutch TMB Study Group. Clinical features of transient monocular blindness and the likelihood of atherosclerotic lesions of the internal carotid artery. *J Neurol Neurosurg Psychiatry* 2001; 71: 247–9.

9 Sharma S, Brown GC, Pater JL, Cruess AF. Does a visible retinal embolus increase the likelihood of hemodynamically significant carotid artery stenosis in patients with acute retinal arterial occlusion? *Arch Ophthalmol* 1998; 116: 1602–6.

10 Mitchell P, Wang JJ, Li W *et al*. Prevalence of asymptomatic retinal emboli in an Australian urban community. *Stroke* 1997; 28: 63–6.

11 Merchut MR, Gupta SR, Naheedy MH. The relation of retinal artery occlusion and carotid artery stenosis. *Stroke* 1988; 19: 1239–42.

12 Ross Russell RW, Page NGR. Critical perfusion of the brain and the retina. *Brain* 1983; 106: 419–27.

13 Mizener JB, Podhajsky P, Hayreh SS. Ocular ischemic syndrome. *Ophthalmology* 1997; 104: 859–64.

14 Droy-Lefaix MT, Szabo ME, Doly N. Ischemia and reperfusion-induced injury in rat retina obtained from normotensive and spontaneously hypertensive rats: effect of free radical scavengers. *Int J Tiss Reac* 1993; 15: 85–91.

15 Golledge J, Wright R, Pugh N, Lane IF. Color-coded Duplex assessment alone before endarterectomy. *Br J Surg* 1996; 83: 1234–7.

16 Kerty E, Eide N, Horven I. Ocular hemodynamic changes in patients with high-grade carotid occlusive disease and development of chronic ocular ischemia. I. Doppler and dynamic tonometry changes. *Acta Ophthalmol Scand* 1995; 73: 66–71.

17 Wiznia RA, Pearson WN. Use of transesophageal echocardiography for the detection of a likely source of embolization to the central retinal artery. *Am J Ophthalmol* 1991; 111: 104–5.

18 Benavente OR, Eliaszaw M, Streifler JY *et al.* Prognosis after transient monocular blindness associated with carotid artery stenosis. *N Engl J Med* 2001; 345: 1084–90.

19 Benavente OR, Streifler JY, Harbison JW, Eliasszaw M, Hashinski VC, Barnett HJM. Differences between retinal TIA and hemispheric TIA of carotid stenosis origin: observations from NASCET. *Neurology* 1992; 42 (Suppl. 3): 341.

20 Kline B. The natural history of patients with amaurosis fugax. *Ophthalomol Clin N Am* 1996; 9: 351–7.

21 Hartmann A, Rundek T, Mast H *et al.* Mortality and causes of death after first ischemic stroke. The Northern Manhattan Stroke Study. *Neurol* 2001; 57: 2000–5.

22 Babikian V, Wijman CA, Koleini B *et al.* Retinal ischemia and embolism. Etiologies and outcomes based on a prospective study. *Cerebrovasc Dis* 2001; 12: 108–13.

23 Goodwin JA, Gorelick PB, Helgason CM. Symptoms of amaurosis fugax in atherosclerotic carotid artery disease. *Neurology* 1987; 37: 829–35.

24 Leao AAP. Spreading depression of activity in cerebral cortex. *J Neurophysiol* 1944; 7: 391–6.

25 Fisher CM. Late-life migraine accompaniments as a cause of unexplained transient ischemic attacks. *Can J Neurol Sci* 1980; 7: 9–17.

26 Wijman CAC, Wolf PA, Case CS *et al.* Migrainous visual accompaniments are not rare in late life. The Framingham Study. *Stroke* 1998; 29: 1539–43.

27 Winterkorn JMS, Kupersmith MJ, Wirtschafter JD, Forman S. Brief report: treatment of vasospastic amaurosis fugax with calcium-channel blockers. *N Engl J Med* 1993; 32: 396–8.

28 Shahar E, Desatnik H, Brand N *et al.* Epileptic blindness in children: a localizing sign of various epileptic disorders. *Clin Neurol Neurosurg* 1996; 98: 237–41.

29 Sadeh M, Goldhammer Y, Kuritky A. Postictal blindness in adults. *J Neurol Neurosurg Psychiatry* 1984; 46: 566–9.

30 Barry E, Sussman NM, Bosley TM, Harner RN. Ictal blindness and status epilepticus amauroticus. *Epilepsia* 1985; 26: 577–84.

31 Hayreh SS. Anterior ischemic optic neuropathy. *Arch Neurol* 1981; 38: 675–8.

32 Beck RW, Servais GE, Hayreh SS. Anterior ischemic optic neuropathy. IX. Cup-to-disc ratio and its role in pathogenesis. *Ophthalmology* 1987; 94: 1503–8.

33 Beck RW, Hayreh SS, Podhajsky P et al. Aspirin therapy in nonarteritic anterior ischemic optic neuropathy. *Am J Ophthalmol* 1997; 123: 212–7.

34 Hayreh SS, Podhajsky P, Zimmerman MB. Role of nocturnal arterial hypotension in optic nerve head ischemic disorders. *Ophthalmologica* 1999; 213: 76–96.

35 Hayreh SS, Joos KM, Podhajsky PA et al. Systemic diseases associated with nonarteritic anterior ischemic optic neuropathy. *Am J Ophthalmol* 1994; 118: 766–80.

36 Ischemic Optic Neuropathy Decompression Trial Research Group. Characteristics of patients with nonarteritic anterior ischemic optic neuropathy eligible for the Ischemic Optic Neuropathy Decompression Trial. *Arch Ophthalmol* 1996; 114: 1366–74.

37 Kawasaki A, Purvin VA, Burgett RA. Hyperhomocysteinemia in young patients with nonarteritic anterior ischemic optic neuropathy. *Br J Ophthalmol* 1999; 83: 1287–90.

38 Ischemic Optic Neuropathy Decompression Trial Research Group. Optic nerve decompression surgery for nonarteritic anterior ischemic optic neuropathy is not effective and may be harmful. *JAMA* 1995; 273: 625–32.

39 Johnson LN, Guy ME, Krohel GB et al. Levodopa may improve vision loss in recent onset, nonarteritic anterior ischemic optic neuropathy. *Ophthalmology* 2000; 107: 521–6.

40 Fry CL, Carter JE, Kanter MC et al. Anterior ischemic optic neuropathy is not associated with carotid artery atherosclerosis. *Stroke* 1993; 24: 539–42.

41 Botelho PJ, Johnson LN, Arnold AC. The effect of aspirin on the visual outcome of nonarteritic anterior ischemic optic neuropathy. *Am J Ophthalmol* 1996; 121: 450–1.

42 Kupersmith MJ, Frohman L, Sanderson M et al. Aspirin reduces the incidence of second eye NAION. A retrospective study. *J Neuroophthalmol* 1997; 17: 1287–90.

43 Rizzo JF, Lessell S. Optic neuritis and ischemic optic neuropathy. Overlapping clinical profiles. *Arch Ophthalmol* 1991; 109: 1668–72.

44 Hayreh SS, Podhajsky PA, Raman R et al. Giant cell arteritis: validity and reliability of various diagnostic criteria. *Am J Ophthalmol* 1997; 123: 285–96.

45 Hunder GG, Bloch DA, Michel BA et al. The American College of Rheumatology 1990 criteria for the classification of giant cell arteritis. *Arthritis Rheum* 1990; 33: 122–8.

46 Hayreh SS, Podhajsky PA, Zimmerman B. Occult giant cell arteritis: ocular manifestations. *Am J Ophthalmol* 1998; 125: 521–6.

47 Achkar AA, Lie JT, Hunder GG et al. How does previous corticosteroid treatment affect the biopsy findings in giant cell (temporal) arteritis? *Ann Intern Med* 1994; 120: 987–92.

48 Liu GT, Glaser JS, Schatz NJ et al. Visual morbidity in giant cell arteritis: clinical characteristics and prognosis for vision. *Ophthalmology* 1994; 101: 1779–85.

49 Cornblath WT, Eggenberger ER. Progressive visual loss from giant cell arteritis despite high dose intravenous methylprednisolone. *Ophthalmology* 1997; 104: 854–8.

50 Bengtsson BA, Malmvall BE. An alternate day corticosteroid regimen in maintenance therapy of giant cell arteritis. *Acta Med Scand* 1981; 209: 347–50.

51 Ferraccioli GF, Di Poi E, Damato R. Steroid sparing therapeutic approaches to polymyalgia rheumatica-giant cell arteritis: state of the art and perspectives. *Clin Exp Rheumatol* 2000; 18: S58–S60.

PART II

Diagnostic Studies

CHAPTER 5

Head CT and MRI Findings in Patients with Transient Ischemic Attacks

Chelsea S. Kidwell, Jeffrey L. Saver

Introduction

Transient ischemic attacks (TIAs) are currently defined as neurological symptoms due to focal cerebral ischemia that resolve completely within 24 h [1]. This definition was originally conceived based on the concept that transient clinical deficits are due to transient ischemia that is not associated with permanent brain injury or infarction. However, rapid advances in computed tomography (CT) and magnetic resonance imaging (MRI) technology in the last 25 years have contributed significantly to our understanding of the pathophysiology of clinically defined TIAs, requiring re-examination of these initial simplistic notions.

CT studies performed in the 1980s first suggested that TIAs may, in fact, be associated with neuroimaging evidence of infarction. In fact, in 1983 Waxman and Toole coined the term 'cerebral infarct with transient signs' (CITS) to describe this newly recognized category of patients who met clinical criteria for TIA but showed a relevant infarct on imaging studies [2]. In the late 1980s and early 1990s, routine MRI studies further clarified the frequency of this association in patients studied with more sensitive neuroimaging techniques. Most recently, the clinical implementation of diffusion-perfusion MRI has provided definitive evidence of acute infarction in some patients in the setting of clinical TIA syndromes and additional insight into the underlying pathophysiology of these syndromes.

Goals of neuroimaging evaluation of TIA

The goals of the modern neuroimaging evaluation of TIA are to (i) obtain evidence of a vascular etiology for the symptoms either directly (evidence of hypoperfusion and/or acute infarction) or indirectly (identification of a presumptive source, such as a large-vessel stenosis, (ii) exclude an alternative non-ischemic etiology, such as tumor, abscess, etc., (iii) acquire data regarding the anatomical and vascular localization of the event, (iv) ascertain the underlying vascular mechanism of the event (e.g. large vessel atherothrombotic, cardioembolic, small- vessel lacunar, etc.), which, in turn, allows selection of the optimal therapy, and (v) identify prognostic outcome categories.

Standard CT

CT studies performed in the 1980s demonstrated that non-ischemic etiologies can be identified in approximately 1–5% of clinical TIAs, including tumor, abscess, and subdural hematoma [3,4]. These early CT studies also revealed that both anatomically relevant and nonrelevant (presumably remote, silent) infarcts may be identified in a significant proportion of TIA patients. While some early reports suggested that ischemic lesions were absent or rare in TIA patients [5,6], later studies, using later generation technology, have clearly shown that this is not the case. Across all CT studies, any infarct has been visualized in 0–68% of patients, and any relevant infarct in 0–28%. The Dutch TIA trial provides representative data from one of the largest analyses of CT findings in TIA patients. Of 606 patients with transient cerebral ischemia, 13% of patients had a relevant infarct and 6% of patients had an irrelevant infarct, for a total rate of any infarction of 19% [7].

Numerous CT studies have reported an increased frequency of lesions with longer duration of the TIA episode [3,8,9]. In the Dutch TIA trial, the investigators found that relevant infarcts occurred more frequently with longer attack duration. This was true both in patients meeting strict criteria for TIA, as well as for the cohort as a whole, which also included patients with reversible ischemic neurologic deficit (RIND) and minor stroke [7,10]. Two additional studies in patients with carotid territory TIAs have supported this association [8,9]. In one report, Bogousslavsky and colleagues studied 57 patients with carotid territory TIAs and found that the likelihood of infarction on CT was > 80% for attacks lasting longer than 45–60 min [9].

Several large-scale clinical trials and case series have shed light on the clinical characteristics associated with the finding of a CT lesion in TIA patients. In the Dutch TIA trial, patients with relevant infarcts were more likely to have a history of hypertension as well as involvement of speech during the attack [10]. In a study of 284 TIA patients, Murros and Evans found that any CT evidence of infarction was significantly associated with increased age and the presence of carotid stenosis [11]. Using data from the NASCET trial, Eliasziw and colleagues found that previous clinically diagnosed stroke, older age, and male sex were all significantly associated with the occurrence of ipsilateral CT-verified infarcts in TIA patients with severe carotid stenosis [12].

Several important brain and vessel imaging characteristics have also been identified in patients with CT-verified lesions. Numerous studies suggested that patients with infarcts in association with clinical TIA are more likely to have large-vessel stenoses [12–14]. In addition, Meagher *et al.* studied 50 TIA patients who underwent both CT imaging and catheter angiography and found that patients with any infarct were more likely to have diminished collateral reserve on angiography [15].

A few investigators have analyzed the distribution and anatomical localization of CT lesions in patients with TIAs. In the Dutch TIA trial, 606 patients had anterior circulation TIAs. Of these, 79 had anatomically relevant infarcts, of which 58% were in small deep penetrator territories and 42% were in larger cortical territories [16]. Calandre and colleagues reported CT abnormalities in 25% of TIA patients, 25% of RIND patients, and 35% of stroke with minimal deficit patients [17]. Across these groups, 68% of infarcts were cortical, 27% hemispheric subcortical, and 5% cerebellar. In a study of 261 TIA patients, Turnbull and colleagues reported that nondominant hemisphere infarcts were twice as common as dominant infarcts and tended to be larger in size [4].

One of the most compelling reasons to distinguish TIA patients with an associated acute infarction on imaging studies from those without acute infarction would be a difference in prognosis between these two groups. While definitive prospective data are lacking at the moment, the Dutch TIA Trial provides some preliminary information. In this trial, the investigators found that evidence of any infarct on CT (in either a relevant or nonrelevant location) significantly increased the risk of a subsequent stroke with a hazard ratio of 1.5, and was also an independent risk factor for subsequent myocardial infarction or vascular death. In addition, diffuse white matter hypodensity was associated with an increased risk of subsequent stroke with a hazard ratio of 1.6 after adjusting for baseline variables [18].

Similarly, Evans and colleagues studied 564 consecutive TIA patients, of whom 350 had CT performed [19]. After controlling for baseline covariates, they found that patients with CT-verified infarcts had significantly shorter survival times than those without CT evidence of infarcts ($P = 0.035$) with an increased risk of death of 109% over a 10-year period following the TIA. However, this study did not assess the risk associated with evidence of a new, appropriately located TIA-related infarct. In contrast, Eliasziw and colleagues did not find an increased risk of ipsilateral stroke associated with CT evidence of an anatomically relevant infarct in a group of TIA patients with severe carotid stenosis treated medically as part of the North American Symptomatic Carotid Endarterectomy Trial [12].

Additional CT techniques: xenon CT, perfusion CT, CT angiography

Very limited data are available regarding xenon CT findings in patients with TIA. In one study, Firlik and colleagues analyzed data from 53 patients presenting with acute hemispheric stroke symptoms who underwent xenon-enhanced CT cerebral blood flow studies within 8 h of symptom onset (and before any clinical improvement) [20]. Eight patients had a complete resolution of symptoms within 24 h. Mean cerebral blood flow (CBF) in the symptomatic vascular territory in these eight patients was significantly greater compared with patients with evolving strokes. The authors concluded that patients with ischemic neurological deficits that will later resolve can be acutely distinguished from patients with evolving cortical infarctions using xenon CT CBF measurements. At the time of writing, we were not able to identify any substantive reports describing perfusion CT changes or CT angiography findings specifically in the TIA population.

Standard MRI

Conventional MRI is more sensitive than standard CT in identifying both new and pre-existing ischemic lesions in TIA patients. Across various studies, MRI has shown evidence of at least one infarct somewhere in the cerebrum in 46–81% of TIA patients [21,22]. Some of these infarcts are in locations that could have accounted for the deficits observed during the TIA. Among patients meeting clinical criteria for TIA, 31–39% demonstrate neuroanatomically relevant infarcts on conventional MRI [21,23]. It is difficult with both conventional MRI and CT to determine what proportion of these appropriately localized infarcts occurred at the time of the index TIA, and what proportion existed prior to the presenting event.

The earliest report of MRI findings in TIA patients came from Awad and colleagues [24]. This group studied 22 patients with both MRI and CT. They found 77% of patients had focal ischemic changes on MRI compared with 32% on CT. However, the majority of lesions did not correlate with symptomatology.

Fazekas and colleagues reported the results of conventional MRI in 62 patients with hemispheric TIAs [21]. Forty-five of these patients also had contrast-enhanced studies. They found that 81% of their cohort had MRI evidence of focal ischemic injury, and that 31% demonstrated evidence of an acute TIA-associated infarct. The definition Fazekas and colleagues employed for acute TIA-associated infarcts was: lesions (i) located in a vascular territory potentially corresponding to the patient's TIA symptoms, (ii) having signal characteristics of appearing hyperintense on T2-weighted scans and isointense or only minimally hypointense on T1-weighted scans, and (iii) showing regional swelling or contrast enhancement. This definition is problematic, as many lesions remote in time may demonstrate this T2/T1 pattern and the accuracy of rater discrimination of swelling for small lesions is uncertain. The majority of infarcts identified as acute (68%) were < 1.5 cm in diameter and 58% were purely cortical. Thirty-seven percent of the acute infarcts were multiple in nature. Contrast enhancement occurred in five of the 45 patients studied, and in two of these patients was essential to the delineation of the acute lesion. Evidence of infarction in these patients was associated with a higher frequency of a history of vascular or cardiac disorders.

Additional insight regarding lesion location and clinical characteristics of patients with TIA-associated lesions in conventional MRI comes from two additional studies. In their study of 64 patients with carotid territory TIAs studied with MRI, Kimura and colleagues found 16 of 41 patients demonstrated contrast enhancement [23]. The majority of contrast-enhancing lesions were cortical (81%). Aphasia or confusional state, hypertension, and presence of an emboligenic cardiac or arterial source were more frequently observed in patients with enhancement. The increased rate of contrast enhancement in this study compared with the Fazekas report may be related to differences in patient characteristics and timing of the MRI studies. Bhadelia et al. studied 100 TIA patients from the Cardiovascular Health Study imaged with standard MRI sequences [22]. Brain infarcts were demonstrated in 46% of the TIA patients compared with 28% of patients without a history of TIA. In stepwise logistic regression analysis, diastolic blood pressure and internal carotid intima-media thickness were predictive of infarction on MRI. These authors also found an increased frequency of cortical infarcts and multiple infarcts in the TIA patients.

Preliminary data regarding neuroimaging prognosis in TIA patients is now available. Walters and colleagues [25] performed serial MRI studies over a 2-year period in 125 TIA patients and compared the results with 75 controls. They found that 47% of the TIA patients demonstrated evidence of new asymptomatic lesions on follow-up imaging compared with 12% of controls. Thirteen TIA patients had new cerebral transient symptoms, of which two had new relevant MRI lesions. In addition, four TIA patients experienced a clinical stroke during the follow-up period (three ischemic events, one intracerebral hemorrhage). Factors that correlated with an increased risk of a new ischemic lesion included diastolic blood pressure, male sex, age, and initial severity of MRI ischemic lesions. Also of note, these authors found that TIA patients had an accelerated rate of cerebral atrophy compared with controls.

Diffusion-weighted imaging

While standard brain imaging techniques, including CT and conventional MRI, are insensitive to dynamic and regionally varying neural parenchymal

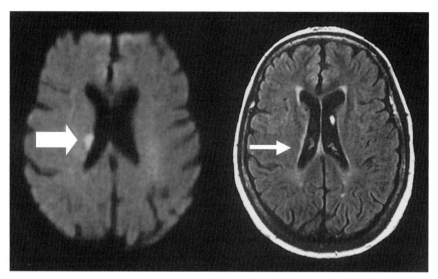

Fig. 5.1 Seventy-five-year-old female with a history of hypertension and atrial fibrillation presented with several hours of left-sided weakness. Diffusion-weighted sequence (right image) shows right periventricular white matter lesion (thick arrow) not visualized on the standard FLAIR sequence (thin arrow). ©UCLA Stroke Center.

responses to tissue ischemia, the novel MRI techniques of diffusion and perfusion imaging permit visualization of these critical tissue processes, and have afforded new insights into the pathophysiology of human cerebral ischemia. Moreover, clinical studies have demonstrated that MRI is of substantial clinical utility in patients with TIAs.

Studies from five groups have now confirmed that diffusion-weighted imaging (DWI) provides a more precise evaluation of ischemic insult in TIA patients compared with standard CT and MRI studies (Figs 5.1 & 5.2) [26–30]. These series show convergent results regarding the frequency of DWI positivity among TIA patients—among the five studies encompassing 202 patients, the aggregate rate of DWI positivity was 44%, ranging from 35 to 48% (Table 5.1) [26–30].

The increased sensitivity of DWI over standard MRI sequences was first demonstrated in a UCLA study, where 20 of 42 TIA patients exhibited diffusion MR abnormalities. Five of the 20 patients with a DWI lesion (25%) did not show a lesion correlate on initial T2-weighted sequences. The remaining 15 patients did exhibit T2-weighted lesion abnormalities in the same regions as DWI alterations.

Detailed data correlating symptom duration with the presence of DWI lesions come from three studies. In the UCLA study, a precise report of TIA duration (all episodes were unequivocally less than 24 h) was available for

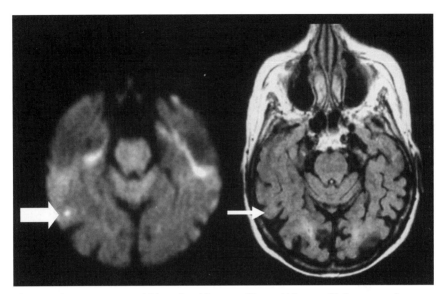

Fig. 5.2 Ninety-two-year-old female with several hours' history of left arm weakness. Diffusion-weighted sequence (right image) shows 1–2-mm right temporal lesion (thick arrow). Follow-up imaging 1 month later does not show resultant infarct on FLAIR sequence (thin arrow). ©UCLA Stroke Center.

Table 5.1 Time intervals and yield of diffusion magnetic resonance imaging (MRI) in transient ischemia attack (TIA) patients: three series

Series	TIA duration (mean), h	Time from TIA onset to MRI (mean), h	Frequency of positive DWI findings on MRI, %
UCLA (*n* = 42)	3.2 h*	17	48
Duke (*n* = 40)	4.8 h	37	35
MGH (*n* = 57)	1.9 h	39	46
Takayama (*n* = 19)	—	—	37
Bisschops (*n* = 44)	—	—	47
Sum (*n* = 202)	—	—	44

*Median duration was 2.0 h.

15 of the 20 patients with DWI abnormalities and 17 of the 22 without DWI abnormalities. Duration of TIA symptoms for patients without a DWI abnormality was mean 3.2 h (± 4.7 h standard deviation), median 0.5 h vs. mean 7.3 h (± 6 h standard deviation), median 4.0 h for patients with a DWI abnormality (*t*-test for difference in means, $P = 0.03$). The percent of patients with a DWI abnormality within various symptom duration intervals increased as the total duration of symptoms increased (Fig. 5.3).

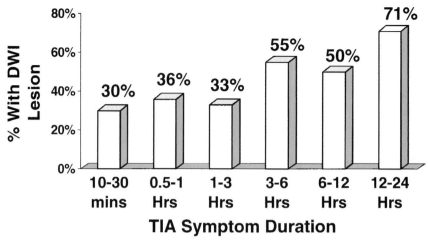

Fig. 5.3 The percent of transient ischemic attack (TIA) patients with a diffusion-weighted imaging (DWI) abnormality within various symptom duration intervals. ©UCLA Stroke Center.

Similarly, the Duke investigators found that, in their cohort, TIAs of longer clinical duration were more likely to be DWI positive. Among DWI-positive patients, mean TIA duration was 7.1 h in the Duke cohort and 7.3 h in the UCLA cohort; in DWI-negative patients mean TIA duration was 3.2 h in both cohorts. In contrast, TIA duration was not a predictor of DWI positivity in the Massachusetts General Hospital (MGH) series. In part, this discrepancy may be due to the briefer average duration of TIAs and the longer interval from TIA offset to MRI in the MGH study.

The UCLA investigators also analyzed the relationship between DWI findings and time from symptom onset to MRI. For the group as a whole, the mean time to MRI study was 17 h (range 1.25–73 h), and did not significantly differ between the DWI-negative patients (mean 15.8 h) and the DWI-positive patients (mean 19.5 h). One patient in the group without DWI lesions was still symptomatic at the time of the MRI, while two in the DWI-positive category were still symptomatic at the time of MRI. Interval from time of resolution of TIA symptoms to time of MRI for patients with a DWI abnormality was mean 12.7 h, median 8.8 h in patients with a DWI abnormality vs. mean 12.9 h, median 5.1 h in patients without a DWI abnormality (rank sums test for difference in medians, $P = 0.7$).

In addition, the UCLA investigators compared diffusion imaging characteristics in patients with DWI lesions vs. patients with completed stroke and found that there were significant differences in the DWI and apparent diffusion coefficient (ADC) signatures between these groups (Table 5.1). Completed stroke patients had larger volumes and greater intensities of ADC and DWI alteration than TIA patients.

The sensitivity and specificity of DWI offer unique precision in characterizing the vascular and anatomical localization of ischemic TIA lesions. This information provides important insights into the underlying etiological mechanism. In the 20 UCLA patients with diffusion MRI abnormalities, DWI signal changes were localized to the brainstem in four patients, the cerebellum in two patients, subcortical hemispheric structures in seven patients, and cortical regions in seven patients. Vascular territories affected were superficial middle cerebral artery in six patients, deep middle cerebral artery in six patients, brainstem perforators in four patients, and posterior cerebral arteries in two patients. In these 20 patients, the final etiological mechanism was felt to be small-vessel lacunar in nine patients, large-vessel atherothrombotic in four patients, and cardioembolic in seven patients.

In the UCLA series, DWI results altered the attending physician's opinion regarding vascular localization in 7/20 patients, anatomical localization in 8/20 patients, and probable TIA mechanism in 6/20 patients. The types of alterations in diagnosis were varied and no single pattern predominated. For example, among etiological diagnoses, of four patients initially suspected to have large-artery atherothrombotic mechanisms, one changed post-DWI to likely cardioembolic and one changed to likely small vessel; of seven initial cardioembolic diagnoses, one changed to likely large-vessel atherothrombotic and one changed to likely small vessel; and of nine initial small vessel diagnoses, one changed to likely large-vessel atherothrombotic and one changed to likely cardioembolic.

The MGH study provided insights into the clinical characteristics of patients with DWI-positive lesion. These investigators found that prior, nonstereotyped TIAs identified stroke etiology, and cortical symptoms were independent clinical predictors of DWI positivity. These clinical factors seem to index larger, more severe ischemic episodes, as does longer duration of clinical deficits, and this underlying physiological factor is likely to be the most critical for the appearance of DWI abnormality. In the UCLA Study, there were no significant differences between patients who demonstrated DWI abnormalities and those who did not in age, sex, and presence of hypertension, diabetes, tobacco use, hypercholesterolemia, or history of prior stroke or TIA.

One particularly noteworthy finding that has evolved from DWI studies in TIA patients is that DWI-positive TIA lesions do not consistently evolve to a completed infarction on follow-up imaging studies. In the UCLA series, all 20 TIA patients demonstrating DWI abnormalities were contacted for a follow-up MRI, and nine of these patients agreed to return for repeat neuroimaging. Three patients were studied with head CT and six with brain MRI 2–7 months post event. Of these nine patients, five (three MRI, two CT) demonstrated a subsequent infarct in the region corresponding to the original DWI abnormality, while four (three MRI, one CT) did not. Five of the 22 patients without a DWI abnormality underwent follow-up imaging (three MRI, two CT), 2 weeks to 15 months post event. None demonstrated a subsequent relevant infarct. In addition, there are two case reports in the literature of DWI lesions associated with TIAs reporting reversibility of the DWI abnormalities on follow-up imaging [31,32]. Of note, however, in the Takayama series of 19 TIA patients, all of the DWI-positive lesions (seven patients) evolved to persistent T2 lesions. This discrepancy may be related to patient characteristics and timing of the imaging studies.

Perfusion-weighted imaging

Scant data are available regarding perfusion-weighted imaging (PWI) findings in patients with clinical TIAs. However, two case reports in the literature provide some insight into the potential role of PWI in the evaluation of TIA. In one report, the initial DWI study was negative while the PWI scan demonstrated a perfusion deficit in a region compatible with the focal symptoms [33]. Despite resolution of the clinical symptoms, the follow-up DWI scan showed a small lesion in the initially hypoperfused area. In the second report, a patient with a prolonged reversible ischemic neurological deficit underwent acute and follow-up diffusion- and perfusion-weighted imaging [32]. The initial PWI scan showed a large PWI lesion with a smaller relatively less conspicuous DWI abnormality. At the time of follow-up imaging, both the clinical and imaging abnormalities had completely resolved.

These two cases suggest that PWI is likely to be even more sensitive than DWI in detecting acute ischemic changes in some TIA patients. Since PWI is able to detect regions of relative hypoperfusion that do not reach the threshold of tissue bioenergetic compromise required to cause a lesion on DWI, a greater number of patients with modest degrees of ischemia may be detected with this technique. The anticipated utility of perfusion MRI is supported by perfusion studies employing other imaging modalities that have demonstrated detectable blood flow abnormalities in a substantial proportion of TIA patients [34,35].

Additional MR techniques: MR spectroscopy and MR angiography

MR spectroscopy is an interesting new application of MRI for the study of patients with TIA. A preliminary report by Giroud and colleagues of five TIA patients found no differences in N-acetylaspartate (NAA)/creatine ratio, but did find an increase in lactate/creatine ratio. More recently, Bisschops and colleagues performed an analysis of 44 TIA patients studied with MR angiography and [1]H-magnetic resonance spectroscopy [28].

They found that the NAA/choline ratio in non-infarcted regions was significantly decreased in the symptomatic hemisphere compared with the asymptomatic hemisphere and control subjects. In the symptomatic hemisphere, the lactate/NAA ratio was significantly increased compared with control subjects. These authors also reported that the TIA patients had normal flow distribution through the circle of Willis and did not have any alterations in flow volume in any of the arteries.

Neuroimaging findings in TIA

These neuroimaging studies, particularly those employing diffusion MRI, provide important new insights into the pathophysiology of TIAs and the clinical utility of these techniques in TIA patients. Across all diffusion MRI series, more than two of every five cerebral TIA patients demonstrated DWI evidence of acute bioenergetic compromise. In the UCLA study, among TIA patients with early DWI abnormalities who had follow-up imaging, approximately one-half exhibited late CT or MRI evidence of established infarction. Together, these data suggest that approximately one-quarter of cerebral TIA patients actually have cerebral infarction with transient signs. A distinct subset of TIA patients, representing about one-fifth of TIA cases, who have early DWI abnormalities but no late evidence of established infarction has now been identified. The delineation of such TIA patients suggests that DWI abnormalities may be reversible in humans if early restoration of blood flow is obtained. This observation has been confirmed, with important additional complexities, by MRI studies in patients undergoing reperfusion after thrombolytic stroke therapy [36].

In TIA patients, the ADC volume, mean ADC value, DWI volume and DWI signal intensity were all significantly less abnormal than in acute stroke patients. These differences support the concept that the cerebral ischemia experienced by patients with TIAs is less in volume and severity than that experienced by patients with clinically completed stroke syndromes.

Both the UCLA and Duke series found a strong statistical correlation between duration of TIA symptoms and presence of a lesion on DWI. This correlation, however, was not absolute. DWI lesions appeared in patients with clinical episodes as brief as 10 min while some patients in the DWI-negative group had symptoms lasting > 12 h. DWI abnormalities do appear to be uncommon, if present at all, in patients with clinical symptoms lasting < 5 min.

In addition to improving our understanding of the underlying pathophysiological processes that occur with TIAs, these data add to a growing body of evidence demonstrating the clinical utility of DWI [37,38]. A variety of studies have demonstrated that the diagnosis of TIA is often difficult, especially for the non-neurologist [39,40]. Kraaijeveld and colleagues found κ measures of interrater agreement of only 0.65 among eight experienced neurologists diagnosing 56 TIA patients and of only 0.31 for determination of the vascular territory involved [41]. The size, appearance and location of DWI lesion(s) in TIA may help guide physicians in determining the underlying etiological mechanism and in choosing the optimal therapeutic regimen to reduce the probability of recurrent TIAs or completed stroke in the future.

In the UCLA study, information obtained from the DWI study led to a change in the suspected anatomical localization, vascular localization, and TIA mechanism in over one-third of patients. In addition to clarifying the site and source of ischemia in patients with clinically definite TIAs, diffusion imaging also can be quite helpful in patients with atypical transient neurological symptoms, when it is unclear whether the event was a TIA vs. migraine, hyperventilation, brief seizure, or other TIA mimic. Although DWI abnormalities have been rarely reported in TIA mimics, a visualized diffusion abnormality in these cases generally provides supportive evidence of the diagnosis of TIA.

The observation that DWI alone was positive in 25% of patients, while 75% had correlative lesions identified retrospectively on T2-weighted imaging underestimates the diagnostic impact of DWI. Even in the patients with T2-visible lesions, the diffusion imaging provided added clinical utility. Many of the T2-positive patients had multiple foci of increased T2 signal, and determining which, if any, T2 foci were new and related to the recent TIA may not have been possible without the DWI sequences. Standard T2-weighted sequences alone are generally incapable of reliably differentiating acute from chronic events.

As noted in the above discussion of CT findings in TIA patients, identifying which patients have a new infarct on imaging may have important prognostic value [42]. Only larger series with long-term follow-up will be able to distinguish if there is a difference in prognosis in TIA patients without diffusion abnormalities, TIA patients with transient diffusion abnormalities but no eventual T2 lesion, and patients with diffusion abnormalities and a subsequent T2 lesion. We concur with the general view advanced by Caplan that all TIA patients are at significant risk of subsequent vascular events, and it is the underlying mechanism rather than the duration of symptoms that is most critical to determine [43]. However, it may be that within each mechanism category, longer duration of a TIA or presence of a DWI abnormality identifies a subgroup at increased risk. How often patients with DWI abnormalities are experiencing ongoing ischemia will need to be clarified by large series of concurrent perfusion studies. The severity and size of the perfusion deficit might also be an indicator of the reversibility of the diffusion abnormality. Finally, the pathological correlates of DWI changes in TIA require investigation, including how often signal abnormalities reflect, at the histopathological level, absence of infarction, incomplete infarction, or complete infarction [44].

Recent studies in animal models and now in human patients with conventionally defined TIAs have identified three unique tissue patterns on diffusion-perfusion MRI, reflecting three somewhat dissimilar ischemic episodes, that can underly clinically similar TIAs:

1 A very brief or low-intensity period of focal ischemia may disrupt synaptic transmission and produce transient neurological deficits without causing early cytotoxic edema or permanent tissue injury. In these cases, perfusion MRI may show focally reduced cerebral blood flow, but both acute diffusion MRI, sensitive to early cytotoxic edema, and late T2 imaging, sensitive to increased water content, a marker of permanent parenchymal injury, will be unrevealing.

2 A somewhat more severe transient ischemic insult may sufficiently disrupt cellular energetic state to impair maintenance of ionic gradients across cell membranes, producing cytotoxic edema, but not cause advanced bioenergetic failure. Early restoration of blood flow may permit cellular re-energization and restoration of ionic gradients, with edema resolution. In this setting, acute perfusion MRI during the episode and diffusion MRI close to the time of the episode will be abnormal, but late T2 imaging will be unrevealing.

3 A more profound ischemic insult may produce loss of cell membrane integrity, in addition to failure of synaptic transmission and cytotoxic edema, with resulting permanent parencyhmal injury. However, early recruitment of alternative neural circuitry and synaptic outgrowth, neuroplasticity and neurorepair, may allow rapid resolution of clinical deficits. In this setting, patients with rapidly transient neurological signs may exhibit early perfusion, early diffusion, and late T2 abnormalities on MRI imaging.

These observations suggest a need to re-examine the utility and accuracy of the current time-based definition of TIA. The concept of a time-based criterion first arose in the 1950s as an imprecise means to distinguish between those cerebral ischemic episodes that caused brain injury and those that did not, in the absence of imaging or other laboratory measures that could directly determine tissue parenchymal status. Proposed time cutoffs varied widely. A 1958 NIH committee on classification of cerebrovascular disease suggested that TIAs could last as long as 1 h [45]. Acheson and Hutchinson, in 1964, also employed a 1-h threshold to distinguish TIA from stroke [46]. However, also in 1964, Marshall employed a 24-h limit in defining TIA, although his data showed that symptoms lasted < 1 h in three-quarters of his patients [47]. In the 1975 revision of the NIH classification document, a 24-h limit for TIAs was adopted [48].

Accumulating evidence suggests that any time cut-off for TIA is inaccurate in reflecting end organ injury. The current 24-h operational definition is especially misleading. Large-scale studies have clarified our understanding of the typical duration of TIAs, showing that most TIAs resolve within

10–60 min rather than lasting several hours [49,50]. Moreover, diffusion MR findings of diffusion change in patients with spells as brief as 10 min challenge the simplistic assumption that, because clinical TIA symptoms rapidly resolve, significant ischemic tissue injury must not occur.

Indeed, MRI studies have demonstrated the untenability of any definition of TIA based solely on clinical manifestations and an arbitrarily assigned time window, rather than tissue changes and physiological processes. While the likelihood of DWI alterations is directly related to the duration of symptoms, some patients with spells as brief as 10 min will show parenchymal changes on diffusion imaging and some with spells exceeding 12 h will show no diffusion alteration. There is not likely to be a fundamental biological difference between a patient whose symptoms last 59 min and a patient whose symptoms last 61 min, or between 23-h 59-min spells and 24-h 1-min spells.

Accordingly, efforts are underway to redefine TIAs using a tissue-based definition that takes into account the fundamental physiological processes indexed by imaging or other laboratory measures, rather than a strict time limit. The UCLA group has proposed the following tissue-based definition:

> A TIA is a brief episode of neurological dysfunction due to focal cerebral ischemia, that is not associated with permanent brain injury. Although most TIAs last 1 min to 2 h, a minority last up to 24 or more hours.

Under this definition, the diagnosis of TIAs may be rendered on clinical grounds alone. For research purposes, it would be useful to have a more detailed, strictly operationalized definition, again based on the presence or absence of tissue injury rather than time interval—this type of definition would incorporate the results of laboratory and neuroimaging tests to stratify the likelihood of a TIA.

The UCLA group has accordingly proposed the following research-orientated tissue-based definition of TIA:

> A TIA is a brief episode of neurological dysfunction, presumed to be due to focal cerebral ischemia, that is not associated with permanent brain injury. Although most TIAs last 1 min to 2 h, a minority last up to 24 or more hours.

• Highly probable TIA: transient neurological dysfunction presumed to be due to focal cerebral ischemia, imaging evidence of focal hypoperfusion during episode, no laboratory/imaging evidence of tissue injury.
• Probable TIA: transient neurological dysfunction presumed to be due to focal cerebral ischemia, perfusion imaging not performed during episode, no laboratory/imaging evidence of tissue injury.
• Possible TIA: transient neurological dysfunction presumed to be due to focal cerebral ischemia, perfusion imaging not performed during episode, no sensitive laboratory/imaging test of tissue injury performed.

This research definition recognizes three levels of strength of evidence for a spell being a TIA. The lowest level is clinical criteria alone. The next level higher is clinical criteria plus a supportive test showing that no parenchymal tissue injury occurred during the spell. The supportive test should be highly sensitive to subtle brain parenchymal injury, such as diffusion MR. Conventional CT and MR are insufficient. Serum biomarkers of brain parenchymal injury, such as the S-100 protein and neuron specific enolase [51,52], may be useful alternative laboratory measures for this definition. The highest level of evidence additionally includes imaging evidence of focal hypoperfusion during the spell. This finding helps to exclude seizures, compressive neuropathies, and other TIA mimics and rules in focal hypoperfusion as the etiology of the episode. Any of the wide variety of perfusion imaging modalities available could provide the data required for this level of evidence, including CT perfusion imaging, xenon CT, perfusion MR, single positron emission tomography (SPECT), positron emission tomography (PET), transcranial Doppler ultrasound, and cerebral angiography.

Conclusion

Neuroimaging studies, particularly diffusion–perfusion-weighted MRI, have fundamentally altered our understanding of the pathophysiology of TIA. The spectrum of ischemic tissue alterations underlying transient clinical symptoms is now understood to variably include synaptic transmission failure, cytotoxic edema, and permanent tissue injury, and these processes are easily delineated in individual patients on MRI. In routine clinical practice, MR permits confirmation of focal ischemia rather than another process as the cause of a patient's deficit, improves accuracy of diagnosis of the vascular localization and etiology of TIA, and assesses the extent of pre-existing cerebrovascular injury. Accordingly, MRI, including diffusion sequences, should now be considered a preferred diagnostic test in the investigation of the patient with potential transient ischemic attacks.

References

1 Special Report from the National Institute of Neurological Disorders and Stroke. Classification of cerebrovascular diseases III. *Stroke* 1990; 21: 637–76.

2 Waxman SG, Toole JF. Temporal profile resembling TIA in the setting of cerebral infarction. *Stroke* 1983; 14: 433–7.

3 Weisberg LA. Computerized tomographic abnormalities in patients with hemispheric transient ischemic attacks. *South Med J* 1986; 79: 804–7.

4 Turnbull IW, Bannister CM. CT observations on the natural history of asymptomatic cerebral infarction following transient ischaemic attacks. *Neurol Res* 1985; 7: 190–3.

5 Madkour O, Elwan O, Hamdy H *et al*. Transient ischemic attacks: electrophysiological (conventional and topographic EEG) and radiological (CCT) evaluation. *J Neurol Sci* 1993; 119: 8–17.

6 Biller J, Laster DW, Howard G, Toole JF, McHenry LC Jr. Cranial computerized tomography in carotid artery transient ischemic attacks. *Eur Neurol* 1982; 21: 98–101.

7 Koudstaal PJ, van Gijn J, Frenken CW *et al*. TIA, RIND, minor stroke: a continuum, or different subgroups? Dutch TIA Study Group. *J Neurol Neurosurg Psychiatry* 1992; 55: 95–7.

8 Kimura K, Minematsu K, Yasaka M, Wada K, Yamaguchi T. The duration of symptoms in transient ischemic attack. *Neurology* 1999; 52: 976–80.

9 Bogousslavsky J, Regli F. Cerebral infarct in apparent transient ischemic attack. *Neurology* 1985; 35: 1501–3.

10 Koudstaal PJ, van Gijn J, Lodder J *et al*. Transient ischemic attacks with and without a relevant infarct on computed tomographic scans cannot be distinguished clinically. Dutch Transient Ischemic Attack Study Group. *Arch Neurol* 1991; 48: 916–20.

11 Murros KE, Evans GW, Toole JF, Howard G, Rose LA. Cerebral infarction in patients with transient ischemic attacks. *J Neurol* 1989; 236: 182–4.

12 Eliasziw M, Streifler JY, Spence JD, Fox AJ, Hachinski VC, Barnett HJ. Prognosis for patients following a transient ischemic attack with and without a cerebral infarction on brain CT. North American Symptomatic Carotid Endarterectomy Trial (NASCET) Group. *Neurol* 1995; 45 (3 Part 1): 428–31.

13 Davalos A, Matias-Guiu J, Torrent O, Vilaseca J, Codina A. Computed tomography in reversible ischaemic attacks: clinical and prognostic correlations in a prospective study. *J Neurol* 1988; 235: 155–8.

14 Grigg MJ, Papadakis K, Nicolaides AN *et al*. The significance of cerebral infarction and atrophy in patients with amaurosis fugax and transient ischemic attacks in relation to internal carotid artery stenosis: a preliminary report. *J Vasc Surg* 1988; 7: 215–22.

15 Meagher E, Grace PA, Bouchier-Hayes D. Are CT infarcts a separate risk factor in patients with transient cerebral ischaemic episodes? *Eur J Vasc Surg* 1991; 5: 165–7.

16 Kappelle LJ, van Latum JC, Koudstaal PJ, van Gijn J. Transient ischaemic attacks and small-vessel disease. Dutch TIA Study Group. *Lancet* 1991; 337: 339–41.

17 Calandre L, Gomara S, Bermejo F, Millan JM, del Pozo G. Clinical–CT correlations in TIA, RIND, and strokes with minimum residuum. *Stroke* 1984; 15: 663–6.

18 van Swieten JC, Kappelle LJ, Algra A, van Latum JC, Koudstaal PJ, van Gijn J. Hypodensity of the cerebral white matter in patients with transient ischemic attack or minor stroke: influence on the rate of subsequent stroke. Dutch TIA Trial Study Group. *Ann Neurol* 1992; 32: 177–83.

19 Evans GW, Howard G, Murros KE, Rose LA, Toole JF. Cerebral infarction verified by cranial computed tomography and prognosis for survival following transient ischemic attack. *Stroke* 1991; 22: 431–6.

20 Firlik AD, Rubin G, Yonas H, Wechsler LR. Relation between cerebral blood flow and neurologic deficit resolution in acute ischemic stroke. *Neurology* 1998; 51: 177–82.

21 Fazekas F, Fazekas G, Schmidt R, Kapeller P, Offenbacher H. Magnetic resonance imaging correlates of transient cerebral ischemic attacks. *Stroke* 1996; 27: 607–11.

22 Bhadelia RA, Anderson M, Polak JF *et al.* Prevalence and associations of MRI-demonstrated brain infarcts in elderly subjects with a history of transient ischemic attack. The Cardiovascular Health Study. *Stroke* 1999; 30: 383–8.

23 Kimura K, Minematsu K, Wada K, Yonemura K, Yasaka M, Yamaguchi T. Lesions visualized by contrast-enhanced magnetic resonance imaging in transient ischemic attacks. *J Neurol Sci* 2000; 173: 103–8.

24 Awad I, Modic M, Little JR, Furlan AJ, Weinstein M. Focal parenchymal lesions in transient ischemic attacks: correlation of computed tomography and magnetic resonance imaging. *Stroke* 1986; 17: 399–403.

25 Walters RJ, Holmes PA, Thomas DJ. Silent cerebral ischaemic lesions and atrophy in patients with apparently transient ischaemic attacks. *Cerebrovasc Dis* 2000; 10: 12–3.

26 Kidwell CS, Alger JR, Di Salle F *et al.* Diffusion MRI in patients with transient ischemic attacks. *Stroke* 1999; 30: 1174–80.

27 Engelter ST, Provenzale JM, Petrella JR, Alberts MJ. Diffusion MR imaging and transient ischemic attacks. *Stroke* 1999; 30: 2762–3.

28 Ay H, Buonanno FS, Schaefer PW *et al.* Clinical and diffusion-weighted imaging characteristics of an identifiable subset of TIA patients with acute infarction. *Stroke* 1999; 30: 235A (Abstract).

29 Takayama H, Mihara B, Kobayashi M, Hozumi A, Sadanaga H, Gomi S. [Usefulness of diffusion-weighted MRI in the diagnosis of transient ischemic attacks]. *No Shinkei* 2000; 52: 919–23.

30 Bisschops RHC, Kappelle LJ, Mali W, van der Grond J. Hemodynamic and metabolic changes in transient ischemic attack patients. *Stroke* 2001; 33: 110–5.

31 Lecouvet FE, Duprez TP, Raymackers JM, Peeters A, Cosnard G. Resolution of early diffusion-weighted and FLAIR MRI abnormalities in a patient with TIA. *Neurology* 1999; 52: 1085–7.

32 Neumann-Haefelin T, Wittsack HJ, Wenserski F *et al.* Diffusion- and perfusion-weighted MRI in a patient with a prolonged reversible ischaemic neurological deficit. *Neuroradiology* 2000; 42: 444–7.

33 Ide C, De Coene B, Trigaux JP *et al.* Discrepancy between diffusion and perfusion imaging in a patient with transient ischaemic attack. *J Neuroradiol* 2001; 28: 118–22.

34 Laloux P, Jamart J, Meurisse H, De Coster P, Laterre C. Persisting perfusion defect in transient ischemic attacks: a new clinically useful subgroup? *Stroke* 1996; 27: 425–30.

35 You DL, Shieh FY, Tzen KY, Tsai MF, Kao PF. Cerebral perfusion SPECT in transient ischemic attack. *Eur J Radiol* 2000; 34: 48–51.

36 Kidwell CS, Saver JL, Mattiello J *et al*. Thrombolytic reversal of acute human cerebral ischemic injury shown by diffusion/perfusion magnetic resonance imaging. *Ann Neurol* 2000; 47: 462–9.

37 Lee LJ, Kidwell CS, Alger J, Starkman S, Saver JL. Impact on stroke subtype diagnosis of early diffusion-weighted magnetic resonance imaging and magnetic resonance angiography. *Stroke* 2000; 31: 1081–9.

38 Lutsep HL, Albers GW, DeCrespigny A, Kamat GN, Marks MP, Moseley ME. Clinical utility of diffusion-weighted magnetic resonance imaging in the assessment of ischemic stroke. *Ann Neurol* 1997; 41: 574–80.

39 Ferro JM, Falcao I, Rodrigues G *et al*. Diagnosis of transient ischemic attack by the non-neurologist. A validation study. *Stroke* 1996; 27: 2225–9.

40 Calanchini PR, Swanson PD, Gotshall RA *et al*. Cooperative study of hospital frequency and character of transient ischemic attacks. IV. The reliability of diagnosis. *JAMA* 1977; 238: 2029–33.

41 Kraaijeveld CL, van Gijn J, Schouten HJ, Staal A. Interobserver agreement for the diagnosis of transient ischemic attacks. *Stroke* 1984; 15: 723–5.

42 Toole JF. The Willis lecture: transient ischemic attacks, scientific method, and new realities. *Stroke* 1991; 22: 99–104.

43 Caplan LR. Are terms such as completed stroke or RIND of continued usefulness? *Stroke* 1983; 14: 431–3.

44 Li F, Liu KF, Silva MD *et al*. Transient and permanent resolution of ischemic lesions on diffusion-weighted imaging after brief periods of focal ischemia in rats: correlation with histopathology. *Stroke* 2000; 31: 946–54.

45 Ad Hoc Committee on Cerebrovascular Disease of the Advisory Council of the National Institute on Neurological Disease and Blindness. A classification of and outline of cerebrovascular diseases. *Neurology* 1958; 8: 395–434.

46 Acheson J, Hutchinson EC. Observations on the natural history of transient cerebral ischaemia. *Lancet* 1964; 2: 871–4.

47 Marshall J. The natural history of transient ischaemic cerebrovascular attacks. *Q J Med* 1964; 33: 309–24.

48 A classification and outline of cerebrovascular diseases. II. *Stroke* 1975; 6: 564–616.

49 Levy DE. How transient are transient ischemic attacks? *Neurology* 1988; 38: 674–7.

50 Dyken ML, Conneally M, Haerer AF *et al*. Cooperative study of hospital frequency and character of transient ischemic attacks. I. Background, organization, and clinical survey. *JAMA* 1977; 237: 882–6.

51 Elting JW, de Jager AE, Teelken AW *et al*. Comparison of serum S-100 protein levels following stroke and traumatic brain injury. *J Neurol Sci* 2000; 181: 104–10.

52 Persson L, Hardemark HG, Gustafsson J *et al*. S-100 protein and neuron-specific enolase in cerebrospinal fluid and serum: markers of cell damage in human central nervous system. *Stroke* 1987; 18: 911–8.

CHAPTER 6

Single-Photon Emission Computed Tomography (SPECT) and Positron Emission Tomography (PET)

Colin P. Derdeyn, William J. Powers

Introduction

Single-photon emission computed tomography (SPECT) and positron emission tomography (PET) are related neuroimaging techniques that allow the non-invasive measurement of regional physiological processes such as cerebral blood flow (PET and SPECT) and oxygen metabolism (PET) in the human brain. The primary application of SPECT and PET in patients with transient ischemic attack (TIA) is the assessment of hemodynamic impairment due to occlusive cerebrovascular disease. Many patients presenting with TIA have significant arterial lesions, such as stenoses or complete occlusions. These lesions have the potential for reducing the perfusion pressure of the brain, depending on the degree of arterial narrowing and the adequacy of collateral sources of blood flow. Information regarding the hemodynamic status of the brain beyond the stenosis or occlusion has proven prognostic value in certain clinical situations and, pending the outcome of clinical trials, may guide therapy in the future.

In this chapter, we will review the physical principles underlying SPECT and PET. We will discuss the physiology of hemodynamic impairment and how it can be assessed with SPECT and PET. Finally, we will review the literature for the current clinical applications for SPECT and PET studies of cerebral hemodynamics in patients with TIAs. At present, data are inadequate to support the routine use of these techniques to guide patient care, although such use is widespread. Investigational applications of SPECT and PET can be separated into three categories. The first lies in prospective studies of hemodynamic impairment as independent risk factors for subsequent stroke in well-defined clinical populations. These populations may include patients with TIAs and extracranial or intracranial athero-sclerotic disease. Other important vascular pathologies include arterial dissection, vasospasm associated with subarachnoid hemorrhage, and venous occlusive disease. These studies shed light on the association between hemodynamic impairment and stroke risk, as well as the frequency of hemodynamic impairment in patients with these different pathological conditions. The second application is as a secondary endpoint to assess the effects of medical or surgical intervention on cerebral hemodynamic status. This literature is extensive, but inconclusive with regard to actual impact on patient outcome. The third investigational application is critically predicated on the two described above. Once an independent association between a hemodynamic factor and stroke risk has been established, and it is proven that an intervention can reverse the hemodynamic abnormality, a clinical trial of the intervention is necessary to determine if the treatment improves the outcome in the subgroup of patients with the hemodynamic abnormality. Two such studies using PET or SPECT are currently underway. Both are randomized clinical trials of surgical revascularization vs. medical therapy for patients' symptomatic atherosclerotic carotid occlusion and SPECT or PET evidence of severe hemodynamic impairment.

Imaging physics

Both SPECT and PET rely on three major components to measure accurately physiological processes in living humans: a radiotracer, a radiation detection system, and a mathematical model relating the detected radiation to the physiological process under study [1,2]. In this section, we will define these components and discuss their inherent advantages and limitations for the study of cerebrovascular physiology in living humans. Readers interested in greater detail are encouraged to refer to texts that treat these subjects in greater detail [2].

Radiotracers are radioactive molecules that are administered in trace quantities, so that they do not affect the physiological process under study. SPECT and PET use fundamentally different radiotracers. SPECT radiotracers decay by emitting a single gamma ray. This gamma ray is also called a photon, hence the term 'single-photon emission' in the SPECT acronym. Gamma rays are similar to X-rays, but have higher energy. The most commonly used gamma-emitting radiotracers for SPECT are radioactive forms of technetium (^{99m}Tc) and iodine (^{123}I). ^{99m}Tc can be produced in a nuclear medicine laboratory using commercially available molybdenum kits. It is commonly bound to different organic molecules and has a half-life of 6 h. ^{123}I is cyclotron-produced and then transported owing to its relatively long half-life (13 h).

In contrast, PET radiotracers are not gamma-emitting. By definition, PET relies on positron-emitting radio-isotopes. Positrons are small nuclear particles with the same mass as an electron, but with a positive charge. After emission, they travel up to a few millimeters within tissue, losing energy, and then ultimately and fatally interacting with an electron. This interaction results in the annihilation of both the positron and the electron and the generation of two high-energy gamma photons of equal energy but headed in opposite directions. The half-lives of these positron-emitting radionuclides range from a few minutes to a few hours. These relatively short half-lives allow high administered radioactivity with less total radiation dose to the patient or subject as well as the ability to perform sequential studies. The limitation of a short half-life is that the radiotracer often has to be prepared very nearby or on site. The most commonly used radiotracers for cerebral hemodynamic studies use ^{15}O-labeled compounds (half-life 120 s) and require an on-site linear accelerator or cyclotron for production.

SPECT and PET also differ fundamentally in their respective radiation detection systems. Most modern SPECT systems use several flat gamma camera heads to detect the gamma rays arising from the study subject. The camera head contains a collimator to absorb photons from the patient that are not arising from the immediate field of view, a large crystal—a scintillation crystal—for the detection of X-ray photons, and a collection of photomultiplier tubes. The scintillation crystal gives off a flash of visible light when it absorbs a gamma ray. The photomultiplier tubes cover the back surface of the scintillation crystal and produce a pulse of electricity in response to the light flash. Electronic circuits use this information to determine the location of each gamma ray interaction in the crystal. The camera heads are rotated around the body to obtain multiple two-dimensional views. These data are reconstructed in tomographic planes using similar algorithms to those used in X-ray computed tomography.

A PET scanner consists of a large number of detector pairs connected by coincidence circuits to identify the simultaneous arrival of the annihilation photons, traveling on opposed, 180° trajectories. The detectors consist of a scintillation crystal and photomultiplier tubes. After correction for attenuation of photons by the head within the scanner bore, the data from all the detector pairs are used to reconstruct a series of linear projections. These projections are combined to produce a two-dimensional reconstruction of the regional radioactivity within the scanner. Scanners with multiple rings of detectors can generate several reconstructed tomographic slices of the imaged volume simultaneously. Three-dimensional acquisitions and reconstructions of data can also be obtained with newer, multiring scanners.

Quantitative SPECT techniques face two potentially limiting problems. First, gamma photons are variably attenuated by tissue; some may travel a long distance through tissue and reach the detector, while another photon from the same location may be absorbed by surrounding tissue. Second, the spatial resolution of external gamma ray detectors is distance dependent: as the distance between the source of gamma rays and the external detector increases, the spatial resolution of detectors decreases [1]. Most existing SPECT systems incorporate empiric or other corrections for attenuation and mathematical adjustments for distance-dependent resolution. PET does not suffer from these two problems. The spatial resolution of a pair of annihilation coincidence detectors is nearly uniform for most of the region found between detectors [1]. The fraction of activity lost to attenuation can be measured individually and accurately corrected for.

A variety of other technical factors affect the ultimate accuracy of the reconstructed SPECT and PET image as a quantitative measure of regional radioactivity. One critical factor is the effect of image resolution on the accuracy of measurement of regional radioactivity. A lack of understanding of this issue can lead to errors in the interpretation of SPECT or PET data. In any tomographic system such as SPECT or PET, detected radiation will be redistributed or smeared over a larger area. The pattern of redistribution is approximately Gaussian for a point source of radiation, with the maximum measured value occurring at the original point. The resolution of the reconstructed image is described in terms of this point spread function and is usually given as the width of the point spread function at one-half its maximum amplitude. This is known as the full width, half maximum (FWHM) of a given detector system. The FWHM therefore describes the degree of smearing of radioactivity in a reconstructed image. The ability of a SPECT or PET scanner to discriminate between two small adjacent structures or accurately measure the activity in a small region will depend on the FWHM of the system as well as the amount and distribution of activity within the region of interest and the surrounding areas.

Because of the smearing or redistribution of detected radioactivity, any given region in the reconstructed image will not contain all the activity actually within the region. Some of the activity will spill over into adjacent areas. Similarly, activity in the surrounding tissue or structures will also be redistributed into the region of interest. This phenomenon is known as the 'partial volume effect'. An important consequence of this principle is that PET will always measure a gradual change in activity where an abrupt change actually exists, such as at the edge of an infarct or hemorrhage. Measurements made at the borders of such lesions will not be accurate, unless sophisticated post-processing techniques are applied [3].

The third requirement for SPECT and PET measurement of cerebrovascular physiology is a mathematical model that quantitatively relates the externally detected regional radioactivity to the physiological variable under study. These models must take into account a number of factors, including the mode of tracer delivery to the tissue, the distribution and metabolism of the tracer within the tissue, the exit of the tracer and metabolites from the tissue, the recirculation of both the tracer and its labeled metabolites, and the amount of tracer and metabolites remaining in the blood. The model must be practically applicable given the amount of radioactivity that can be safely administered to human subjects. Finally, the validity of all the underlying assumptions and possible sources of error for each model when applied to the study of both normal physiology and disease states must be clearly understood. Ideally, each technique used in the study of cerebrovascular physiology should be rigorously validated by paired comparison with an accepted 'gold standard' under the specific conditions for which it will be used.

Physiology of cerebral hemodynamic impairment

Cerebral perfusion pressure (CPP) is defined as the difference between mean arterial pressure and the venous back-pressure or intracranial pressure, since venous back-pressure is usually negligible. For patients with arterial occlusive disease, the perfusion pressure is essentially equal to the mean arterial pressure. Arterial lesions, such as stenoses or complete occlusions, can result in a significant reduction in the pressure in the distal arterial territory [4,5]. The degree of reduction will depend on the degree of stenosis and, most importantly, the adequacy of collateral sources of blood flow. For example, some patients with complete occlusion of a carotid artery have normal perfusion pressure in the distal hemisphere because of circle of Willis collaterals [6].

Direct measurements of CPP in humans are not practical, and therefore indirect methods of assessment have been developed [7]. These methods are based on the normal compensatory hemodynamic and metabolic responses of the cerebral circulation to reduced perfusion pressure. Our knowledge of these responses is primarily from studies involving acute and global reductions in mean arterial pressure in animal models and humans. The extent that they are valid in humans with chronic regional reductions in CPP is not completely defined and remains an active area of ongoing investigation. Emerging empirical evidence, discussed in later sections, shows that the presence of some of these compensatory responses predicts an increased risk of stroke in patients with cerebrovascular disease.

Two compensatory mechanisms to acute reductions in CPP have been established in both animals and humans: autoregulation and increased oxygen extraction fraction (OEF) [8,9]. As CPP falls within the autoregulatory range, cerebral blood flow (CBF) is maintained at near normal levels by reflex vasodilatation of resistance arterioles, a phenomenon known as autoregulation (Fig. 6.1) [8,10]. CBF falls only at a slight rate through the autoregulatory range [11,12]. Consequently, as the metabolic

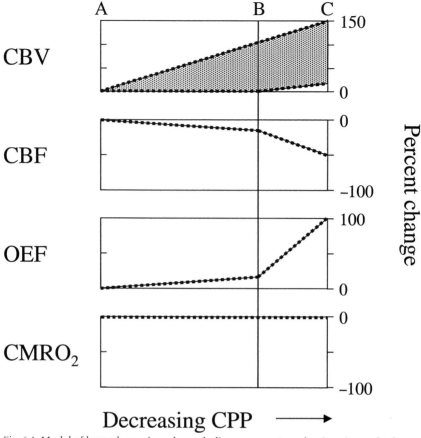

Fig. 6.1 Model of hemodynamic and metabolic responses to reductions in cerebral perfusion pressure. Point A represents baseline. The distance between points A and B represents the autoregulatory range. The distance between points B and C represents exceeded autoregulatory capacity where cerebral blood flow (CBF) falls passively as a function of pressure. Point C represents the exhaustion of compensatory mechanisms to maintain normal oxygen metabolism and the onset of true ischemia. Cerebral blood volume (CBV) may not change [13,32] or may increase [31,77,78] within the autoregulatory range (between A and B). Once autoregulatory capacity is exceeded (between B and C), CBV may increase slightly (10–20%) [13,32], remain elevated [77,78] or continue to increase (up to 150%) [31]. CBF falls slightly, down to 18%, through the autoregulatory range (between A and B) [11,79]. Once autoregulatory capacity is exceeded, CBF falls passively as a function of pressure down to 50% of baseline values (between B and C). Oxygen extraction fraction (OEF) increases slightly, up to 18%, with the reductions in CBF through the autoregulatory range (between A and B) [13]. After autoregulatory capacity is exceeded and flow falls up to 50% of baseline, OEF may increase up to 100% from baseline [80]. CMRO2: The cerebral metabolic rate for oxygen consumption remains unchanged throughout this range of cerebral perfusion pressure (CPP) reduction (between A and C), due to both autoregulatory vasodilatation and increased OEF [78,80]. Reprinted with permission from Derdeyn *et al.* Variability of cerebral blood volume and oxygen extraction: stages of hemodynamic impairment revisited. *Brain* 2002; 125: 595–607.

rate for oxygen in the brain remains constant and the delivery of oxygen to the brain (CBF multiplied by the arterial oxygen content of the blood) is reduced, there is a slight increase in oxygen extraction by the brain tissue at the lower limits of the autoregulatory range [13]. With further reductions in CPP beyond the autoregulatory capacity, CBF will fall passively as a function of pressure. OEF will increase steeply to support oxygen metabolism and tissue function [4,9,14]. Oxygen extraction fraction can increase to up to 80% from a normal baseline of 30%. Further reductions in CPP reductions beyond the ability of OEF to compensate for reduced CBF will lead to true ischemia, with an insufficient delivery of oxygen to meet metabolic demands. Cellular energy failure will result and permanent injury may ensue, depending on the degree and duration of the ischemia.

Assessment of cerebral hemodynamics

Identification of these compensatory mechanisms in humans with cerebrovascular disease relies on non-invasive imaging techniques, such as PET and SPECT. A single measurement of blood flow is not indicative of hemodynamic status for two reasons. First, nearly normal flow can be maintained with autoregulatory vasodilatation—normal flow does not exclude reduced perfusion pressure—and second, reduced CBF may be due to reduced metabolic demand. This may occur remote from the site of ischemic injury, such as with crossed cerebellar diaschisis [15–17] or after a lacunar infarction (Fig. 6.2). Reduced CBF does not automatically indicate reduced perfusion pressure, therefore. Consequently, three basic strategies have been developed for the *in vivo* assessment of hemodynamic impairment in humans. The first two are intended to detect pre-existing autoregulatory vasodilatation. The third relies on direct measurements of oxygen extraction.

The first strategy relies on paired CBF measurements with the initial measurement obtained at rest and the second measurement obtained following a cerebral vasodilatatory stimulus. Hypercapnia, acetazolamide, and physiological tasks such as hand movement have all been used as vasodilatatory stimuli. Normally, each will result in a robust increase in CBF. If the CBF response is muted or absent, preexisting autoregulatory cerebral vasodilatation due to reduced cerebral perfusion pressure is inferred (Fig. 6.3). The blood flow responses to these vasodilatatory stimuli have been categorized into several grades of hemodynamic impairment: (i) reduced augmentation (relative to the contralateral hemisphere or normal controls); (ii) absent augmentation (same value as baseline); and (iii) paradoxical reduction in regional blood flow compared with baseline measurement. This final category, also called the 'steal' phenomenon, can only be identified with quantitative CBF techniques [18].

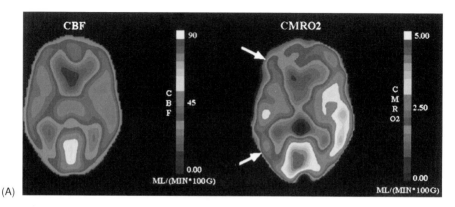

(A)

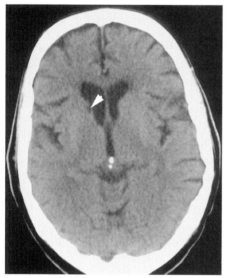

(B)

Fig. 6.2 Lacunar infarction causing hemispheric reduction in metabolism (Fig. 6.2A, CMRO2, right image, white arrows) and flow (Fig. 6.2A, CBF, left image). This patient had a normal computed tomography (CT) scan and normal CMRO2 on a prior positron emission tomography (PET) examination. Repeat PET study (shown here) demonstrated interval development of reduced hemispheric CMRO2 and cerebral blood flow (CBF). A repeat CT scan showed a new, clinically silent lacunar infarction in the head of the caudate nucleus (B, white arrowhead).

Quantitative or qualitative (relative) measurements of CBF can be made using a variety of SPECT and PET methods. CBF is defined as the volume of blood delivered to a defined mass of tissue per unit time, usually expressed in milliliters of blood per 100 g of brain per minute [ml/[100 g · min)]. Most of the commonly employed SPECT techniques employ a variety of compounds that are nearly completely extracted from the blood on their first pass through the cerebral circulation and trapped in the tissue. Commonly used first-pass compounds include ^{99m}Tc-labeled ethylene cysteine dimmer (^{99m}Tc-ECD) and hexamethylpropyleneamine oxime (^{99m}Tc-HMPAO), as well as iodine-133-labeled N-isopropyl-p-[^{123}I]-iodoamphetamine (^{123}I-IMP) (Fig. 6.3). The amount of measured activity in different regions linearly reflects the regional CBF at the time of injection.

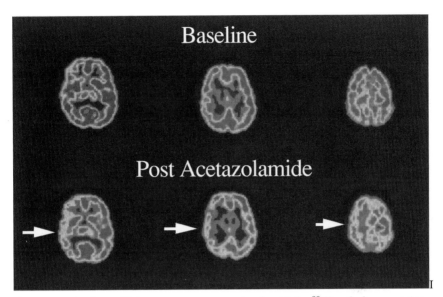

Fig. 6.3 Impaired vasodilatatory response to acetazolamide by ^{99m}Tc ethylene cysteine dimmer (ECD) single-photon emission computed tomography (SPECT). This is an 18-year-old woman angiographic evidence of Moya Moya phenomena affecting the right distal internal carotid artery. Baseline SPECT study (top row) shows symmetric activity between the hemispheres, indicating no difference in relative cerebral blood flow (CBF). After vasodilatatory challenge with acetazolamide (lower row), there is a reduction in CBF in the right middle cerebral artery territory (white arrows), relative to CBF in the contralateral hemisphere. Images courtesy of Ronald van Heertum MD, Columbia University College of Physicians and Surgeons.

With the long half-life of these compounds, scanning can be performed hours after injection and the acquisition can be prolonged to increase counting statistics. Relative CBF compared with other brain regions can be determined simply as the ratio of regional radioactivity. When combined with an arterial time–activity curve obtained at the time of injection, quantitative CBF values can be calculated. Some inaccuracies due to imperfect tissue-trapping occur. SPECT CBF measurements can also be obtained with inhalation of xenon-133 [19,20]. Xenon-133 is a freely diffusible gas and washes out of the tissue quickly. Pulmonary concentrations of xenon-133 are often used instead of arterial time–activity curves for the calculation of quantitative CBF. PET methods can use intravenously injected ^{15}O-labeled water or inhaled ^{15}O-labeled carbon dioxide to measure absolute or relative values of CBF [21–23]. Inhaled ^{15}O-labeled carbon dioxide is rapidly converted to ^{15}O-labeled water in the blood by carbonic anhydrase. These scans are obtained either immediately after a bolus injection (for water) or in a steady-state situation over several minutes (for carbon dioxide). Both PET methods provide accurate measurements of low values of CBF but underestimate high flows due to incomplete first-pass extraction of water. Thus, they are appropriate for studies of ischemia or hypoperfusion. These problems can be overcome using ^{15}O-labeled butanol, as it is completely extracted. PET images obtained using either the ^{15}O-labeled water or ^{15}O-labeled carbon dioxide methods can be used for both relative and absolute CBF measurements. The radioactivity in the images is linearly proportional to CBF, so relative CBF can be calculated from regional radioactivity ratios. As with SPECT, quantitative CBF is obtained using arterial time–activity data.

The paired CBF measurements used to assess for vasodilatatory capacity may be relative or quantitative. A common term in the literature for the provocative tests of vasodilatatory capacity is 'cerebrovascular reserve' (CVR). With absolute measurements of CBF, this is frequently calculated as: CVR (%) = $100 \times (CBF_{post\ stimulus} - CBF_{baseline})/CBF_{baseline}$. Because of the tomographic nature of the CBF measurements, CVR can be calculated regionally for different arterial territories. When relative CBF techniques are used, a change in a calculated asymmetry index is often used to determine vasodilatatory capacity [24]. This is the amount of measured activity in one brain region expressed as a percentage of the amount of activity in the contralateral, normal brain region or in the unaffected cerebellum. The change in the index after vasodilatatory challenge relative to baseline asymmetry is calculated.

The second strategy of hemodynamic assessment uses either the measurement of regional cerebral blood volume (CBV), alone, or in combination with measurements of CBF in the resting brain in order to detect the presence of autoregulatory vasodilatation (Fig. 6.4). CBV is defined as the volume of intravascular blood within a defined mass of tissue and is generally expressed as ml of blood per 100 g of brain. SPECT techniques generally use ^{99m}Tc-labeled albumin or red cells [25,26]. CBV can be measured by PET with either trace amounts of $C^{15}O$ or ^{11}CO [27]. Both carbon monoxide tracers label the red blood cells. Blood volume is calculated using a correction factor for the difference between peripheral vessel and cerebral vessel hematocrit. The CBV/CBF ratio (or, inversely, the CBF/CBV ratio), mathematically equivalent to the vascular mean transit time, may be more sensitive than CBV alone for the identification of autoregulatory vasodilatation [13]. It may be less specific, however, [28]. The CBV/CBF ratio may increase in low flow conditions with normal perfusion pressure, such as hypocapnia. One issue that remains controversial is to what extent autoregulatory vasodilatation of arterioles gives rise to measurable increases in the cerebral blood volume [29]. Experimental data have produced conflicting results [30–32]. The identification of increased CBV in patients with carotid occlusion almost certainly reflects autoregulatory vasodilatation, however, [29].

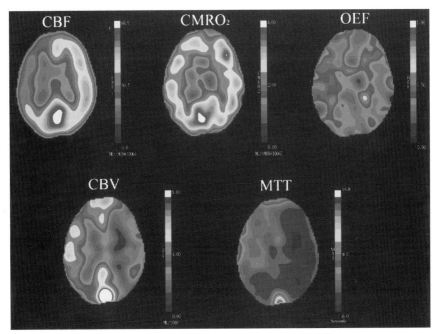

Fig. 6.4 Severe hemodynamic impairment: increased oxygen extraction fraction (OEF). This positron emission tomography (PET) scan shows increased cerebral blood volume (CBV)—indicating autoregulatory vasodilation (CBV) in a patient with unilateral carotid occlusion. Mean vascular transit time (MTT), mathematically equal to the ratio of CBV to cerebral blood flow (CBF) and another indicator of autoregulatory vasodilatation, is also increased. This is insufficient to maintain flow, however, and flow is reduced (CBF, arrows). In this situation, the brain can increase the fraction of oxygen extracted from the blood (OEF) in order to maintain normal oxygen metabolism (CMRO2) and brain function.

The last strategy relies on direct measurements of OEF to identify patients with regions of increased oxygen extraction (Fig. 6.4). At present, regional measurements of OEF can be made only with PET using ^{15}O-labeled radiotracers. A scan is obtained after inhalation of ^{15}O-labeled oxygen. Both steady-state and bolus inhalational methods have been successfully employed and validated [22,33–35]. Quantitative measurements of OEF by either PET method require independent measurements of CBF and CBV [22,23,35,36]. The quantitative value for the regional oxygen metabolism (CMRO$_2$) can then be calculated from an equation using OEF, CBF and arterial oxygen content. A count-based method of relative OEF estimation has also been successfully used [33,37]. This method does not require an arterial line for time–activity data or a CBV scan to correct for intravascular, unextracted labeled oxygen.

The regional analysis of the hemodynamic images generated by the techniques described above is variable. The raw, unprocessed images consist of actual counts of measured radioactivity. These images are often smoothed with a filtering algorithm to produce images that are visually interpretable. When quantitative measurements of CBF, CBV, or OEF are desired, the images are processed using mathematical programs to convert the measured counts into hemodynamic or metabolic values for each pixel in the image. Other data are also required for metabolic processing, including arterial time–activity data, as well as other physiological information such as hematocrit and arterial oxygen content for some calculations. Regions of interest encompassing many pixels are drawn by hand on the images or placed using stereotactic coordinates. The accuracy of measurements in small regions is affected by the statistical distribution of radioactivity (noise), image resolution, and partial volume effects. To reduce these problems, data from several regions within a vascular territory, such as the middle cerebral artery, may be averaged. The decision regarding whether a region is abnormal may be made by comparing the measured counts or values from a particular region with similar regional data from normal control subjects, or from the normal contralateral hemisphere. Investigators have used many different approaches for these analyses, including absolute values, or hemispheric ratios of absolute or relative values. The boundaries of the normal range can be set by using 95% confidence limits from normal control subjects or by the actual range of values observed in the normal subjects.

Association of hemodynamic impairment with clinical and imaging findings

There appear to be a few clinical and imaging findings that are highly predictive of severe hemodynamic impairment. The sensitivity of these findings is often poor, however: most patients with severe hemodynamic impairment do not have them. For example, the clinical syndromes of limb-shaking or postural TIAs, while stongly associated with hemodynamic impairment [38,39], are rare. Few patients with severe hemodynamic impairment have these symptoms, however. Similarly, the findings of linear white matter infarcts in the centrum semiovale or corona radiata are specific, but relatively insensitive, indicators of abnormal hemodynamics in patients with carotid artery occlusion [40–42]. The same is true for angiographic and other anatomical imaging studies. These methods identify the presence and degree of stenosis or occlusion and the patterns of collateral flow. However, this information simply demonstrates the highways of cerebral blood flow and not the traffic. There are significant associations between different patterns of collateral flow and hemodynamic impairment, but the ability of these tests to identify reliably individual patients with severe hemodynamic compromise is poor [43]. Several studies have examined the relationship between hemodynamic abnormalities and patterns of collateral flow. Associations between certain patterns, such as extensive pial collateralization or absence of circle of Willis collaterals, and severe hemodynamic impairment have been reported in large series of patients [43–45]. Some findings, such as pial collateral flow to the insula, appear to highly specific, but insensitive [43], while others, such as absent circle of Willis, appear to be sensitive, but not specific markers of hemodynamic impairment [45].

Association of hemodynamic impairment with stroke risk

Most TIAs involve the carotid territory [46,47]. Patients presenting with TIAs commonly have stenotic or completely occlusive lesions of the carotid artery or its branches. In a consecutive series, Bogousslavksy *et al.* found > 75% stenosis or occlusion of the carotid artery in 29% of 250 patients presenting with carotid TIAs and studied by catheter angiography [48].

Many TIAs and strokes are due to arterial emboli arising from atherosclerotic plaque [49]. However, there is emerging evidence that the presence of reduced perfusion pressure (hemodynamic compromise) is an independent risk factor for ischemic stroke [50–52]. It is possible that there is a synergistic effect between an active, embologenic plaque and severe hemodynamic impairment in producing a permanent ischemic injury—embolic material may be more likely to cause permanent damage in brain tissue that is already maximally compensating for pre-existing low pressure [52–54].

The relative role of hemodynamic and embolic factors in the pathogenesis of stroke in patients with stenosis of the common carotid artery bifurcation may be a moot point, as surgical endarterectomy is proven to be an effective treatment for the reduction in stroke risk, regardless of the presumed mechanism [55]. Currently, there are no proven effective treatments for many patients with other lesions, such as those with complete occlusion of the carotid artery or intracranial arterial stenosis or occlusion. Rational development of preventative treatments in these patients depends on an understanding of the importance of hemodynamic factors in the pathogenesis of stroke.

Several SPECT and PET studies have evaluated the association of hemodynamic impairment with subsequent ischemic stroke in patients with cerebrovascular disease [51,52,56–59]. As these imaging tests are indirect techniques, empiric proof is required to demonstrate that any of these hemodynamic or metabolic abnormalities is an independent risk factor for subsequent stroke [7]. Many of the published investigations relating hemodynamic impairment to stroke risk have significant methodological flaws, limiting the conclusions that can be drawn from them [7]. For example, many studies have included both symptomatic and asymptomatic patients, as well as patients with stenoses and occlusions. The risk of stroke in these different populations may be quite variable. In addition, none of these studies has separately analyzed their data for patients presenting with TIAs. Consequently, there are few data regarding the frequency of hemodynamic impairment in patients presenting with TIA and different degrees and locations of arterial stenosis and occlusion.

SPECT studies

Three prospective studies have used SPECT techniques to investigate hemodynamic stroke risk in patients with occlusive cerebrovascular disease, with variable results. All three studies included patients with prior TIAs and strokes. No subgroup analysis for patients with TIAs was reported for any of the three. The two studies with negative results both used ^{123}I-IMP SPECT measurements of relative cerebral blood flow before and after acetazolamide injection. In the study by Hasegawa et al., 51 symptomatic and asymptomatic patients with different lesions—stenoses and occlusions of intra- and extra-cranial arteries, were followed for a mean of 18.5 months [56]. Twenty of the 51 patients had reduced vasodilatatory capacity. No strokes occurred during the follow-up period. In the second study, by Yokota and several authors from the previous study, 105 symptomatic patients with severe stenosis or occlusion of the internal carotid or proximal middle cerebral artery were studied [57]. The number of patients presenting with TIA was not reported. Fifty-five patients had evidence of a reduced blood flow response to acetazolamide by ^{123}I-IMP SPECT. Ten ipsilateral strokes occurred during a median follow-up period of 2.7 years—five in the 55 patients with reduced vasodilatatory capacity and five in the 50 patients with normal vasodilatatory capacity.

The single positive study used ^{133}Xe SPECT to measure absolute CBF before and after injection of acetazolamide [58]. They enrolled 77 symptomatic patients, including 42 with TIAs, and complete occlusion of the internal carotid artery ($n = 62$) or middle cerebral artery ($n = 15$). They categorized their patients into four groups: (1) normal CBF and normal CVR in the middle cerebral artery territory; (2) normal CBF and reduced CVR; (3) reduced CBF and reduced CVR; and (4) reduced CBF and normal CVR. Sixteen total and seven ipsilateral strokes occurred during a mean follow-up period of 3.5 years. Six total and four ipsilateral strokes occurred in the 11 patients in group 3. The risk of total and ipsilateral stroke was significantly higher in these patients than in the other three groups combined.

PET studies

As with the SPECT data, published PET studies of cerebral hemodynamic impairment and stroke risk have not separately analyzed data for patients presenting with TIA. Three studies have been reported, one negative study using measurements of CBV and CBF and two positive studies using OEF measurements. In this section we will present the data from these three studies, followed by re-analysis of our data from the St Louis Carotid Occlusion Study (STLCOS) for patients presenting with TIA.

Powers *et al.* reported hemodynamic and stroke-risk data on 30 retrospectively identified symptomatic patients with severe carotid stenosis or occlusion [60]. All had normal head computed tomographic examinations after presenting with TIA or minor stroke. Nine patients had normal CBV/CBF ratios and normal OEF. One of these nine patients suffered an ipsilateral stroke within a year of presentation. One of the 16 patients with increased CBV/CBF ratios had an ipsilateral stroke. None of the five patients with increased OEF suffered an ipsilateral stroke.

Two studies have investigated the relationship between OEF and stroke risk. Both reported a positive association. Yamauchi reported 52 symptomatic patients with stenoses and occlusions of the carotid artery and intracranial arteries [51]. Twelve patients were censored because of surgical revascularization. At 1 year, two of the 33 patients with normal OEF had suffered an ipsilateral stroke, compared with four of seven with increased OEF. The difference in stroke occurrence was statistically significant ($P = 0.005$). No multivariate analysis was performed. The strongest evidence for an association between increased OEF and stroke risk was provided by the STLCOS [52]. This was a blinded, prospective study of 81 patients with symptomatic carotid occlusion that also specifically assessed the impact of other risk factors. Increased OEF was identified in 39 of the 81 patients on study enrollment. During a mean follow-up period of 3.2 years, 11 of the 13 total ipsilateral strokes occurred in the 39 patients with increased OEF. The risk of all stroke and ipsilateral ischemic stroke in symptomatic patients with increased OEF was significantly higher than in those with normal OEF (log rank $P = 0.005$ and $P = 0.004$, respectively). Multivariate analysis of 17 baseline stroke risk factors confirmed the independence of this relationship. The age-adjusted relative risk conferred by increased OEF was 6.0 [95% confidence interval (CI) 1.7, 21.6] for all stroke and 7.3 (95% CI 1.6, 33.4) for ipsilateral ischemic stroke.

These two studies differed in the OEF methodology used to determine hemodynamic status. Yamauchi *et al.* used absolute measurements of OEF. Re-analysis of their data after 5 years of follow-up showed significance only when absolute hemispheric OEF values were used, not for hemispheric ratios of absolute values [59]. We investigated the use of the three different techniques of OEF analysis—absolute OEF, hemispheric ratios of absolute OEF, and hemispheric ratios of the count-based OEF method [61]. We compared their performance for the prediction of stroke risk for our STLCOS data. All three methods were predictive of stroke risk, depending on the threshold value used to separate normal from abnormal. The count-based method appeared to be the most sensitive and specific of the three methods by receiver–operating curve analysis.

Of the 81 symptomatic patients enrolled in the STLCOS, 33 presented with TIAs. Twelve of these 33 patients presented with amaurosis fugax and the remaining 21 with cerebral TIAs. Increased OEF was identified in nine of the 21 patients with cerebral TIAs and in three of the 12 patients with ocular TIAs. Three ipsilateral strokes occurred during a mean follow-up period of 2.2 years. All three patients had increased OEF and cerebral TIAs. The risk of ipsilateral stroke in patients with increased OEF and any TIA ($P = 0.01$) or cerebral TIA ($P = 0.03$) was significantly greater than in patients with normal OEF by the log rank statistic. The Kaplan–Meier plot of stroke risk for patients with any TIA is shown in Fig. 6.5.

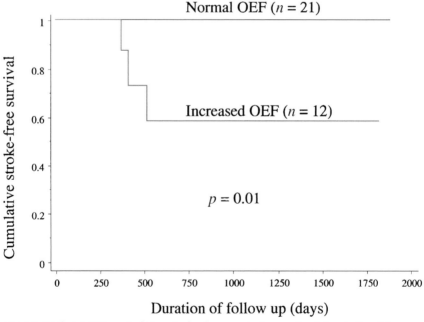

Fig. 6.5 Kaplan–Meier cumulative stroke-free survival curve for St Louis Carotid Occlusion Study (STLCOS) transient ischemic attack (TIA) patients. No strokes were observed during follow-up in the 21 symptomatic patients with normal oxygen extraction fraction (OEF) on enrollment. Three strokes occurred in the 12 patients with increased OEF ($P = 0.01$).

Changes in hemodynamic status over time

Both SPECT and PET have also been used to investigate the changes in hemodynamic status over time in patients with chronic hemodynamic impairment. Both vasodilatatory capacity and OEF and CBF can improve over time, presumably due to improved flow through collateral channels. Whether all patients are capable of this improvement is not clear. Animal studies of experimental carotid occlusion have shown an improvement in vasodilatatory capacity over time and an increase in diameter of collateral vessels [62,63]. Hasegawa and colleagues reported improvement in vasoreactivity in three of 20 patients with atherosclerotic cerebrovascular disease studied with ^{123}I-IMP SPECT and an acetazolamide challenge [56]. Repeat PET studies were performed in 10 patients with increased OEF enrolled in the STLCOS [64]. These patients were selected from the 28 patients with increased OEF and no interval stroke. Follow-up PET was performed between 12 and 59 months after enrollment. The ratio of ipsilateral to contralateral OEF improved from a mean of 1.16 to 1.08 ($P = 0.022$). This improvement was a function of time: greater reductions were seen with longer duration of follow-up ($P = 0.023$, $r = 0.707$). The ratio of ipsilateral to contralateral CBF improved from 0.81 to 0.85 ($P = 0.021$). No change in CBV or $CMRO_2$ was observed. The absolute cerebral metabolic rate for glucose metabolism was reduced in the ipsilateral hemisphere ($P = 0.001$ compared with normal controls) but the ratio of $CMRO_2$/CMRGlc was normal, indicating no increase in glycolytic metabolism in the patients with chronic hypoperfusion.

Secondary endpoint studies

SPECT and PET measurements of hemodynamic factors have been used as secondary endpoints to assess the effects of medical or surgical intervention on cerebral hemodynamic status. This literature is extensive, but inconclusive with regard to actual impact on patient outcome. In addition, none of these studies has separated patients with TIAs from those with stroke.

Superficial temporal artery to middle cerebral artery (STA-MCA) bypass is an effective means of improving hemodynamic and metabolic status in patients with atherosclerotic occlusion of the common carotid, internal carotid, or middle cerebral artery. The operation consistently improves OEF in patients with increased OEF at baseline [65–67]. The ratio of CBV to CBF, an indicator of autoregulatory vasodilatation, may remain abnormal in some of these patients [67,68]. However, as discussed above, the specificity of this ratio for autoregulatory vasodilatation is unclear. Improvement in both CBF and vasodilatatory capacity measured by SPECT after STA-MCA bypass surgery has also been reported [69].

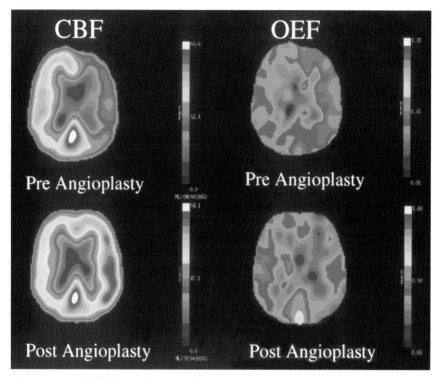

Fig. 6.6 Reversal of abnormal increased oxygen extraction fraction (OEF) after angioplasty for a symptomatic intracranial internal carotid artery stenosis. The top row of images (immediately before angioplasty) shows the reduction of cerebral blood flow (CBF) and compensatory increase in OEF in the hemisphere distal to the stenosis. The lower row of images acquired 36 h after angioplasty shows the improvement in CBF and OEF. Reprinted with permission from Derdeyn *et al. Neurosurgery* 2001; 48: 436–440 [73].

Similarly, the ability of carotid endarterectomy to improve hemodynamic status has also been amply documented [70–72]. Angioplasty and stenting is also effective in this regard (Fig. 6.6) [73]. One area of active research regarding carotid revascularization procedures and hemodynamics is the prediction and management of post-procedural hyperperfusion hemorrhage [74]. These events tend to occur in patients with severe hemodynamic impairment, high-grade stenoses, and recent ischemic symptoms. They may be related to an impairment in autoregulatory capability due to long-standing reductions in CPP and chronic autoregulatory vasodilatation. The ability of PET or SPECT to predict hyperperfusion hemorrhage reliably has not been proven.

Clinical therapeutic trials

The presence of increased OEF has been proven as an independent predictor of subsequent stroke in patients with symptomatic carotid occlusion in two rigorous prospective studies [51,52]. Extracranial–intracranial (EC/IC) bypass surgery can effectively reverse this hemodynamic abnormality [65,67,75,76]. A randomized trial of EC/IC bypass limited to patients with increased OEF is currently underway: the Carotid Occlusion Surgery Study (W. J. Powers and W. Clarke). The goal of this study is to test the hypothesis that surgical anastomosis of the superficial temporal artery to the middle cerebral artery when added to best medical therapy can reduce by 40%, despite perioperative stroke and death, subsequent ipsilateral ischemic stroke (fatal and nonfatal) at 2 years in patients with recently (≤ 120 days) symptomatic internal carotid artery occlusion and ipsilateral increased OEF measured by PET. We will test this hypothesis by conducting a randomized, nonblinded, controlled trial in 372 patients randomized to surgery or best medical therapy. A similar trial is ongoing in Japan—the Japanese EC/IC Bypass Trial (JET, Ogawa, principal investigator), using SPECT to identify patients for randomization.

Conclusion

SPECT and PET provide unique information regarding the hemodynamic status of patients with TIAs and occlusive arterial lesions. These tools have been used extensively in a variety of different clinical investigations and have proven prognostic value in certain specific clinical situations involving patients with TIAs and complete occlusion of a carotid artery. Presently the major research applications of SPECT and PET can be grouped into three categories: natural history studies of hemodynamic impairment and stroke risk, secondary endpoint studies of different interventions on hemodynamic impairment, and clinical trials of therapy for specific patient populations at risk of stroke due to hemodynamic factors. If these trials are successful, these tools will become important in guiding therapy in selected patients with TIA.

References

1 Derdeyn CP, Powers WJ. Positron emission tomography: experimental and clinical applications. In: HH Batjer, ed. *Cerebrovascular Disease*. Philadelphia: Lippincott-Raven, 1997: 239–53.
2 van Heertum RL, Tikofsky RS, eds. *Functional Cerebral SPECT and PET Imaging*, 3rd edn. New York: Lippincott Williams Wilkins, 2000.
3 Videen TO, Dunford-Shore JE, Diringer MN, Powers WJ. Correction for partial volume effects in regional blood flow measurements adjacent to hematomas

in humans with intracerebral hemorrhage: implementation and validation. *J Comput Assist Tomogr* 1999; 23: 248–56.

4 Boysen G. Cerebral hemodynamics in carotid surgery. *Acta Neurologica Scand* 1973; 49 (Suppl. 52): 3–86.

5 Deweese JA, May AG, Lipchik EO, Rob CG. Anatomic and hemodynamic correlations in carotid artery stenosis. *Stroke* 1970; 1: 149–57.

6 Gibbs JM, Wise RJS, Leendeers KL, Jones T. Evaluation of cerebral perfusion reserve in patients with carotid artery occlusion. *Lancet* 1984; 1: 310–4.

7 Derdeyn CP, Grubb RL Jr, Powers WJ. Cerebral hemodynamic impairment: methods of measurement and association with stroke risk. *Neurology* 1999; 53: 251–9.

8 Rapela CE, Green HD. Autoregulation of canine cerebral blood flow. *Circ Res* 1964; 15: I205–I211.

9 Kety SS, King BD, Horvath SM, Jeffers WA, Hafkenschiel JH. The effects of an acute reduction in blood pressure by means of differential spinal sympathetic block on the cerebral circulation of hypertensive patients. *J Clin Invest* 1950; 29: 402–7.

10 MacKenzie ET, Farrar JK, Fitch W, Graham DI, Gregory PC, Harper AM. Effects of hemorrhagic hypotension on the cerebral circulation: I. Cerebral blood flow and pial arteriolar caliber. *Stroke* 1979; 10: 711–8.

11 Dirnagl U, Pulsinelli W. Autoregulation of cerebral blood flow in experimental focal brain ischemia. *J Cereb Blood Flow Metab* 1990; 10: 327–36.

12 Kontos HA, Wei EP, Navari RM, Levasseur JE, Rosenblum WI, Patterson JL. Responses of cerebral arteries and arterioles to acute hypotension and hypertension. *Am J Physiol* 1978; 243: H371–H383.

13 Schumann P, Touzani O, Young AR, Baron J-C, Morello R, MacKenzie ET. Evaluation of the ratio of cerebral blood flow to cerebral blood volume as an index of local cerebral perfusion pressure. *Brain* 1998; 121: 1369–79.

14 Lennox WG, Gibbs FA, Gibbs EL. Relationship of unconsciousness to cerebral blood flow and to anoxemia. *Arch Neurol Psych* 1935; 34: 1001–13.

15 Lenzi GL, Frackowiak RS, Jones T. Cerebral oxygen metabolism and blood flow in human cerebral ischemic infarction. *J Cereb Blood Flow Metab* 1982; 2: 321–35.

16 Martin WR, Raichle ME. Cerebellar blood flow and metabolism in cerebral hemisphere infarction. *Ann Neurol* 1983; 14: 168–76.

17 Pantano P, Baron JC, Samson Y, Bousser MG, Derouesne C, Comar D. Crossed cerebrellar diaschisis. Further studies. *Brain* 1986; 109: 677–94.

18 Lassen NA, Palvolgyi R. Cerebral steal during hypercapnia and the inverse reaction during hypocapnia observed with the [133]xenon technique in man. *Scand J Clin Lab Invest* 1968; 22 (Suppl. 102): 13D (Abstract).

19 Lassen NA, Hoedt-Rasmussen K, Sorenson SC *et al*. Regional cerebral blood flow in man determined by krypton. *Neurology* 1963; 13: 719–27.

20 Celsis P, Goldman T, Henriksen L, Lassen NA. A method for calculating regional cerebral blood flow from emission computed tomography of inert gas concentrations. *J Comput Assist Tomogr* 1981; 5: 641–5.

21 Raichle ME, Martin WRW, Herscovitch P, Mintun MA, Markham J. Brain blood flow measured with intravenous H215O. II. Implementation and validation. *J Nucl Med* 1983; 24: 790–8.

22 Videen TO, Perlmutter JS, Herscovitch P, Raichle ME. Brain blood volume, blood flow, and oxygen utilization measured with O-15 radiotracers and positron emission tomography: revised metabolic computations. *J Cereb Blood Flow Metab* 1987; 7: 513–6.

23 Frackowiak RSJ, Lenzi G-L, Jones T, Heather JD. Quantitative measurement of regional cerebral blood flow and oxygen metabolism in man using O-15 and positron emission tomography: theory, procedure, and normal values. *J Comput Assist Tomogr* 1980; 4: 727–36.

24 Hirano T, Minematsu K, Hasegawa Y, Tanaka Y, Hayashida K, Yamaguchi T. Acetazolamide reactivity on I-IMP single photon emission computed tomography in patients with major cerebral artery occlusive disease: correlation with positron emission tomography parameters. *J Cereb Blood Flow Metab* 1994; 14: 763–70.

25 Sakai F, Nakazawa K, Tazaki Y *et al*. Regional cerebral blood volume and hematocrit measured in normal human volunteers by single-photon emission computed tomography. *J Cereb Blood Flow Metab* 1985; 5: 207–13.

26 Vlasenko A, Petit-Taboue MC, Bouvard G, Morello R, Derlon JM. Comparative quantitation of cerebral blood volume: SPECT versus PET. *J Nucl Med* 1997; 38: 919–24.

27 Martin WR, Powers WJ, Raichle ME. Cerebral blood volume measured with inhaled C15O and positron emission tomography. *I Cereb Blood Flow Metab* 1987; 7: 421–6.

28 Grubb RL Jr, Raichle ME, Eichling JO, Ter-Poossian MM. The effects of changes in PaCO2 on cerebral blood volume, blood flow, and vascular mean transit time. *Stroke* 1974; 5: 630–9.

29 Derdeyn CP, Videen TO, Yundt KD *et al*. Variability of cerebral blood volume and oxygen extraction fraction: stages of hemodynamic impairment revisited. *Brain* 2002; 125: 595–607.

30 Tomita M, Gotoh F, Kobari M *et al*. Autoregulatory response in cerebral vasculature versus low perfusion hyperemia following middle cerebral artery occlusion in cats. *J Cereb Blood Flow Metab* 1985; 5 (Suppl.): S405–S406.

31 Ferrari M, Wilson DA, Hanley DF, Traystman RJ. Effects of graded hypotension on cerebral blood flow, blood volume, and mean transit time in dogs. *Am J Physiol* 1992; 262: H1908–H1914.

32 Zaharchuk G, Mandeville JB, Bogdanov AA, Weissleder R, Rosen BR, Marota JJA. Cerebrovascular dynamics of autoregulation and hypoperfusion: an MRI study of CBF and changes in total and microvascular cerebral blood volume during hemorrhagic hypotension. *Stroke* 1999; 30: 2197–205.

33 Jones T, Chesler DA, Ter-Pogossian MM. The continuous inhalation of Oxygen-15 for assessing regional oxygen extraction in the brain of man. *Br J Radiol* 1976; 49: 339–43.

34 Baron JC, Steinling M, Tanaka T, Cavalheiro E, Sousaline F, Collard P. Quantitative measurement of CBF, oxygen extraction fraction (OEF) and CMRO2 with the O-15 continuous inhalation technique and positron emission tomography (PET): experimental evidence and normal values in man. *J Cereb Blood Flow Metab* 1981; 1 (Suppl. 1): S5–S6.

35 Mintun MA, Raichle ME, Martin WRW, Herscovitch P. Brain oxygen utilization measured with O-15 radiotracers and positron emission tomography. *J Nuc Med* 1984; 25: 177–87.

36 Lammertsma AA, Wise RJS, Heather JD *et al.* Correction for the presence of intravascular Oxygen-15 in the steady-state technique for measuring regional oxygen extraction ratio in the brain: 2. Results in normal subjects and brain tumor and stroke patients. *J Cereb Blood Flow Metab* 1983; 3: 425–31.

37 Derdeyn CP, Videen TO, Simmons NS *et al.* Count-based PET method for predicting stroke in patients with symptomatic carotid occlusion. *Radiology* 1999; 212: 499–506.

38 Powers WJ, Tempel LW, Grubb RL Jr, Raichle ME. Clinical correlates of cerebral hemodynamics. *Stroke* 1987; 18: 284.

39 Levine RL, Lagreye HL, Dobkin JA *et al.* Cerebral vasocapacitance and TIAs. *Neurology* 1989; 39: 25–9.

40 Waterston JA, Brown MM, Butler P, Swash M. Small deep cerebral infarcts associated with occlusive internal carotid artery disease. A hemodynamic phenomenon? *Arch Neurol* 1990; 47: 953–7.

41 Yamauchi H, Fukuyama H, Yamaguchi S, Miyoshi T, Kimura J, Konishi J. High-intensity area in the deep white matter indicating hemodynamic compromise in internal carotid artery occlusive disorders. *Arch Neurol* 1991; 48: 1067–71.

42 Derdeyn CP, Khosla AS, Videen TO *et al.* Patterns of cerebral infarction with severe hemodynamic impairment. *Radiology* 2001; 220: 195–201.

43 Derdeyn CP, Shaibani A, Moran CJ, Cross DT Jr, Grubb RL Jr, Powers WJ. Lack of correlation of angiographic findings and severe hemodynamic compromise in patients with carotid occlusion. *Stroke* 1999; 30: 1025–32.

44 van Everdingen KJ, Visser GH, Klijn CJM, Kappelle LJ, van der Grond J. Role of collateral flow on cerebral hemodynamics in patients with unilateral internal carotid artery occlusion. *Ann Neurol* 1998; 44: 167–76.

45 Vernieri F, Pasqualetti P, Matteis M *et al.* Effect of collateral blood flow and cerebral vasomotor reactivity on the outcome of carotid artery occlusion. *Stroke* 2001; 32: 1552–8.

46 Dennis MS, Bamford JM, Sandercock PA, Warlow CP. Incidence of transient ischemic attacks in Oxfordshire, England. *Stroke* 1989; 20: 333–9.

47 Sempere AP, Duarte J, Cabezas C, Clavería LE. Incidence of transient ischemic attacks and minor ischemic strokes in Segovia, Spain. *Stroke* 1996; 27: 667–71.

48 Bogousslavsky J, Hachinski VC, Boughner DR, Fox AJ, Vinuela F, Barnett HJ. Cardiac and arterial lesions in transient ischemic attacks. *Arch Neurol* 1986; 43: 223–8.

49 Caplan LR. Brain embolism, revisited. *Neurology* 1993; 43: 1281–7.

50 Klijn CJM, Kappelle LJ, Tulleken CAF, van Gijn J. Symptomatic carotid artery occlusion: a reappraisal of hemodynamic factors. *Stroke* 1997; 28: 2084–93.

51 Yamauchi H, Fukuyama Y, Nagahama Y *et al*. Evidence of misery perfusion and risk for recurrent stroke in major cerebral arterial occlusive diseases from PET. *J Neurol Neurosurg Psychiatry* 1996; 61: 18–25.

52 Grubb RL Jr, Derdeyn CP, Fritsch SM *et al*. The importance of hemodynamic factors in the prognosis of symptomatic carotid occlusion. *JAMA* 1998; 280: 1055–60.

53 Omae T, Mayzel-Oreg O, Li F, Sotak CH, Fisher M. Inapparent hemodynamic insufficiency exacerbates ischemic damage in a rat microembolic stroke model. *Stroke* 2000; 31: 2494–9.

54 Derdeyn CP. Physiological neuroimaging: emerging clinical applications. *JAMA* 2001; 285: 3065–8.

55 North American Symptomatic Carotid Endarterectomy Trial (NASCET) Collaborators. Beneficial effect of carotid endarterectomy in symptomatic patients with high-grade carotid stenosis. *N Engl J Med* 1991; 325: 445–53.

56 Hasegawa Y, Yamaguchi T, Tsuchiya T, Minematsu K, Nishimura T. Sequential change of hemodynamic reserve in patients with major cerebral artery occlusions or severe stenosis. *Neuroradiology* 1992; 34: 15–21.

57 Yokota C, Hasegawa Y, Minematsu K, Yamaguchi T. Effect of acetazolamide reactivity and long-term outcome in patients with major cerebral artery occlusive disease. *Stroke* 1998; 29: 1743–4 [letter].

58 Kuroda S, Houkin K, Kamiyama H, Mitsumori K, Iwasaki Y, Abe H. Long-term prognosis of medically treated patients with internal carotid or middle cerebral artery occlusion: can acetazolamide test predict it? *Stroke* 2001; 32: 2110–6.

59 Yamauchi H, Fukuyama H, Nagahama Y *et al*. Significance of increased oxygen extraction fraction in five-year prognosis of major cerebral arterial occlusive disease. *J Nucl Med* 1999; 40: 1992–8.

60 Powers WJ, Tempel LW, Grubb RL Jr. Influence of cerebral hemodynamics on stroke risk: one year follow up of 30 medically treated patients. *Ann Neurol* 1989; 25: 325–30.

61 Derdeyn CP, Videen TO, Grubb RL Jr, Powers WJ. Comparison of PET oxygen extraction fraction methods for the prediction of stroke risk. *J Nucl Med* 2001; 42: 1195–7.

62 Coyle P, Panzenbeck MJ. Collateral development after carotid artery occlusion in Fischer 344 rats. *Stroke* 1990; 21: 316–21.

63 De Ley G, Nshimyumuremyi JB, Leusen J. Hemispheric blood flow in the rat after unilateral carotid common carotid occlusion: evaluation with time. *Stroke* 1985; 16: 69–73.

64 Derdeyn CP, Yundt KD, Videen TO, Grubb RL Jr, Carpenter DA, Powers WJ. Compensatory mechanism to chronic hypoperfusion in patients with carotid occlusion. *Stroke* 1999; 30: 1019–24.

65 Gibbs JM, Wise RJ, Thomas DJ, Mansfield AO, Russell RW. Cerebral hemodynamic changes after extracranial-intracranial bypass surgery. *J Neurol Neurosurg Psychiatry* 1987; 50: 140–50.

66 Powers WJ, Grubb RL Jr, Raichle ME. Clinical results of extracranial-intracranial bypass surgery in patients with hemodynamic cerebrovascular disease. *J Neurosurg* 1989; 70: 61–7.

67 Takagi Y, Hashimoto N, Iwama T, Hayashida K. Improvement of oxygen metabolic reserve after extracranial-intracranial bypass surgery in patients with severe hemodynamic insufficiency. *Acta Neurochir (Wien)* 1997; 139: 52–6.

68 Powers WJ, Press GA, Grubb RL Jr, Gado M, Raichle ME. The effect of hemodynamically significant carotid artery disease on the hemodynamic status of the cerebral circulation. *Ann Int Med* 1987; 106: 27–35.

69 Kume N, Hayashida K, Iwama T, Cho I, Matsunaga N. Use of 123I-IMP brain SPET to predict outcome following STA-MCA bypass surgery: cerebral blood flow but not vasoreactivity is a predictive parameter. *Eur J Nucl Med* 1998; 25: 1637–42.

70 Uno M, Harada M, Nagahiro S. Quantitative evaluation of cerebral metabolites and cerebral blood flow in patients with carotid stenosis. *Neurol Res* 2001; 23: 573–80.

71 Lishmanov Y, Shvera I, Ussov W, Shipulin V. The effect of carotid endarterectomy on cerebral blood flow and cerebral blood volume studied by SPECT. *J Neuroradiol* 1997; 24: 155–62.

72 Cikrit DF, Dalsing MC, Harting PS *et al.* Cerebral vascular reactivity assessed with acetazolamide single photon emission computer tomography scans before and after carotid endarterectomy. *Am J Surg* 1997; 174: 193–7.

73 Derdeyn CP, Cross DT 3rd, Moran CJ, Dacey RG Jr. Reversal of focal misery perfusion after intracranial angioplasty: case report. *Neurosurgery* 2001; 48: 436–9.

74 Baker CJ, Mayer SA, Prestigiacomo CJ, Van Heertum RL, Solomon RA. Diagnosis and monitoring of cerebral hyperfusion after carotid endarterectomy with single photon emission computed tomography: case report. *Neurosurgery* 1998; 43: 157–60.

75 Baron JC, Bousser MG, Rey A, Guillard A, Comar D, Castaigne P. Reversal of focal 'misery perfusion syndrome' by extra-intracranial artery bypass in hemodynamic cerebral ischemia. A case study with 0–15 positron emission tomography. *Stroke* 1981; 12: 454–9.

76 Powers WJ, Martin WR, Herscovitch P, Raichle ME, Grubb RL Jr. Extracranial-intracranial bypass surgery: hemodynamic and metabolic effects. *Neurology* 1984; 34: 1168–74.

77 Grubb RL Jr, Phelps ME, Raichle ME, Ter-Pogossian MM. The effects of arterial blood pressure on the regional cerebral blood volume by X-ray fluorescence. *Stroke* 1973; 4: 390–9.

78 Grubb RL Jr, Raichle ME, Phelps ME, Ratcheson RA. Effects of increased intracranial pressure on cerebral blood volume, blood flow, and oxygen utilization in monkey. *J Neurosurg* 1975; 43: 385–98.

79 Heistad DD, Kontos HE. Cerebral circulation. In: Shepherd JT, Abboud FM, eds. *Handbook of Physiology*, Vol. 3. Bethesda: American Physiological Society, 1983: 137–82.

80 McHenry LC Jr, Fazekas JF, Sullivan JF. Cerebral hemodynamics of syncope. *Am J Med Sci* 1961; 80: 173–8.

Cerebrovascular Ultrasound

Janet L. Wilterdink

Ultrasound principles

Cerebrovascular imaging makes use of two ultrasound techniques: B-mode imaging and Doppler ultrasound. B-mode imaging or real-time brightness-modulated sonography images tissue and vessel structure in a two-dimensional gray scale display. The display is generated from the amplitude of reflected sound waves which are modified by tissues with different acoustic impedance. Axial resolution and lateral resolution depend on the emitted ultrasound frequency and in general are insufficient to quantify accurately the degree of arterial narrowing. The B-mode image is used to guide the Doppler ultrasound examination and to provide information about vessel anatomy and plaque characteristics.

Doppler ultrasound employs the Doppler principle: the shift in frequency of sound waves reflected from red blood cells moving within a vessel is proportional to their velocity. The Doppler spectrum therefore is a waveform of arterial blood flow in real time. Specific characteristics of the Doppler spectrum help to identify the artery of its origin. For example, the internal carotid artery (ICA) has a low-impedance high-capacitance spectrum characterized by smooth systolic upstroke and presence of diastolic flow. These distinguish it from the high-resistance spectrum which characterizes the external carotid artery (ECA) (Fig. 7.1). Because velocity is inversely proportional to lumen diameter, focal increases in blood cell velocity suggest focal narrowing. Quantification of arterial narrowing is most reliably obtained by criteria that utilize elevations in peak systolic velocity, end diastolic velocity, mean velocity, or some combination thereof, as measured by the Doppler spectrum.

Color Doppler flow imaging superimposes a two-dimensional color-coded real-time Doppler image of intravascular blood flow on the gray scale B-mode image of vessel anatomy, with the degree of color saturation correlating with the flow velocity (Fig. 7.2). Color flow imaging does not clearly improve test accuracy but does improve the efficiency and probably the reproducibility of the test by making anatomy easier to

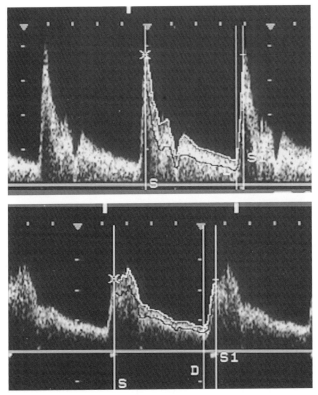

Fig. 7.1 Doppler spectral waveforms. (Above) External carotid artery, a high resistance signal characterized by abrupt systolic upstroke, rapid declination and low diastolic flow. (Below) Internal carotid artery, a capacitance signal characterized by a more gradual systolic upstroke and decline and more diastolic flow.

visualize and directing the technician to high-yield areas in the artery for Doppler sampling.

Carotid duplex ultrasound

Carotid duplex ultrasound (CDUS), as its name suggests, combines the two ultrasound modalities of B-mode imaging and Doppler waveform analysis described above to examine the cervical carotid arteries.

Carotid atherosclerosis

The most important role of CDUS in a patient with transient ischemic attack (TIA) is to identify carotid atherosclerotic plaque as the cause for

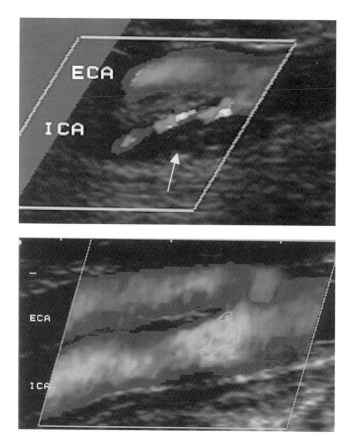

Fig. 7.2 Color Doppler images of diseased carotid bifurcations. (Above) Severe stenotic narrowing by echolucent plaque (arrow). The color Doppler image quickly directs the technician to the high-velocity flow jet within the lumen. (Below) Mild stenotic narrowing. In this case the areas of highest color saturation (shown here as brightest white) direct the technician toward areas of Doppler sampling that will contain the highest velocities, allowing for consistent, reproducible results.

the TIA and thereby identify patients who will benefit from carotid endarterectomy to prevent further sequelae.

Atherosclerotic plaque with narrowing of the carotid bifurcation is believed to be causative in 15–25% of patients with anterior circulation TIA or stroke [1–4]. The pathogenesis of most TIA or stroke resulting from cervical atherosclerosis is believed to result from embolization of material from the atherosclerotic plaque surface. Therefore, while severe carotid disease is often described as 'hemodynamically significant', flow limitation *per se* is believed to cause the minority of ischemic symptoms

Table 7.1 Influence of percent stenosis on stroke risk and risk reduction from surgery in NASCET [8–10]

% Stenosis	Annual ipsilateral stroke rate in medical group*	Relative risk reduction from carotid endarterectomy, %
90–99	0.21	75
80–89	0.17	63
70–79	0.11	63
50–69	0.041	29
30–49	0.035	20†

*Calculated from 2 and 5 years cumulative incidence rates using $-1/a$ ($\ln(1-b)$) where a = years followed and b = cumulative incidence rate.
†Nonsignificant.

resulting from carotid disease. All patients with TIA whose symptoms are potentially referable to the territory of the ICA should be evaluated for atherosclerotic carotid disease, as no subsets of clinical symptoms or signs, such as carotid bruit, are reliable in either selecting or excluding patients for such evaluation [5].

While CDUS provides much information about the carotid plaque, including plaque content and surface characteristics, it is the degree of carotid narrowing that best correlates with pathological findings and other imaging modalities (conventional and magnetic resonance angiography). More importantly, the degree of carotid narrowing influences prognosis; data correlating degree of stenosis and stroke risk are well established in both asymptomatic and symptomatic individuals [6,7]. The North American Symptomatic Carotid Endarterectomy Trial (NASCET) not only confirmed the relationship between degree of stenosis and stroke risk (Table 7.1), but also found that the benefit of carotid endarterectomy, as measured by relative risk reduction of recurrent stroke, also increased with increasing stenosis [8–10]. These data allow sophisticated analysis of risk and benefit in patients with TIA who are found to have an ipsilateral carotid stenosis between 50 and 99%.

Given the importance of degree of carotid narrowing to clinical decision making, the sensitivity, specificity, and accuracy of CDUS in this regard are critical. Analysis of CDUS results in the carotid endarterectomy trials drew attention to the widely varying performance of CDUS in this regard [11,12]. This theme continues to be echoed in the plethora of studies reported in the literature since. Interpretation of this literature, however, is complicated by the different CDUS criteria used, different angiographic (or other gold standard) criteria used, variable adjustment for verification and other forms of bias, and whether CDUS sensitivity for a specific 'cut-off point' of stenosis (e.g. less than vs. greater than 70%) was measured or whether for the entire range of stenoses. Older studies may also be limited by older technology. Results have also improved in more recent years by the recognized need for individual, laboratory-specific, on-going validation of CDUS criteria.

Commonly used CDUS criteria include peak systolic velocity (PSV) in the ICA, end diastolic velocity (EDV) in the ICA and/or the ratio of the PSVs in the ICA to the common carotid artery (CCA). The latter has the theoretical advantage of taking into account hemodynamic changes and/or equipment-specific variables that might influence recorded blood velocities within the carotid system that are unrelated to focal narrowing [13]. However, variations in velocity along the CCA can make this technique subject to variability as well [14]. While systematic investigation by two groups suggest that ICA PSV is the single best criterion [15,16], others find that ICA to CCA PSV ratios work best in their laboratory [17,18], while still others use combined PSV and EDV criteria [19]. These differences probably reflect the technique and experience of the ultrasonographer as well as the equipment used [20–22]. Individual laboratory validation studies should be done to determine their site-specific best CDUS criteria for categorizing disease severity.

The performance of CDUS criteria will necessarily be specific to the angiographic criterion for measurement of stenosis which is used for its validation. The most commonly used angiographic criterion for this purpose is that used by NASCET investigators, as this criterion is easily applied, reproducible, and has been correlated with clinical outcomes with and without surgery. This method compares the residual lumen diameter at the most stenotic site with that in the normal ICA distal to the stenosis [23]. Close to 90% or better sensitivity and specificity of CDUS in identifying categories of surgical disease as so defined appear to be widely achievable [24–31]. However, this quality of performance cannot be taken for granted and results may fall far short, in part because not all laboratories do the recommended audits and validation studies [31–36].

Laboratories also may choose criteria which elevate sensitivity over either specificity or accuracy in order to produce the best clinical outcome for patients [28,37]. This type of analysis requires that criteria be specific to clinical scenario as the relative importance of sensitivity and specificity is different for asymptomatic and symptomatic patients. For example, because failure to identify a > 70% stenosis in a symptomatic patient carries a high excess stroke and death risk of almost 17%, a high sensitivity (few false negatives) of the test criterion is more important than either specificity or accuracy to the patient's outcome. Using published outcome data and receiver–operator characteristic analysis, test criteria can be developed that maximize patient outcome for the specific clinical situation [37–39].

Not surprising, given the wide spectrum of CDUS performance reported in the literature, are the differing opinions whether CDUS can be used alone to select patients for endarterectomy [25,40–44], or whether it should be used instead to select patients for conventional angiography for definitive diagnosis of disease severity [32–34,45,46]. Many have concluded that concordant CDUS and magnetic resonance angiography results are sufficiently accurate to avoid invasive testing [45,47,48], while others argue that magnetic resonance angiography contributes little to nothing over CDUS results [29,41]. It is logical to conclude that this decision depends not only on locally measured CDUS sensitivity and specificity but also on local performance of magnetic resonance angiography and local risks of conventional angiography.

Plaque characteristics, whether visualized by CDUS, angiography, or pathological specimens, have long interested investigators in their potential for identifying unstable lesions that have a high risk of causing imminent stroke. However, clinical investigations have been somewhat disappointing. Surface characteristics, most notably carotid plaque ulceration, seen on pathological specimens have correlated quite variably with symptomatic vs. nonsymptomatic lesions [49]. Correlation of plaque ulceration seen on CDUS with that seen pathologically is also imperfect [50–52]. Similarly, ultrasound characteristics of plaque content such as intraplaque hemorrhage and lipid cores, both represented on B-mode ultrasound as echolucent regions within the plaque (Fig. 7.2), have been found by some but not others to predict either pathological findings, symptomatic status or prognosis [49,52–57]. Both ulceration and echolucency are more common in more severely stenotic lesions, perhaps explaining why neither of these findings appear more compelling in determining prognosis than does percentage stenosis [58,59]. Higher resolution imaging and efforts to standardize interpretation of plaque characteristics may make these investigations more consistently fruitful in the future [60].

Non-atherosclerotic disease of carotid bifurcation

Non-atherosclerotic disease of the cervical carotid system is far less common and therefore contributes a much lower percentage to the overall burden of stroke and TIA. Nonetheless, as the treatment and prognosis are quite different for these entities, it is important for the clinician to be aware of them and their ultrasound characteristics. These include Takayasu's arteritis, radiation angiopathy, carotid artery dissection and fibromuscular dysplasia.

In general the duplex findings in non-atherosclerotic diseases are nonspecific, difficult to distinguish clearly from the more common atherosclerotic narrowing, and require further, more diagnostic imaging with magnetic resonance and/or conventional angiography. However, certain

CDUS patterns may be noteworthy. For example in Takayasu's arteritis, CDUS findings typically include a long segment of diffuse, homogeneous, circumferential vessel wall thickening in the proximal CCA, often sparing the internal and external carotid arteries [61,62]. This contrasts with the more usual eccentric appearance of narrowing by atherosclerosis which is most common in the ICA at the level of the bifurcation. Fibromuscular disease, in contrast, typically involves the cervical ICA more distally, at the C1, C2 level, often too high for high-quality duplex examination, while radiation arteropathy will vary depending upon the level of radiation therapy [63,64].

Carotid artery dissection may have distinctive findings on CDUS including a tapered lumen distal to the bulb, a floating intimal flap, a double lumen and/or intralumenal membrane [65–67]. When such findings are found they may be diagnostic, but often the CDUS examination reveals only nonspecific abnormalities of narrowing or occlusion, or may even be unremarkable [67,68]. However, when the diagnosis is made, whether by CDUS or conventional or magnetic resonance angiography, CDUS may be helpful in following such lesions; the Doppler spectrum normalizes over weeks to months in about two-thirds of patients [67,68].

Giant call arteritis most commonly affects the branch arteries of the ECA, including the superficial temporal artery and occipital arteries, giving rise to TIA of the eye (amaurosis fugax) or permanent blindness. Less commonly, cerebral TIA or stroke may occur when the cervical internal carotid and vertebral arteries are involved. The most common site of involvement is just before these arteries become intracranial. Giant cell arteritis is suspect in elderly individuals with TIA who have a prodrome of headache and systemic symptoms of arthralgias, malaise, fatigue, and weight loss. With a sensitivity of 73% and specificity of 100%, color duplex ultrasonography of the temporal arteries shows a characteristic dark halo around the lumen, believed to represent arterial wall edema, in patients with temporal arteritis [69].

Pitfalls of CDUS

The many advantages of CDUS include that it is non-invasive, relatively inexpensive, well tolerated and potentially portable. It is equally important for the clinician to be aware of limitations and potential pitfalls in CDUS diagnosis of carotid atherosclerosis. First, it is less accurate at quantifying degrees of stenosis < 50%; this is less problematic for the clinician because at present there is no clinical imperative for quantifying these lower degrees of stenoses.

More problematic is distinguishing carotid occlusion from highly stenosed but still patent arteries. This is a clinically important distinction as both prognosis and management of these lesions differ. CDUS diagnoses carotid occlusion by failing to identify a signal from that artery. This has inherent problems. Confidence in the diagnosis can be improved by finding other ultrasound abnormalities, such as the presence of collateral flow patterns on transcranial Doppler, and longitudinal pulsation of the artery. 'Internalization' of the ECA may either help the technician or present another opportunity for diagnostic confusion. This phenomenon occurs when the ECA supplies collateral flow to the ipsilateral cerebral hemisphere when the ICA is occluded; hence the ECA waveform takes on characteristics of—and the artery may be misidentified as—a normal ICA. Techniques of temporal tapping (transmission of tapping over the superficial temporal artery are reflected downstream in the ECA) and observation of external carotid artery branches usually prevents the technician from making this error. Nonetheless, severe but non-occlusive narrowing may be found in 5–15% of arteries when CDUS has diagnosed carotid occlusion [70–73]. While magnetic resonance angiography has similar difficulties in differentiating the nearly from the completely occluded artery, combining the two tests may reduce the error rate [48]. Further complicating this issue is the fact that on occasion, the 'gold standard' angiography may misclassify an artery as completely occluded when CDUS correctly indicates patency [71,74].

Increased blood flow velocities are not specific to arterial narrowing and at times represent increased collateral flow. When the carotid artery contralateral to the diseased artery provides collateralization via the anterior communicating artery, elevated velocities seen in that cervical carotid artery may lead the technician to mistakenly diagnose or overestimate stenosis there [75–77].

Clearly, the expertise and experience of ultrasonographer is critical to the accurate performance of CDUS [20,22]. Equipment also influences test results [21]. Because the test results rely so heavily on the technician and the machine used, validation studies with adjustment of diagnostic criteria should be regularly performed in individual laboratories [12,20,22,31,35,78–80]. This is a standard for ultrasound laboratory accreditation, yet accreditation is not widely required, audits are not universally performed and the performance of a given laboratory may be unknown to the clinician relying on its test results.

Vertebral duplex ultrasound

The elements of the vertebral duplex ultrasound examination and interpretation are similar to those for CDUS, but it is more challenging. The vertebral artery is more difficult to image than the carotid as it lies deeper and runs through the C1–C6 vertebral processes which block ultrasound transmission (Fig. 7.3). The low lying origin of the vertebral artery, which is the predominant site of cervical vertebral artery stenosis, is difficult to

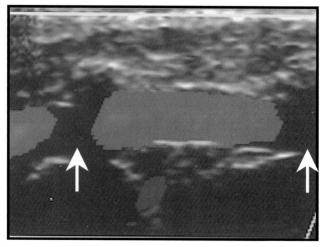

Fig. 7.3 Color Doppler image of a normal appearing vertebral artery. Flow is discontinuously seen between the vertebral processes (arrows).

visualize, especially on the left where it is seen in only 70–86% of patients [81–84]. Limited imaging also makes it difficult to distinguish congenital hypoplasia or aplasia from disease. It should be remembered also that increased flow velocities within the vertebral system may also result from increased collateral blood flow in the presence of a flow-limiting stenosis in the carotid system.

The contribution of proximal vertebral atherosclerosis to TIA and stroke is poorly quantified. Cervical vertebral disease is less common and less severe than carotid disease; and is also less likely to be symptomatic than intracranial vertebrobasilar disease [85]. At present, limitations in the vertebral duplex examination preclude quantification of vertebral artery stenoses, although sensitivity for detection of disease > 50% has been reported to be as high as 80%, albeit in very experienced hands [86].

Similar to CDUS and carotid dissection, the ultrasound findings for vertebral dissection, while often abnormal (75–86%), are uncommonly specifically diagnostic [87–89]. The diagnosis is more surely made by magnetic resonance or conventional angiography. Cases are described where the more specifically diagnostic bilumenal blood flow is seen, but these are the exception rather than the rule [88,90]. However, when abnormalities are found on ultrasound, it may be a useful modality for following the patient for resolution [89,91].

Vertebral duplex ultrasound has more success in detecting flow alterations due to subclavian steal syndrome [92]. This phenomenon occurs as a result of obstruction of the proximal subclavian artery or brachiocephalic trunk and may produce vertebrobasilar TIAs often in association with upper

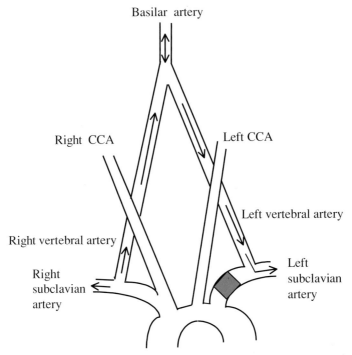

Fig. 7.4 Schematic demonstrating subclavian steal phenomemon. With obstruction in the left subclavian artery, the duplex examination will reveal normal anterograde blood flow in the right vertebral artery and either manifest or latent retrograde blood flow (coded blue on color flow imaging) in the left vertebral artery.

extremity activity (Fig. 7.4). On ultrasound, retrograde flow in the ipsilateral vertebral artery may be manifest, occurring without activation procedures, or it may be latent, occurring in response to post-ischemic hyperemia of the upper extremity. The latter may be reproduced in the laboratory allowing for real-time imaging of vertebral artery flow alterations. Vertebral artery flow reversals may also be evaluated by transcranial Doppler [93]. Subclavian steal is usually a benign syndrome; most (85%) are asymptomatic, and 50% of those with vertebrobasilar TIAs remit spontaneously [94,95].

A small number of patients experience vertebrobasilar TIAs due to mechanical compression of the vertebral arteries by the vertebrae during extremes of rotation, flexion or extension. The vertebral duplex examination is an ideal diagnostic modality for this syndrome, as vertebral artery flow alterations may be reproduced by head-turning maneuvers performed during the ultrasound examination [96–98].

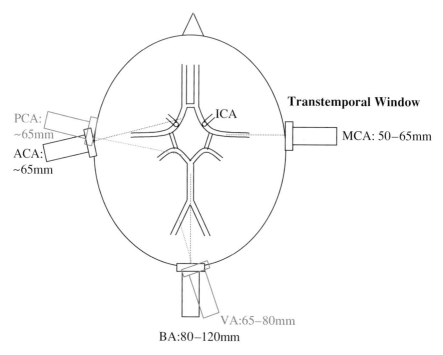

Fig. 7.5 Schematic demonstrating fundamental technique of the transcranial Doppler (TCD) examination. Arteries are insonated through 'bone windows'. Shown here are the temporal and transoccipital windows. Arteries in each window are identified by probe position, depth of insonation and direction of arterial blood flow (see Fig. 7.6). MCA, Middle cerebral artery; ACA, anterior cerebral artery; PCA, posterior cerebral artery; VA, vertebral artery; BA, basilar artery.

Transcranial Doppler ultrasound

In transcranial Doppler (TCD) ultrasound, low-frequency pulsed Doppler ultrasound allows acquisition of Doppler waveforms through 'bone windows' in the skull but does not allow B-mode imaging. The transorbital window allows access to the ophthalmic artery and carotid siphon, the temporal window, the middle, anterior and posterior cerebral arteries, and the occipital window, the vertebral and basilar arteries. Within each window, vessels are identified by direction of blood flow, depth of insonation, probe position, and spectral waveform characterisitics (Fig. 7.5). So-called transcranial Doppler imaging which makes use of color-coded Doppler techniques described earlier increases confidence in vessel identification. It is important for the clinician to be aware that limited segments of these intracranial arteries are available to TCD examination. Moreover, temporal bone window thickening occurs in 5–25% of patients, limiting access to the middle, anterior and posterior cerebral arteries [99–103], and in many individuals only a portion of the basilar artery can be isonated [104].

Intracranial atherosclerosis

An important role for TCD in the TIA patient is to identify large-artery atherosclerosis within the insonated arteries as the cause of stroke [105,106]. Intracranial atherosclerosis is increasingly recognized as an important cause of stroke, especially in other countries and within minority groups within the USA (blacks, Asians and women) in whom it contributes an overall higher burden to ischemic stroke than it does for white males [107,108]. The impetus for identifying intracranial atherosclerosis in TIA patients will be furthered by the development of stroke prevention treatments (such as angioplasty) specific to this disease, but even now its diagnosis may spare patients from having invasive, risky and/or expensive tests, in search for alternative diagnoses.

As with duplex ultrasound of the cervical arteries, the diagnosis of arterial narrowing is made using standardized criteria of increased blood flow velocities which are specific to the artery in question. Similarly too, the diagnosis of arterial occlusion is made by undetectable signals, which is even more problematic in this 'blind' examination. Unlike the plethora of studies which compare CDUS and angiography, validation studies for TCD are quite limited. These studies are challenged by the fact that the performance of the 'gold standard' angiography is more limited intracranially than extracranially, as it is more difficult to obtain unobstructed images of the diseased artery in more than one plane. There is also even less unanimity regarding TCD criteria for diagnosis or classification of intracranial stenosis, with PSV, EDV, and mean flow velocity and other more subjective parameters all used. For diagnosing intracranial atherosclerotic disease of varying severity, the range of reported sensitivities are 73–100% and specificities 89–99% [99,102,103,109–113]. These studies are limited in some cases by retrospective definitions of interpretation criteria and other methodological flaws. A true understanding of TCD's utility in diagnosing this disease awaits further study.

Cervical carotid atherosclerosis

TCD is also complementary to CDUS for the diagnosis of severe cervical ICA disease. TCD may detect collateral flow patterns downstream to severe ICA disease that both increase confidence in the CDUS findings and may be useful to the surgeon in planning carotid endarterectomy (Fig. 7.6 and Table 7.2). The prevalence of collateral flow patterns seen on TCD increases

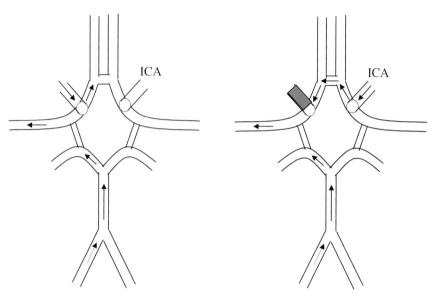

Fig. 7.6 Schematic of the circle of Willis demonstrating transcranial Doppler (TCD) evaluation of collateral blood flow patterns. On the left, normal direction of blood flow is depicted in the arteries at the sites of TCD examination. On the right, distal to the left internal carotid artery (ICA) occlusion, collateral blood flow to the left hemisphere is being supplied by the contralateral ICA via the anterior communicating artery. The TCD examination will show flow reversal in the insonated portion of the left anterior cerebral artery (ACA) and increased blood flow velocities in the right ACA.

Table 7.2 Collateral flow patterns seen on transcranial Doppler (TCD) downstream from severe internal carotid artery stenosis or occlusion

Source of collateral flow	TCD findings	References
Contralateral internal carotid artery via the anterior communicating artery	Reversed flow direction in the ipsilateral ACA Increased velocity in the contralateral ACA	[102, 114, 118, 120, 153–155]
Ipsilateral external carotid artery via the ophthalmic artery	Reversed flow direction in the ipsilateral ophthalmic artery	[102, 118, 120, 153, 156–159]
Either vertebral artery	Increased blood flow velocities in the vertebral and basilar arteries and/or proximal PCA Detection of posterior communicating artery blood flow	[102,120,155,160]

ACA, Anterior cerebral artery; PCA, posterior cerebral artery.

Table 7.3 Hemodynamic transcranial Doppler findings distal to severe carotid narrowing

Absent ophthalmic artery [120,161]
Absent carotid siphon signal [118,120]
Diminished MCA pulsatility [102, 118, 120, 155, 158, 162]
Decreased velocity MCA (absolute or relative to contralateral side) [114, 154, 158, 162, 163]
Decreased velocity ophthalmic artery [157]
Diminished MCA flow acceleration [102,118,120,157,164]

MCA, Middle cerebral artery.

with the degree of narrowing, being most common distal to complete arterial occlusion. Extracranial carotid compression may increase the sensitivity of TCD to detect collateral flow patterns but requires special experience and may be risky or contraindicated in some patients [114–117]. Other TCD findings downstream from carotid narrowing reflect slow or altered flow and usually require 80–100% proximal narrowing to become significantly prevalent (Table 7.3). The use of these TCD findings individually or as part of a TCD 'battery' has a sensitivity for detecting > 70% ICA stenosis of 79–95% and may improve the sensitivity and specificity of the ultrasound examination over CDUS alone in the diagnosis of severe carotid disease [118–120].

Cerebrovascular reactivity refers to changes in blood flow velocity seen on TCD in response to hypercapnea and/or administration of acetazolamide. This is not a routine part of the TCD examination. However, findings of decreased cerebrovascular reactivity in patients with symptomatic but not asymptomatic cervical carotid stenosis suggest that it may have a future role in selecting high-risk patients for carotid endarterectomy [121,122].

Acute cerebral ischemia

TCD findings may help predict prognosis in patients who present early with acute neurological deficit consistent with TIA or stroke. The presence of middle cerebral artery (MCA) occlusion or blood flow velocity reduction is associated with lower rate of early clinical improvement, particularly if this finding persists [123–126]. A low-resistance MCA waveform on TCD may also suggest the presence of leptomeningeal collateral flow, a pattern which has been associated with less severe neurological deficits [126,127]. Investigators are studying the efficacy of TCD in selecting patients for and monitoring patients after thrombolytic therapy [105,125,128].

Advances and future applications in cerebrovascular ultrasound

Microemboli detection by Doppler ultrasound refers to the appearance of high-intensity transient signals (HITS) within the Doppler spectrum. Investigators have correlated the frequency of HITS to symptomatic vs. asymptomatic carotid lesions [129,130], high-grade vs. low-grade carotid lesions [131], the presence vs. absence of cardioembolic source [132–134], the recency of symptoms [134–137], and treatment [138]. Microemboli are seen at higher rates during vascular procedures such as carotid endarterectomy, carotid angioplasty, cardiac catheterization, cardioversion and bypass surgery, and in some studies predict cerebrovascular complications [83,129,139–143]. Bilateral vs. unilateral microemboli may distinguish between large artery vs. cardiac embolic sources [144]. In one small series it appeared predictive of future ischemic events in already symptomatic patients with high-grade ICA stenosis [145]. These investigations suggest that monitoring for emboli may have a future role in defining high-risk lesions and identifying patients for specific treatments, but a specific clinically useful role has not yet been defined.

Power Doppler ultrasound provides an image of carotid arterial blood flow in either two or three dimensions. Power Doppler displays the strength of the Doppler signal reflecting the density of moving red blood cells rather than their velocity as in color flow imaging. It has superior signal-to-noise ratio and has the advantage over other ultrasound techniques of providing an image when both the ultrasound image and detection of Doppler flow are impeded by dense calcification. For characterizing stenoses between 50 and 99% it has not been shown to be superior to duplex scanning [30,146–148]. It may offer advantages for characterizing lower degrees of stenosis, but there is no clinical imperative for doing so at the present time [30]. Other authors have found this modality to improve the capability of CDUS to distinguish between nearly occluded and occluded ICAs [149]. Surgeons may find the image detail provided by power Doppler useful in planning surgery [147,150].

Contrast enhancement may be provided to the ultrasound examination by intravenously administered agents containing micro air bubbles that increase the echogenicity of arterial blood flow. The use of these contrast agents may enhance the ability of duplex ultrasound to determine patency in arteries that otherwise appear occluded [149,151]. This has not been found to be the case by others [152]. Contrast may also improve the rate of successful insonation through the temporal windows by TCD and the yield of detecting disease [123,128].

References

1 Bogousslavsky J, Van Melle G, Regli F. The Lausanne Stroke Registry: analysis of 1,000 consecutive patients with first stroke. *Stroke* 1988; 19: 1083–92.

2 Mead GE, Shingler H, Farrell A, O'Neill PA, McCollum CN. Carotid disease in acute stroke. *Age Aging* 1998; 27: 677–82.

3 Kolominsky-Rabas PL, Weber M, Gefeller O, Neundoerfer B, Heuschmann PU. Epidemiology of ischemic stroke subtypes according to TOAST criteria: incidence, recurrence, and long-term survival in ischemic stroke subtypes: a population-based study. *Stroke* 2001; 32: 2735–40.

4 Grau A, Weimar C, Buggle F *et al.* Risk factors, outcome, and treatment in subtypes of ischemic stroke: the German stroke data bank. *Stroke* 2001; 32: 2559–66.

5 Mead GE, Wardlaw JM, Lewis SC, McDowall M, Dennis MS. Can simple clinical features be used to identify patients with severe carotid stenosis on Doppler ultrasound? *J Neurol Neurosurg Psychiatry* 1999; 66: 16–9.

6 Chambers BR, Norris JW. Outcome in patients with asymptomatic neck bruits. *N Engl J Med* 1986; 315: 860–5.

7 Autret A, Pourcelot L, Saudeau D *et al.* Stroke risk in patients with carotid stenosis. *Lancet* 1987; 1: 888–90.

8 North American Symptomatic Carotid Endarterectomy Trial collaborators. Beneficial effect of carotid endarterectomy in symptomatic patients with high-grade carotid stenosis. *N Engl J Med* 1991; 325: 445–53.

9 Barnett HJM. Lessons from symptomatic carotid stenosis of interest in considering asymptomatic disease. In: Bernstein EF, Callow AD, Nicolaides AN, Shifrin EG, eds. *Cerebral Revascularization*. London: Medical-Orion Publishing Co., 1993: 483–7.

10 Barnett HJ, Taylor DW, Eliasziw M *et al.* Benefit of carotid endarterectomy in patients with symptomatic moderate or severe stenosis. *N Engl J Med* 1998; 339: 1415–25.

11 Eliasziw M, Rankin RN, Fox AJ *et al.* Accuracy and prognostic consequences of ultrasonography in identifying severe carotid artery stenosis. *Stroke* 1995; 26: 1747–52.

12 Howard G, Baker WH, Chambless LE *et al.* An approach for the use of Doppler ultrasound as a screening tool for hemodynamically significant stenosis (despite heterogeneity of Doppler performance). A multicenter experience. *Stroke* 1996; 27: 1951–7.

13 Ranke C, Creutzig A, Becker H, Trappe HJ. Standardization of carotid ultrasound: a hemodynamic method to normalize for interindividual and interequipment variability. *Stroke* 1999; 30: 402–6.

14 Lee VS, Hertzberg BS, Workman MJ *et al.* Variability of Doppler US measurements along the common carotid artery: effects on estimates of internal carotid arterial stenosis in patients with angiographically proved disease. *Radiology* 2000; 214: 387–92.

15 Hunink MGM, Polak JF, Barlan MM, O'Leary DH. Detection and quantification of carotid artery stenosis: efficacy of various Doppler velocity parameters. *Am J Roentgenol* 1993; 160: 619–25.

16 Schwartz SW, Chambless LE, Baker WH *et al.* Consistency of Doppler parameters in predicting arteriographically confirmed carotid stenosis. *Stroke* 1997; 28: 343–7.

17 Winkelaar GB, Chen JC, Salvian AJ, *et al.* New duplex ultrasound scan criteria for managing symptomatic 50% or greater carotid stenosis. *J Vasc Surg* 1999; 29: 986–94.

18 Soulez G, Therasse E, Robillard P *et al.* The value of internal carotid systolic velocity ratio for assessing carotid artery stenosis with Doppler sonography. *Am J Roentgenol* 1999; 172: 207–12.

19 Chen JC, Salvian AJ, Taylor DC *et al.* Predictive ability of duplex ultrasonography for internal carotid artery stenosis of 70%–99%: a comparative study. *Ann Vasc Surg* 1998; 12: 244–7.

20 Alexandrov, AV, Vital D, Brodie DS, Hamilton P, Grotta JC. Grading carotid stenosis with ultrasound. An interlaboratory comparison. *Stroke* 1997; 28: 1208–10.

21 Fillinger MF, Baker RJJ, Zwolak RM *et al.* Carotid duplex criteria for a 60% or greater angiographic stenosis: variation according to equipment. *J Vasc Surg* 1996; 24: 856–64.

22 Criswell BK, Langsfeld M, Tullis MJ, Marek J. Evaluating institutional variability of duplex scanning in the detection of carotid artery stenosis. *Am J Surg* 1998; 176: 591–7.

23 North American Symptomatic Carotid Endarterectomy Trial Steering Committee. North American Symptomatic Carotid Endarterectomy Trial. Methods, patient characteristics and progress. *Stroke* 1991; 22: 711–20.

24 Carpenter JP, Lexa FJ, Davis JT. Determination of duplex Doppler ultrasound criteria appropriate to the North American Symptomatic Carotid Endarterectomy Trial. *Stroke* 1996; 27: 695–9.

25 Dinkel HP, Moll R, Debus S. Color flow Doppler ultrasound of the carotid bifurcation: can it replace routine angiography before carotid endarterectomy? *Br J Radiol* 2001; 74: 590–4.

26 Neschis DG, Lexa FJ, Davis JT, Carpenter JP. Duplex criteria for determination of 50% or greater carotid stenosis. *J Ultrasound Med* 2001; 20: 207–15.

27 Huston J, Iyer SS III, James EM *et al.* Redefined duplex ultrasonographic criteria for diagnosis of carotid artery stenosis. *Mayo Clin Proc* 2000; 75: 1133–40.

28 Grant EG, Duerinckx AJ, El Saden SM *et al.* Ability to use duplex US to quantify internal carotid arterial stenoses: fact or fiction? *Radiology* 2000; 214: 247–52.

29 Jackson MR, Chang AS, Robles HA *et al.* Determination of 60% or greater carotid stenosis: a prospective comparison of magnetic resonance angiography and duplex ultrasound with conventional angiography. *Ann Vasc Surg* 1998; 12: 236–43.

30 Muller M, Ciccotti P, Reiche W, Hagen T. Comparison of color-flow Doppler scanning, power Doppler scanning, and frequency shift for assessment of carotid artery stenosis. *J Vasc Surg* 2001; 34: 1090–5.

31 Elmore JR, Franklin DP, Thomas DD, Youkey JR. Carotid endarterectomy: the mandate for high quality duplex. *Ann Vasc Surg* 1998; 12: 156–62.

32 New G, Roubin GS, Oetgen ME *et al.* Validity of duplex ultrasound as a diagnostic modality for internal carotid artery disease. *Catheter Cardiovasc Interv* 2001; 52: 9–15.

33 Bain DJ, Fergie N, Quin RO, Greene M. Role of arteriography in the selection of patients for carotid endarterectomy. *Br J Surg* 1998; 85: 768–70.

34 Dippel DW, de Kinkelder A, Bakker SL *et al.* The diagnostic value of color duplex ultrasound for symptomatic carotid stenosis in clinical practice. *Neuroradiology* 1999; 41: 1–8.

35 Perkins JM, Galland RB, Simmons MJ, Magee TR. Carotid duplex imaging: variation and validation. *Br J Surg* 2000; 87: 320–2.

36 Qureshi AI, Suri MF, Ali Z *et al.* Role of conventional angiography in evaluation of patients with carotid artery stenosis demonstrated by Doppler ultrasound in general practice. *Stroke* 2001; 32: 2287–91.

37 Wilterdink JL, Feldmann E, Easton JE, Ward R. Performance of carotid ultrasound in evaluating candidates for carotid endarterectomy is optimized by an approach based on clinical outcome rather than accuracy. *Stroke* 1996; 27: 1094–8.

38 McNeil B, Keeler E, Adelstein S. Primer on certain elements of medical decision making. *N Engl J Med* 1975; 293: 211–5.

39 Wilterdink JL, Feldmann E, Easton JD, Ward R. Carotid Duplex ultrasound (CDUS) interpretation in asymptomatic carotid endarterectomy candidates: a patient-outcome rather than accuracy-based approach. *Neurology* 1995; 45: A224.

40 Zierler RE. Vascular surgery without arteriography: use of Duplex ultrasound. *Cardiovasc Surg* 1999; 7: 74–82.

41 Erdoes LS, Marek JM, Mills JL *et al.* The relative contributions of carotid duplex scanning, magnetic resonance angiography, and cerebral arteriography to clinical decision making: a prospective study in patients with carotid occlusive disease. *J Vasc Surg* 1996; 23: 950–6.

42 Hood DB, Mattos MA, Mansour A *et al.* Prospective evaluation of new duplex criteria to identify 70% internal carotid artery stenosis. *J Vasc Surg* 1996; 23: 254–61.

43 Ballotta E, Da Giau G, Abbruzzese E *et al.* Carotid endarterectomy without angiography: can clinical evaluation and duplex ultrasonographic scanning alone replace traditional arteriography for carotid surgery workup? A prospective study. *Surgery* 1999; 126: 20–7.

44 Golledge J, Ellis M, Sabharwal T *et al.* Selection of patients for carotid endarterectomy. *J Vasc Surg* 1999; 30: 122–30.

45 Worthy SA, Henderson J, Griffiths PD, Oates CP, Gholka A. The role of duplex sonography and angiography in the investigation of carotid artery disease. *Neuroradiology* 1997; 39: 122–6.

46 Johnston DC Goldstein LB. Clinical carotid endarterectomy decision making: noninvasive vascular imaging versus angiography. *Neurology* 2001; 56: 1009–15.

47 Back MR, Wilson JS, Rushing G *et al*. Magnetic resonance angiography is an accurate imaging adjunct to duplex ultrasound scan in patient selection for carotid endarterectomy. *J Vasc Surg* 2000; 32: 429–38; discussion 439–40.

48 Friese S, Krapf H, Fetter M *et al*. Ultrasonography and contrast-enhanced MRA in ICA-stenosis: is conventional angiography obsolete? *J Neurol* 2001; 248: 506–13.

49 Bassiouny HS, Davis H, Massawa N *et al*. Critical carotid stenoses: morphologic and chemical similarity between symptomatic and asymptomatic plaques. *J Vasc Surg* 1989; 9: 202–12.

50 Comerota AJ, Katz ML, White JV, Grosh JD. The preoperative diagnosis of the ulcerated carotid atheroma. *J Vasc Surg* 1990; 11: 505–10.

51 Bluth EI, McVay LV 3rd, Merritt CR, Sullivan MA. The identification of ulcerative plaque with high resolution duplex carotid scanning. *J Ultrasound Med* 1988; 7: 73–6.

52 Widder B, Paulat K, Hackspacher J *et al*. Morphological characterization of carotid artery stenoses by ultrasound duplex scanning. *Ultrasound Med Biol* 1990; 16: 349–54.

53 Belcaro G, Laurora G, Cesarone MR *et al*. Ultrasonic classification of carotid plaques causing less than 60% stenosis according to ultrasound morphology and events. *J Cardiovasc Surg* 1993; 34: 287–94.

54 Schulte-Altedorneburg G, Droste DW, Haas N *et al*. Preoperative B-mode ultrasound plaque appearance compared with carotid endarterectomy specimen histology. *Acta Neurol Scand* 2000; 101: 188–94.

55 Liapis CD, Kakisis JD, Kostakis AG. Carotid stenosis: factors affecting symptomatology. *Stroke* 2001; 32: 2782–6.

56 Gronholdt ML, Nordestgaard BG, Schroeder TV, Vorstrup S. Sillesen H. Ultrasonic echolucent carotid plaques predict future strokes. *Circulation* 2001; 104: 68–73.

57 Bendick PJ, Glover JL, Hankin R *et al*. Carotid plaque morphology: correlation of duplex sonography with histology. *Ann Vasc Surg* 1988; 2: 6–13.

58 Polak JF, O'Leary DH, Kronmal RA *et al*. Sonographic evaluation of carotid artery atherosclerosis in the elderly: relationship of disease severity to stroke and transient ischemic attack. *Radiology* 1993; 188: 363–70.

59 Svindland A, Torvik A. Atherosclerotic carotid disease in asymptomatic individuals. An histological study of 53 cases. *Acta Neurol Scand* 1988; 78: 506–17.

60 Hartmann A, Mohr JP, Thompson JL, Ramos O, Mast H. Interrater reliability of plaque morphology classification in patients with severe carotid artery stenosis. *Acta Neurol Scand* 1999; 99: 61–4.

61 Bond JR, Charboneau JW, Stanson AW. Takayasu's arteritis. Carotid duplex sonographic appearance, including color Doppler imaging. *J Ultrasound Med* 1990; 9: 625–9.

62 Sun Y, Yip PK, Jeng JS, Hwang BS, Lin WH. Ultrasonographic study and long-term follow-up of Takayasu's arteritis. *Stroke* 1996; 27: 2178–82.

63 Cheng SW, Ting AC, Lam LK, Wei WI. Carotid stenosis after radiotherapy for nasopharyngeal carcinoma. *Arch Otolaryngol Head Neck Surg* 2000; 126: 517–21.

64 Russo CP, Smoker WR. Nonatheromatous carotid artery disease. *Neuroimaging Clin N Am* 1996; 6: 811–30.

65 de Bray JM, Lhoste P, Dubas F, Emile J, Saumet JL. Ultrasonic features of extracranial carotid dissections: 47 cases studied by angiography. *J Ultrasound Med* 1994; 13: 659–64.

66 Treiman GS, Treiman RL, Foran RF *et al.* Spontaneous dissection of the internal carotid artery: a nineteen-year clinical experience. *J Vasc Surg* 1996; 24: 597–605.

67 Steinke W, Rautenberg W, Schwartz A, Hennerici M. Noninvasive monitoring of internal carotid artery dissection. *Stroke* 1994; 25: 998–1005.

68 Sturzenegger M, Mattle HP, Rivoir A, Baumgartner RW. Ultrasound findings in carotid artery dissection: analysis of 43 patients. *Neurology* 1995; 45: 691–8.

69 Schmidt WA, Kraft HE, Vorpahl K, Volker L, Gromnica-Ihle EJ. Color duplex ultrasonography in the diagnosis of temporal arteritis. *N Engl J Med* 1997; 337: 1336–42.

70 Lee DH, Gao FQ, Rankin RN, Pelz DM, Fox AJ; Duplex and color Doppler flow sonography of occlusion and near occlusion of the carotid artery. *Am J Neuroradiol* 1996; 17: 1267–74.

71 Hetzel A, Eckenweber B, Trummer B *et al.* Color-coded duplex sonography of preocclusive carotid stenoses. *Eur J Ultrasound* 1998; 8: 183–91.

72 Mansour MA, Mattos MA, Hood DB *et al.* Detection of total occlusion, string sign, and preocclusive stenosis of the internal carotid artery by color-flow duplex scanning. *Am J Surg* 1995; 170: 154–8.

73 Berman SS, Devine JJ, Erdoes LS, Hunter GC. Distinguishing carotid artery pseudo-occlusion with color-flow Doppler. *Stroke* 1995; 26: 434–8.

74 Samson RH, Showalter DP, Yunis JP, Buselli K, Perna T. Color flow scan diagnosis of the carotid string may prevent unnecessary surgery. *Cardiovasc Surg* 1999; 7: 236–41.

75 Busuttil SJ, Franklin DP, Youkey JR, Elmore JR. Carotid duplex overestimation of stenosis due to severe contralateral disease. *Am J Surg* 1996; 172: 144–7.

76 Fujitani RM, Mills JL, Wang LM, Taylor SM. The effect of unilateral internal carotid arterial occlusion upon contralateral duplex study: criteria for accurate interpretation. *J Vasc Surg* 1992; 16: 459–67.

77 Fischer M, Alexander K. Influence of contralateral obstructions on Doppler-frequency spectral analysis of ipsilateral stenoses of the carotid arteries. *Stroke* 1985; 16: 846–8.

78 Elgersma OE, van Leersum M, Buijs PC *et al.* Changes over time in optimal duplex threshold for the identification of patients eligible for carotid end-arterectomy. *Stroke* 1998; 29: 2352–6.

79 Curley PJ, Norrie L, Nicholson A, Galloway JM, Wilkinson AR. Accuracy of carotid duplex is laboratory specific and must be determined by internal audit. *Eur J Vasc Endovasc Surg* 1998; 15: 511–4.

80 Kuntz KM, Polak JF, Whittemore AD, Skillman JJ, Kent KC. Duplex ultrasound criteria for the identification of carotid stenosis should be laboratory specific. *Stroke* 1997; 28: 597–602.

81 Kuhl V, Tettenborn B, Eicke BM, Visbeck A, Meckes S. Color-coded duplex ultrasonography of the origin of the vertebral artery: normal values of flow velocities. *J Neuroimaging* 2000; 10: 17–21.

82 Bartels E, Flugel KA. Advantages of color Doppler imaging for the evaluation of vertebral arteries. *J Neuroimaging* 1993; 3: 229–33.

83 Davis PC, Nilsen B, Braun IF, Hoffman JCJ. A prospective comparison of duplex sonography vs angiography of the vertebral arteries. *Am J Neuroradiol* 1986; 7: 1059–64.

84 Trattnig S, Schwaighofer B, Hubsch P, Schwarz M, Kainberger F. Color-coded Doppler sonography of vertebral arteries. *J Ultrasound Med* 1991; 10: 221–6.

85 Fisher CM, Gore I, Okabe N, White PD. Atherosclerosis of the carotid and vertebral arteries-extracranial and intracranial. *J Neuropathol Exp Neurol* 1965: 24: 455–76.

86 Ackerstaff RG, Hoeneveld H, Slowikowski JM *et al.* Ultrasonic duplex scanning in atherosclerotic disease of the innominate, subclavian and vertebral arteries. A comparative study with angiography. *Ultrasound Med Biol* 1984; 10: 409–18.

87 Lu CJ, Sun Y, Jeng JS *et al.* Imaging in the diagnosis and follow-up evaluation of vertebral artery dissection. *J Ultrasound Med* 2000; 19: 263–70.

88 Sturzenegger M, Mattle HP, Rivoir A, Rihs F, Schmid C. Ultrasound findings in spontaneous extracranial vertebral artery dissection. *Stroke* 1993; 24: 1910–21.

89 Hoffmann M, Sacco RL, Chan S, Mohr JP. Noninvasive detection of vertebral artery dissection. *Stroke* 1993; 24: 815–9.

90 Cals N, Devuyst G, Jung DK *et al.* Uncommon ultrasound findings in traumatic extracranial vertebral artery dissection. *Eur J Ultrasound* 2001; 12: 227–31.

91 Bartels E, Flugel KA. Evaluation of extracranial vertebral artery dissection with duplex color-flow imaging. *Stroke* 1996; 27: 290–5.

92 Kaneko A, Ohno R, Hattori K *et al.* Color-coded Doppler imaging of subclavian steal syndrome. *Intern Med* 1998; 37: 259–64.

93 Klingelhofer J, Conrad B, Benecke R, Frank B. Transcranial Doppler ultrasonography of carotid-basilar collateral circulation in subclavian steal. *Stroke* 1988; 19: 1036–42.

94 Ackermann H, Diener HC, Seboldt H, Huth C. Ultrasonographic follow-up of subclavian stenosis and occlusion: natural history and surgical treatment. *Stroke* 1988; 19: 431–5.

95 Hennerici M, Klemm C, Rautenberg W. The subclavian steal phenomenon: a common vascular disorder with rare neurologic deficits. *Neurology* 1988; 38: 669–73.

96 Haynes M, Milne N. Color duplex sonographic findings in human vertebral arteries during cervical rotation. *J Clin Ultrasound* 2001; 29: 14–24.

97 Brautaset NJ. Provokable bilateral vertebral artery compression diagnosed with transcranial Doppler. *Stroke* 1992; 23: 288–91.

98 Sturzenegger M, Newell DW, Douville C, Byrd S, Schoonover K. Dynamic transcranial Doppler assessment of positional vertebrobasilar ischemia. *Stroke* 1994; 25: 1776–83.

99 Hennerici M, Rautenberg W, Schwartz A. Transcranial doppler ultrasound for the assessment of intracranial arterial flow velocity—Part 2. Evaluation of intracranial arterial disease. *Surg Neurol* 1987; 27: 523–32.

100 Alexandrov AV, Demchuk AM, Wein TH, Grotta JC. Yield of transcranial Doppler in acute cerebral ischemia. *Stroke* 1999; 30: 1604–9.

101 Baumgartner RW, Mattle HP, Aaslid R. Transcranial color-coded duplex sonography, magnetic resonance angiography, and computed tomography angiography: methods, applications, advantages, and limitations. *J Clin Ultrasound* 1995; 23: 89–111.

102 Demchuk AM, Christou I, Wein TH *et al.* Accuracy and criteria for localizing arterial occlusion with transcranial Doppler. *J Neuroimaging* 2000; 10: 1–12.

103 Rorick MB, Nichols FT, Adams RJ. Transcranial doppler correlations with angiography in detection of intracranial stenosis. *Stroke* 1994; 25: 1931–4.

104 Mull M, Aulich A, Hennerici M. Transcranial Doppler ultrasonography versus arteriography for assessment of the vertebrobasilar circulation. *J Clin Ultrasound* 1990; 18: 539–49.

105 Egido JA, Sanchez C. Neurosonology in cerebral ischemia: future application of transcranial Doppler in acute stroke. *Cerebrovasc Dis* 2001; 11 (Suppl. 1): 15–9.

106 Wijamn CA, McBee NA, Keyl PM *et al.* Diagnostic impact of early transcranial Doppler ultrasonography on the TOAST classification subtype in acute cerebral ischemia. *Cerebrovasc Dis* 2001; 11: 317–23.

107 Caplan LR, Gorelick PB, Hier DB. Race, sex and occlusive cerebrovascular disease: a review. *Stroke* 1986; 17: 648–55.

108 Leung SY, Ng TH, Yuen ST, Lauder IJ, Ho FC. Pattern of cerebral atherosclerosis in Hong Kong Chinese. Severity in intracranial and extracranial vessels. *Stroke* 1993; 24: 779–86.

109 Baumgartner RW, Mattle HP, Schroth G. Assessment of ≥ 50% and < 50% intracranial stenoses by transcranial color-coded duplex sonography. *Stroke* 1999; 30: 87–92.

110 Cher LM, Chambers BR, Smidt V. Comparison of transcranial doppler with DSA in vertebrobasilar ischaemia. *Clin Exp Neurol* 1992; 29: 143–8.

111 Babikian V, Sloan MA, Tegeler CH *et al*. Transcranial Doppler validation pilot study. *J Neuroimaging* 1993; 3: 242–9.

112 Ley-Pozo J, Ringelstein EB. Noninvasive detection of occlusive disease of the carotid siphon and middle cerebral artery. *Ann Neurol* 1990; 28: 640–7.

113 de Bray JM, Missoum A, Dubas F, Emile J, Lhoste P. Dectection of vertebrovasilar intracranial stenoses: transcranial Doppler sonography versus angiography. *J Ultrasound Med* 1997; 16: 213–8.

114 Schneider P, Rossman M, Bernstein E *et al*. Effect of internal carotid artery occlusion on intracranial hemodynamics. Transcranial Doppler evaluation and clinical correlation. *Stroke* 1988; 19: 589–93.

115 Schneider PA, Ringelstein EB, Rossman ME *et al*. Importance of cerebral collateral pathways during carotid endarterectomy. *Stroke* 1988; 19: 1328–34.

116 Bass A, Krupski WC, Dilley RB, Bernstein EF, Otis SM. Comparison of transcranial and cervical continuous-wave Doppler in the evaluation of intracranial collateral circulation. *Stroke* 1990; 21: 1584–8.

117 Khaffaf N, Karnik R, Winkler WB, Valentin A, Slany J. Embolic stroke by compression maneuver during transcranial Doppler sonography. *Stroke* 1994; 25: 1056–7.

118 Wilterdink JL, Feldmann E, Furie KL, Bragoni M, Benavides JG. Transcranial doppler ultrasound battery reliably identifies severe internal carotid artery stenosis. *Stroke* 1997; 28: 133–6.

119 Wilterdink JL, Furie KL, Benavides J, Cabral PJ, Feldmann E. Combined transcranial and carotid Duplex ultrasound optimizes screening for carotid artery stenosis. *Can J Neurol Sci* 1993; 20: S205.

120 Christou I, Felberg RA, Demchuk AM *et al*. A broad diagnostic battery for bedside transcranial Doppler to detect flow changes with internal carotid artery stenosis or occlusion. *J Neuroimaging* 2001; 11: 236–42.

121 Silvestrini M, Troisi E, Matteis M, Cupini LM, Caltagirone C. Transcranial Doppler assessment of cerebrovascular reactivity in symptomatic and asymptomatic severe carotid stenosis. *Stroke* 1996; 27: 1970–3.

122 Yonas H, Smith HA, Durham SR, Pentheny SL, Johnson DW. Increased stroke risk predicted by compromised cerebral blood flow reactivity. *J Neurosurg* 1993; 79: 483–9.

123 Goertler M, Kross R, Baeumer M *et al*. Diagnostic impact and prognostic relevance of early contrast-enhanced transcranial color-coded duplex sonography in acute stroke. *Stroke* 1998; 29: 955–62.

124 Christou I, Burgin WS, Alexandrov AV, Grotta JC. Arterial status after intravenous TPA therapy for ischaemic stroke. A need for further interventions. *Int Angiol* 2001; 20: 208–13.

125 Demchuk AM, Burgin WS, Christou I *et al*. Thrombolysis in brain ischemia (TIBI) transcranial Doppler flow grades predict clinical severity, early

recovery, and mortality in patients treated with intravenous tissue plasminogen activator. *Stroke* 2001; 32: 89–93.

126 Ringelstein EB, Biniek R, Weiller C *et al.* Type and extent of hemispheric brain infarctions and clinical outcome in early and delayed middle cerebral artery recanalization. *Neurology* 1992; 42: 289–98.

127 El-Mitwalli A, Saad M, Christou I, Malkoff M, Alexandrov AV. Clinical and sonographic patterns of tandem internal carotid artery/middle cerebral artery occlusion in tissue plasminogen activator-treated patients. *Stroke* 2002; 33: 99–102.

128 Postert T, Braun B, Meves S *et al.* Contrast-enhanced transcranial color-coded sonography in acute hemispheric brain infarction. *Stroke* 1999; 30: 1819–26.

129 Golledge J, Gibbs R, Irving C *et al.* Determinants of carotid microembolization. *J Vasc Surg* 2001; 34: 1060–4.

130 Markus HS, Thomson ND, Brown MM. Asymptomatic cerebral embolic signals in symptomatic and asymptomatic carotid artery disease. *Brain* 1995; 118: 1005–11.

131 Eicke BM, von Lorentz J, Paulus W. Embolus detection in different degrees of carotid disease. *Neurol Res* 1995; 17: 181–4.

132 Georgiadis D, Lindner A, Manz M *et al.* Intracranial microembolic signals in 500 patients with potential cardiac or carotid embolic source and in normal controls. *Stroke* 1997; 28: 1203–7.

133 Markus HS, Droste DW, Brown MM. Detection of asymptomatic cerebral embolic signals with Doppler ultrasound. *Lancet* 1994; 343: 1011–2.

134 Tong DC, Albers GW. Transcranial Doppler-detected microemboli in patients with acute stroke. *Stroke* 1995; 26: 1588–92.

135 Siebler M, Kleinschmidt A, Sitzer M, Steinmetz H, Freund HJ. Cerebral microembolism in symptomatic and asymptomatic high-grade internal carotid artery stenosis. *Neurology* 1994; 44: 615–8.

136 van Zuilen EV, Moll F, Vermeulen FE *et al.* Detection of cerebral microemboli by means of transcranial Doppler monitoring before and after carotid endarterectomy. *Stroke* 1995; 26: 210–3.

137 Forteza AM, Babikian VL, Hyde C, Winter M, Pochay V. Effect of time and cerebrovascular symptoms of the prevalence of microembolic signals in patients with cervical carotid stenosis. *Stroke* 1996; 27: 687–90.

138 Siebler M, Sitzer M, Rose G, Bendfeldt D, Steinmetz H. Silent cerebral embolism caused by neurologically symptomatic high-grade carotid stenosis. Event rates before and after carotid endarterectomy. *Brain* 1993; 116: 1005–15.

139 Braekken SK, Russell D, Brucher R, Abdelnoor M, Svennevig JL. Cerebral microembolic signals during cardiopulmonary bypass surgery. Frequency, time of occurrence, and association with patient and surgical characteristics. *Stroke* 1997; 28: 1988–92.

140 Stygall J, Kong R, Walker JM *et al.* Cerebral microembolism detected by transcranial Doppler during cardiac procedures. *Stroke* 2000; 31: 2508–10.

141 Markus HS, Clifton A, Buckenham T, Brown MM. Carotid angioplasty. Detection of embolic signals during and after the procedure. *Stroke* 1994; 25: 2403–6.

142 Jansen C, Ramos LM, van Heesewijk JP *et al.* Impact of microembolism and hemodynamic changes in the brain during carotid endarterectomy. *Stroke* 1994; 25: 992–7.

143 Gaunt ME, Martin PJ, Smith JL *et al.* Clinical relevance of intraoperative embolization detected by transcranial Doppler ultrasonography during carotid endarterectomy: a prospective study of 100 patients. *Br J Surg* 1994; 81: 1435–9.

144 Grosset DG, Georgiadis D, Abdullah I, Bone I, Lees KR. Doppler emboli signals vary according to stroke subtype. *Stroke* 1994; 25: 382–4.

145 Censori B, Partziguian T, Casto L, Camerlingo M, Mamoli A. Doppler microembolic signals predict ischemic recurrences in symptomatic carotid stenosis. *Acta Neurol Scand* 2000; 101: 327–31.

146 Koga M, Kimura K, Minematsu K, Yamaguchi T. Diagnosis of internal carotid artery stenosis greater than 70% with power Doppler duplex sonography. *Am J Neuroradiol* 2001; 22: 413–7.

147 Keberle M, Jenett M, Beissert M *et al.* Three-dimensional power Doppler sonography in screening for carotid artery disease. *J Clin Ultrasound* 2000; 28: 441–51.

148 Schmidt P, Sliwka U, Simon SG, Noth J. High-grade stenosis of the internal carotid artery assessed by color and power Doppler imaging. *J Clin Ultrasound* 1998; 26: 85–9.

149 Furst G, Saleh A, Wenserski F *et al.* Reliability and validity of noninvasive imaging of internal carotid artery pseudo-occlusion. *Stroke* 1999; 30: 1444–9.

150 Bendick PJ, Brown OW, Hernandez D, Glover JL, Bove PG. Three-dimensional vascular imaging using Doppler ultrasound. *Am J Surg* 1998; 176: 183–7.

151 Ferrer JM, Samso JJ, Serrando JR *et al.* Use of ultrasound contrast in the diagnosis of carotid artery occlusion. *J Vasc Surg* 2000; 31: 736–41.

152 Hofstee DJ, Hoogland PH, Schimsheimer RJ, de Weerd AW. Contrast enhanced color duplex for diagnosis of subtotal stenosis or occlusion of the internal carotid artery. *Clin Neurol Neurosurg* 2000; 102: 9–12.

153 Babikian VL. Transcranial Doppler evaluation of patients with ischemic cerebrovascular disease. In: Babikian VL, Wechsler LR, eds. *Transcranial Doppler Ultrasonography.* St Louis: Mosby-Year Book, Inc., 1993: 87–104.

154 Cantelmo N, Babikian V, Johnson W *et al.* Correlation of transcranial Doppler and noninvasive tests with angiography in the evaluation of extracranial carotid disease. *J Vasc Surg* 1990; 11: 786–92.

155 Lindegaard KF, Bakke SJ, Grolimund P *et al.* Assessment of intracranial hemodynamics in carotid artery disease by transcranial Doppler ultrasound. *J Neurosurg* 1985; 63: 890–8.

156 Reynolds PS, Greenberg JP, Lien LM *et al.* Ophthalmic artery flow direction on color flow duplex imaging is highly specific for severe carotid stenosis. *J Neuroimaging* 2002; 12: 5–8.

157 Paivansalo M, Riihelainen K, Rissanen T, Suramo I, Laatikainen L. Effect of an internal carotid stenosis on orbital blood velocity. *Acta Radiol* 1999; 40: 270–5.

158 Hedera P, Bujdakova J, Traubner P, Pancak J. Stroke risk factors and development of collateral flow in carotid occlusive disease. *Acta Neurol Scand* 1998; 98: 182–6.

159 Schneider P, Rossman M, Bernstein E, Ringelstein E, Otis S. Noninvasive assessment of cerebral collateral blood supply through the ophthalmic artery. *Stroke* 1991; 22: 31–6.

160 Baumgartner RW, Baumgartner I, Mattle HP, Schroth G. Transcranial color-coded duplex sonography in the evaluation of collateral flow through the circle of Willis. *Am J Neuroradiol* 1997; 18: 127–33.

161 Wilterdink JL, Brooks JM, Furie KL, Feldmann EF. Absent ophthalmic artery signal ipsilateral to severe carotid disease. *J Neuroimaging* 1993; 3: 75.

162 Kelley R, Namon R, Juang S, Lee S, Chang J. Transcranial Doppler ultrasonography of the middle cerebral artery in the hemodynamic assessment of internal carotid artery stenosis. *Arch Neurol* 1990; 47: 960–4.

163 Schneider P, Rossman M, Torem S *et al.* Transcranial Doppler in the management of extracranial cerebrovascular disease: *J Vasc Surg* 1988; 7: 223–31.

164 Kelley RE, Namon RA, Mantelle LL, Chang JY. Sensitivity and specificity of transcranial Doppler ultrasonography in the detection of high grade carotid stenosis. *Neurology* 1993; 43: 1187–91.

CHAPTER 8

Cardiac Diagnostic Studies

Marco R. Di Tullio, Shunichi Homma

Introduction

Embolism from a cardiac source is thought to account for 15–20% of all ischemic strokes. Cardioembolism is also likely to account for a substantial proportion of strokes of otherwise undetermined origin, or 'cryptogenic' strokes, which often have clinical and neuroimaging features compatible with or suggestive of embolism, in the absence of a clearly defined source. Although separate data are not easily available, it is conceivable that cardioembolic sources account for a substantial proportion of transient ischemic attacks (TIA), under the assumption that stroke and TIA share similar etiological mechanisms.

The search for cardiac embolic sources for stroke/TIA has its cornerstone in the use of diagnostic cardiac ultrasound studies, also known as echocardiography. Transthoracic echocardiography (TTE) has long been the most widely used technique to search for cardiac embolic sources. In the last 10 years, however, transesophageal echocardiography (TEE) has complemented, and often replaced, TTE as the preferred technique for such diagnosis. TEE is considerably more sensitive than TTE for this purpose [1,2], and it is estimated that the search of embolic sources currently accounts for approximately one-quarter of all clinical indications for TEE.

The present chapter will review the use of TTE and TEE for the diagnosis of cardioembolic sources for stroke/TIA, and some of the therapeutic and preventive advances that the wide application of these diagnostic modalities has allowed. Cardiac abnormalities that are an established source of ischemic stroke/TIA will be reviewed, along with some newer putative risk factors, whose causative role for stroke/TIA, and the related therapeutic options, are under investigation.

Transthoracic vs. transesophageal echocardiography

Although less sensitive than (TEE) for the diagnosis of cardioembolic sources [1,2], TTE still maintains a role in the diagnostic work-up of patients with ischemic stroke. This technique provides information on cardiac anatomy and function, such as the presence of aortic or mitral valve pathology or left ventricular dysfunction, which may prove important for the diagnosis. It is also capable of detecting some cardiac embolic sources (such as left ventricular thrombus), and is a good screening test for others (patent foramen ovale, atrial septal aneurysm).

In the last 10 years, the introduction and widespread use of TEE has resulted in great improvements in the detection of potential cardiac source of embolus, providing higher sensitivity than TTE for some diagnoses [patent foramen ovale (PFO), small valvular vegetations, atrial septal aneurysm]. TEE has also offered an unprecedented opportunity to identify other potential embolic sources previously not suspected (left atrial appendage thrombus and spontaneous echo-contrast, aortic arch atheromas, valve strands). Overall, TEE increases the likelihood of identifying a cardiac embolic source in stroke or TIA patients by two- to four-fold [1,2]. TTE is a good screening technique, and its use is important to exclude overt cardiac abnormalities, even in patients who have other potential explanations for their cerebrovascular event. On the other hand, TEE should be preferred in patients in whom the cerebral event mechanism remains unknown after a thorough diagnostic work-up, and in those in whom the likelihood of an abnormality not detectable by TTE is high (such as left atrial appendage thrombus in atrial fibrillation, or aortic arch plaques in elderly patients with diffuse atherosclerotic disease).

In the following paragraphs, the contribution of TTE and TEE to the detection of cardioembolic sources will be discussed, both for established sources and for newly discovered ones.

Atrial fibrillation

Atrial fibrillation carries a risk of stroke of about 5% per year, which is two to seven times greater than that of subjects in normal sinus rhythm [3–5]. When atrial fibrillation is associated with rheumatic heart disease (especially mitral stenosis), the risk increases by up to 17 times [6]. Among the conditions associated with an increased risk of cerebrovascular events, atrial fibrillation is one of the greatest offenders, and it is estimated that one out of six of all strokes occurs in patients with atrial fibrillation [7]. The prevalence of atrial fibrillation in the population increases with age (up to 6% and more after the age of 80 years) [2,8], with consequent parallel increase in the associated risk of cerebrovascular events. At any age, the risk of stroke further increases, up to 10–12% per year [9,10], when atrial fibrillation coexists with such risk factors as congestive heart failure, coronary artery disease, diabetes mellitus, arterial hypertension and history of prior thromboembolism. On the other hand, atrial fibrillation in the absence of organic heart disease or risk factors (so called 'lone' atrial fibrillation) appears to carry significantly lower risk, especially in younger patients (approximately 1.3% per year) [10].

Chronic, sustained atrial fibrillation has traditionally been considered to carry the highest risk for stroke/TIA. Recently, however, it has become clear that intermittent, or paroxysmal, atrial fibrillation also carries a substantial risk [11], and similar preventive strategies should therefore be applied to both conditions.

The mechanism by which atrial fibrillation increases the risk of stroke/TIA is the increased predisposition to thrombus formation in the left atrium, with consequent increased risk of embolism. Several clinical trials have shown a benefit of treatment with warfarin and, to a lesser extent, aspirin for the prevention of thromboembolic complications. Adjusted-dose warfarin, aiming for an International Normalized Ratio (INR) of 2.0–3.0, has been proven superior to low-dose warfarin plus aspirin in patients at high risk of thromboembolic complications (identified by one of four criteria: systolic blood pressure > 160 mmHg, previous embolic events, congestive heart failure or fractional shortening < 25% on echocardiogram, female gender over age 75). In the Study on Prevention in Atrial Fibrillation (SPAF) III, stroke incidence was four times greater in patients who received combined low-dose treatment compared with those on adjusted-dose warfarin treatment (7.9% vs. 1.9% per year) [12]. For patients with lower risk, treatment with aspirin 325 mg/day was associated with a relatively low incidence of embolic episodes (2.2% per year, 2.0% being strokes), with the notable exception of patients with a history of hypertension, who had a greater embolic event rate (3.6% per year). Recently, risk-based guidelines for stroke prevention have been jointly issued by the American Heart Association, the American College of Cardiology and the European Society of Cardiology [13]. According to these guidelines, adjusted-dose anticoagulation with INR between 2.0 and 3.0 is recommended in high-risk patients (patients over 75 years of age, especially women; patients over the age of 60 with diabetes mellitus or coronary artery disease; all patients with risk factors for thromboembolism such as heart failure, left ventricular ejection fraction < 35%, history of hypertension, prior thromboembolism, rheumatic heart disease, prosthetic heart valves, thrombus detected by echocardiography). Patients with rheumatic heart disease or prosthetic valves require stronger anticoagulation (INR between 2.5 and 3.5 or higher). Patients at lower risk (age 60–75 years and no risk factors with thromboembolism) can be treated with aspirin 325 mg/day.

TTE is a useful test in patients with atrial fibrillation, allowing the evaluation of the mitral valve and of the dimension of the left atrium, whose dilatation is associated with increased frequency of thrombus formation. TTE can also allow the detection of thrombus in the body of the left atrium (Fig. 8.1). However, most thrombi in patients within atrial fibrillation

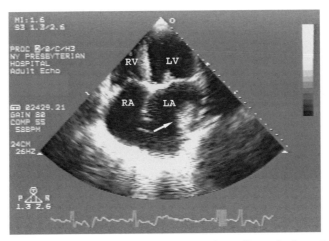

Fig. 8.1 Apical four-chamber view by transthoracic echocardiography in patient with atrial fibrillation. A large thrombus (arrow) is seen on the posterolateral wall of the left atrium. LV, Left ventricle; RV, right ventricle; LA, left atrium; RA, right atrium.

form within the appendage of the left atrium, which is rarely visualized by TEE. This, along with the possibility to visualize spontaneous echo-contrast (SEC) in the atrium, makes TEE a much more sensitive diagnostic technique in patients with atrial fibrillation (see paragraph on left atrial appendage thrombus and SEC).

Left ventricular thrombus

Myocardial infarction (MI) and dilated cardiomyopathy are the conditions most frequently associated with left ventricular thrombus formation. TTE is commonly used for the detection of left ventricular thrombus (Fig. 8.2), and allows the visualization of thrombi of a few millimeters in thickness. Its sensitivity for this diagnosis is not inferior to that of TEE, even because most ventricular thrombi tend to form in the apical region of the ventricle, which may or may not be adequately visualized by TEE in all patients. Therefore, the use of TEE to search for a left ventricular thrombus should be reserved to patients with suboptimal TTE views.

In the first month following an acute MI, the incidence of stroke is between 2% and 3%, with half of the events occurring in the first 5 days after the cardiac event [14]. The risk of stroke/TIA is considered to be elevated in the first 3–6 months, later declining to pre-MI levels. Residual left ventricular dysfunction, atrial fibrillation, a history of systemic or pulmonary embolism, arterial hypertension and prior stroke all increase the stroke risk [14]. The risk of stroke/TIA is mainly related to the formation

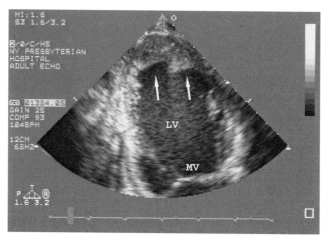

Fig. 8.2 Large apical mural thrombus (arrows) by transthoracic echocardiography, apical two-chamber view. Spontaneous echo-contrast (smoke haze) is also visible within the ventricle. LV, Left ventricle; MV, mitral valve.

of thrombus in the infarcted area, and its subsequent embolization to the brain. Anterior wall infarction carries a much higher rate of thrombus formation than inferior wall infarction. The rate of thrombus formation following anterior infarction is estimated at 25–30%, compared with approximately 5% after inferior infarction. However, some data also exist that do not support an association between infarction location and stroke risk [15], suggesting than mechanisms other than thrombus formation (arrhythmias, ventricular dysfunction) may also contribute to the increased risk of cerebral events post-MI.

TTE is widely used to search for left ventricular thrombus in patients post-MI. Morphological features of the thrombus such as size, protrusion and mobility can be assessed, which are important to evaluate the thromboembolic potential. For high-risk patients, prophylaxis with warfarin aiming for an INR of 2.0–3.0 is recommended [16]. The duration of anticoagulation is generally limited to the first 6 months, and aspirin is generally administered after that time. Long-term anticoagulation can be considered in patients at persistently high risk. In the ASPECT trial, systemic anticoagulation resulted in a 40% reduction in stroke risk over 3 years, although with an increase in the frequency of major hemorrhagic complications [17]. Long-term anticoagulation appears especially beneficial in patients with decreased left ventricular ejection fraction, who have especially high risk of cerebrovascular events [18].

Only sparse information is available on the frequency of thrombus formation and the incidence of cerebral embolization in patients with dilated cardiomyopathy. The frequency of embolic events is generally thought to parallel the deterioration in left ventricular function, but in the Study of Left Ventricular Dysfunction (SOLVD) [19] this relationship was observed only in women. Although data from randomized clinical trials are lacking, systemic anticoagulation with an INR of 2.0–3.0 is generally recommended in patients with previous episodes of thromboembolism, documented left ventricular thrombus, or atrial fibrillation [20]. Aspirin may be an effective therapeutic alternative in patients with dilated cardiomyopathy, but without these additional risk factors [18].

Valvular vegetations

Infective endocarditis is by far the most common etiology of vegetations on the aortic and mitral valves. Endocarditis is associated with a 20–40% chance of embolic events, 65% of which involve the central nervous system [21]. Almost one-quarter of patients with acute endocarditis and at least one vegetation on TEE will have a cerebral embolic event [22], and the risk is especially high when the mitral valve is involved [21–23].

TTE, although very specific for the diagnosis of endocarditis, has sensitivity of only 50–60%. TEE is much more sensitive for this diagnosis [24], besides allowing the evaluation of vegetation morphological characteristics (Fig. 8.3) that increase the risk of embolization (size > 10 mm, mobility, texture, and involvement of more than one leaflet) [22,23,25,26]. The embolic potential of various microorganisms appears to be similar [25], with the possible exception of an increased risk from *Staphylococcus aureus* [23].

The risk of cerebral embolization from endocarditis is highest in the initial day and decreases rapidly after the institution of effective antibiotic

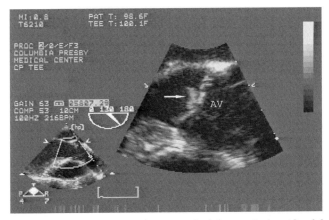

Fig. 8.3 Detail of valvular vegetation (arrow) on the left ventricular side of the aortic valve (AV) by transesophageal echocardiography.

treatment [25], from 13 per 1000 patient-days during the first week to 1.3 per 1000 patient-days after 2 weeks of treatment [21]. Surgery is usually reserved for complications such as intractable congestive heart failure, cardiac abscess, recurrent embolization or persistently positive blood cultures despite antibiotic treatment [21]. Early surgery is also warranted in the case of fungal endocarditis, and often for infections by *Pseudomonas aeruginosa*, Brucella and Coxiella species [21].

Early surgery may also be indicated in patients with prosthetic valve endocarditis, especially when the microorganism involved is *S. aureus* [21]. However, surgery for acute prosthetic endocarditis is a high-risk procedure with considerable morbidity and mortality, especially in the case of mitral involvement [27].

TEE is of special importance for the diagnosis of prosthetic valve endocarditis. In the case of endocarditis in the mitral position, vegetations tend to form on the atrial side of the prosthesis (Fig. 8.4A,B), which is not well visualized by TTE because of the interposition of the prosthesis itself between the ultrasound beam and the vegetation. TEE should therefore be obtained in all patients with suspected prosthetic valve endocarditis.

Cardiac tumors

Although rare (< 0.2% of unselected autopsy series) [28], primary cardiac tumors, and especially myxomas and papillary fibroelastoma, are associated with high frequency of embolic events. Approximately 75% of all cardiac tumors are benign, and 50% of those are myxomas. Three out of four myxomas originate from the left atrium, and especially from the fossa ovalis area of the interatrial septum [29]. Due to this preferential location, myxomas tend to embolize to the systemic circulation, and especially to the brain. It is estimated that 30–40% of all myxomas will embolize [29], to the cerebral circulation in > 50% of cases. Embolization may be caused by tumor fragmentation, or secondary to superimposed thrombus formation and dislodgement. Morphological features of the myxoma affect the embolic risk, as large, mobile myxomas are more likely to embolize, as are myxomas whose surface consists of many fine, villous excrescences, than myxomas with polypoid aspect [29]. Although TTE can identify large myxomas with great accuracy, TEE is invaluable for the detection of small tumors and for the definition of the aforementioned morphological characteristics of the tumor. Surgical resection of the tumor to prevent embolization is recommended in all cases of myxomas, and especially when high-risk morphological appearance is observed.

Papillary fibroelastomas are also frequently associated with cerebral embolism. Embolic events are often the first clinical manifestation of these tumors, due to their preferential location on highly mobile valve leaflets.

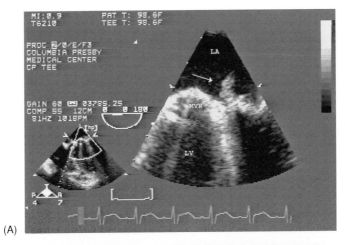

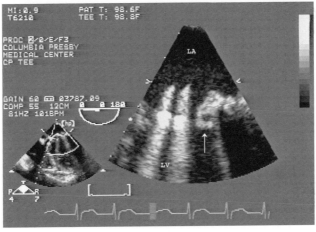

Fig. 8.4 Vegetation on a mechanical prosthesis in a patient status post mitral valve replacement (MVR). (A) During systole, the vegetation is seen attached to the atrial aspect of the mitral annulus. (B) During diastole, the vegetation prolapses through the prosthesis and into the left ventricle. LA, Left atrium; LV, left ventricle.

Surgical resection is indicated for fibroelastomas, with oral anticoagulation usually reserved to cases in which surgery is contraindicated [30].

Malignant primary tumors of the heart, such as angiosarcoma and rhabdomyosarcoma, are rare. Metastatic cardiac tumors are 20–40 times more frequent than primary tumors [29]. For the assessment of the associated embolic risk, the same considerations made for benign tumors on the usefulness of TEE and TTE apply. TEE is also invaluable in the assessment of tumor extension to adjacent structures and blood vessels, which may be critical for the decision about surgical treatment.

Left atrial appendage thrombus and spontaneous echo-contrast

As mentioned earlier, most thrombi in patients with atrial fibrillation form in the atrial appendage, an antero-lateral recess that is infrequently visualized by TTE, but is imaged in all patients by TEE (Fig. 8.5).

A thrombus in the left atrial appendage (Fig. 8.6) is present in 10–20% of patients with atrial fibrillation undergoing TEE [31]. The prevalence of

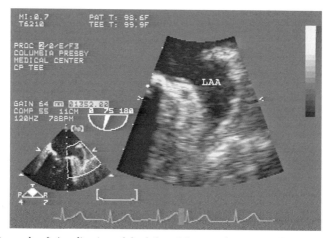

Fig. 8.5 Example of visualization of the left atrial appendage (LAA) by transesophageal echocardiography.

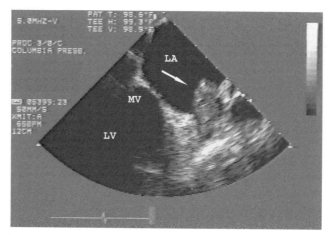

Fig. 8.6 Left atrial appendage thrombus (arrow) by transesophageal echocardiography. LV, Left ventricle; LA, left atrium; MV, mitral valve.

thrombus is higher in patients with chronic atrial fibrillation (27%), but is also substantial in atrial fibrillation of less than 3 days duration (14%) [31]. In patients with atrial fibrillation and a recent embolic event, a prevalence of up to 40% has been reported [32]. In the case of patients presenting with a recent embolic episode, frequency of thrombus between chronic and intermittent atrial fibrillation appears to be similar [31].

Mitral stenosis, severe left ventricular dysfunction, left atrial dilatation, or the presence of a prosthetic mitral valve are all associated with an increased frequency of thrombus in the left atrial appendage [33].

A thrombus in the left atrial appendage increases the risk of cerebrovascular events by three times [34]. TEE is invaluable to diagnose the presence of thrombus and therefore guide the treatment. Oral anticoagulation with warfarin is associated with thrombus resolution in up to 80% of cases [35].

Patients with left atrial thrombus are at high risk of stroke/TIA after electrical cardioversion of atrial fibrillation, as restoration of the contractile activity of the appendage may dislodge a pre-existing thrombus. Prophylactic anticoagulation for at least 3 weeks before cardioversion is usually adopted, followed by several more weeks of treatment after the restoration of sinus rhythm. Recently, TEE has been used to shorten the duration of anticoagulation precardioversion. In patients with no thrombus on TEE, cardioversion can be safely performed after a few days of anticoagulation, also reducing the incidence of bleeding complications [36]. However, anticoagulation following the cardioversion is necessary, as thrombus may form during a period of 'stunning' of the atrium, and embolize once the normal atrial activity resumes.

SEC, or swirling, smoke-like echodensities seen within a cardiac chamber, signals the presence of stagnant blood flow. Although SEC can occasionally be seen by TTE in the left ventricle of patients with severely reduced ventricular function (Fig. 8.2), its detection in the left atrium is difficult by TTE because of the considerable distance between the ultrasound transducer and the atrium. Because of the proximity of the esophagus to the left atrium, and of the higher frequency of the transducer used, TEE is very sensitive in detecting SEC in the left atrium. SEC is present in over 50% of patients undergoing TEE for atrial fibrillation [37]. SEC is rarely observed in normal sinus rhythm (approximately 2% of patients undergoing TEE), and almost invariably in the presence of a significantly dilated left atrium with depressed function [38]. SEC predisposes to thrombus formation [34], and is associated with a three- to four-fold increase in risk of ischemic stroke/TIA [34,37].

Oral anticoagulation decreases the risk of stroke associated with SEC [34,37]. In the SPAAF III trial [34], adjusted-dose warfarin treatment with an INR of 2.0–3.0 was associated with a stroke incidence of 4.5% per year, compared with 18.2% per year for treatment with low-dose warfarin plus aspirin. Adjusted-dose warfarin was also associated with reduced thrombus formation in patients with spontaneous echocontrast (4% vs. 15%).

Proximal aortic atheromas

The presence of large atheromas in the proximal portion of the aorta has been shown to be associated with an increased risk of cerebral embolic events in patients over the age of 60 years. In a large autopsy study [39], patients who had died from ischemic stroke had a significantly higher frequency of ulcerated atheromas in the proximal portion of the aorta than patients who had died from other neurological diseases (26% vs. 5%). TEE was then used to search for these atheromas *in vivo*. Several TEE-based studies, using a case–control [40–42] or a prospective cohort design [43,44], have confirmed the role of aortic atheromas as risk factors for cerebrovascular events. The increase in stroke risk in these studies has varied as a consequence of different definitions of atheroma and different study populations, ranging from 2.6-fold to nine-fold. Large or mobile arch atheromas have also been shown to increase the risk of cerebral embolic events in patients undergoing cardiopulmonary bypass, or other invasive procedures on the ascending aorta, such as cardiac catheterization or intra-aortic balloon pump placement.

The risk of cerebrovascular events has been related to the thickness of the atheroma, with 4 mm or 5 mm chosen as threshold of increased risk in different studies [40–43]. The transverse portion of the aorta, or aortic arch, has been extensively studied, because it is the area from which the head vessels depart. This region can at times be visualized by TTE using a suprasternal or supraclavicular approach (Fig. 8.7), but TEE is far more sensitive for the detection of small atheromas in the region. By TEE, the thickness of the atheroma can easily be measured (Fig. 8.8), which can be used for risk stratification. Also, the presence of complex morphological features, such as ulceration (Fig. 8.9) and mobile components (Fig. 8.10A,B) can be studied. The assessment of atheroma morphology is of prognostic importance, since the presence of ulceration or superimposed mobile thrombus has been shown to increase the risk of cerebrovascular events by up to 17 times [44]. On the other hand, the presence of calcification within a plaque has been associated with decreased embolic risk [45].

Preventive measures to decrease the risk of cerebrovascular events in patients with aortic atheromas are largely based on preliminary evidence, in the absence of prospective randomized clinical trials. Some authorities recommend that systemic anticoagulation with warfarin, aimed at achieving an INR between 2.0 and 3.0, should be used in patients with ulcerated or mobile atheromas [34], which carry higher embolic risk. The need for systemic anticoagulation is more controversial in the case of noncomplex atheromas, although some data exist supporting its usefulness in plaques

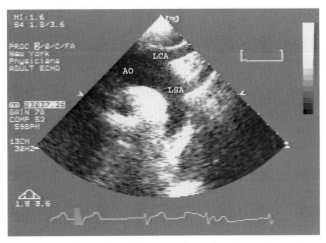

Fig. 8.7 Visualization of the aortic arch by transthoracic echocardiography, suprasternal view. The proximal portion of the aorta (AO) is visualized. The take-off of the left carotid artery (LCA) and of the left subclavian artery (LSA) is seen.

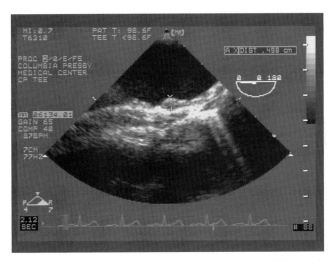

Fig. 8.8 Measurement of atheroma thickness in the mid portion of the aortic arch. The thickness (0.498 cm) is displayed in the upper right corner.

over 4 mm in thickness [45]. Surgical removal has been attempted for atheromas with large mobile components, but this operation has high risk of cerebral embolization [46], and should be reserved for highly selected cases. Preventive treatment with lipid-lowering or antiplatelet agents, although conceivably useful to stabilize the plaque and inhibit platelet

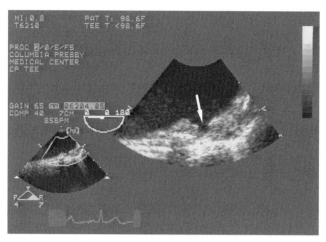

Fig. 8.9 Magnified view of a complex arch atheroma. A large ulceration (arrow) is seen on the lumenal surface.

aggregation on it, has not been adequately tested in randomized, controlled clinical trials.

Patent foramen ovale and atrial septal defect

A PFO is present in 20–25% of normal adults. A PFO may act as a conduit for paradoxical embolization, or embolization to the systemic arterial circulation of fragments of a thrombus originating in the systemic venous circulation.

PFO has been shown to be associated with an increased risk of cerebrovascular events, especially those that occur in the absence of other apparent explanations (cryptogenic strokes) [47,48], often seen in people below the age of 55 years [47]. Paradoxical embolization is considered to be the mechanism for stroke or TIA occurring in patients with PFO and no other obvious causes. However, the only direct demonstration of paradoxical embolization as the culprit mechanism is the presence of thrombus in the PFO (Fig. 8.11), which is an occasional finding. In the majority of cases, embolization through a PFO is diagnosed on the basis of the combined information provided by the clinical picture, compatible neuroimaging evidence, absence of other potential causes, and presence of predisposing conditions (deep venous thrombosis, Valsalva-like maneuvers preceding the event, etc.). Additional elements can corroborate the diagnosis of paradoxical embolization through the PFO. Large PFO size (> 2 mm) has been shown to be associated with increased frequency of cryptogenic stroke [49], and with a greater frequency of superficial infarcts, suggestive of embolic mechanism, on brain imaging

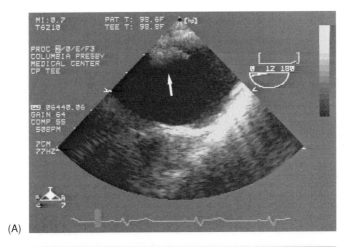

(A)

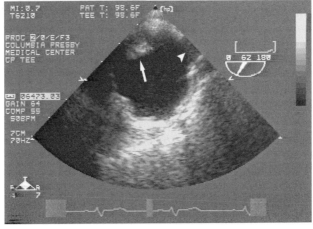

(B)

Fig. 8.10 Large complex atheroma of the aortic arch. (A) In horizontal plane, a large atheroma is visible (arrow), which was highly mobile in real-time imaging. (B) The corresponding longitudinal view shows the spatial relationship between the atheroma (arrow) and the take-off of the left subclavian artery (arrowhead).

[50]. The presence of a deep venous thrombosis [51], or of an associated prothrombotic state may lend further support to the diagnosis of paradoxical embolization.

A PFO is usually diagnosed by TTE with aerated saline injection, documenting the passage of microbubbles from the right to the left cardiac chambers. TTE represents a good screening test for PFO presence, although its sensitivity is only 65–70% of that of TEE with contrast injection [52]. The difference in sensitivity affects especially the ability of TTE to detect small PFOs [52], whose importance as risk factors for cerebral ischemia

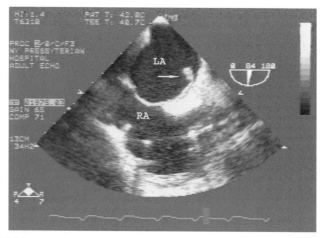

Fig. 8.11 Mobile thrombus (arrow) at the end of a funnel-shaped patent foramen ovale by transesophageal echocardiography (longitudinal view). LA, Left atrium; RA, right atrium.

may be lower [52]. TEE, however, provides additional information on PFO size and morphology that is not obtainable by TTE. The actual separation of the two components of the interatrial septum (septum primum and septum secundum) can be clearly visualized in at least 70% of patients with PFO [52], especially with the aid of Valsalva maneuver or cough to increase the right-sided pressures (Fig. 8.12A,B).

Moreover, with contrast-TTE the exact location of a small shunt (PFO vs. intrapulmonary shunt) may be difficult to distinguish. With TEE, the actual shunt location is visualized, and the quantification of its magnitude is more accurate (Fig. 8.13). Therefore, while contrast-TTE is a good screening test to identify relatively large PFOs, TEE is more sensitive for smaller PFO detection, and should be performed when the assessment of PFO morphology and degree of shunt is important, e.g. when entertaining the possibility of surgical or transcatheter PFO closure.

The preventive measures to adopt in patients with cerebral ischemic events and a PFO are largely empiric. Warfarin or aspirin have been used, with stroke or TIA recurrence rates ranging from 4.7% to 6.7% per year [53–55] in studies with different patient populations and nonrandomized treatment assignment. In a recently published study on cryptogenic stroke patients below 55 years of age [56], the recurrence rate of stroke/TIA on aspirin treatment was low (2.3% at 4 years). The relative efficacy of warfarin and aspirin in a large population of stroke patients unselected by age has been tested in the randomized PFO in Cryptogenic Stroke Study (PICSS), a multicenter study on 630 stroke patients undergoing TEE sponsored by the National Institute of Neurological Disorders and Stroke

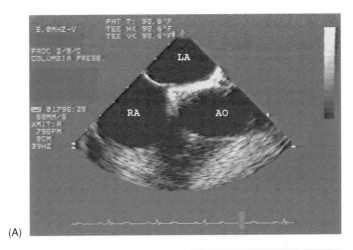

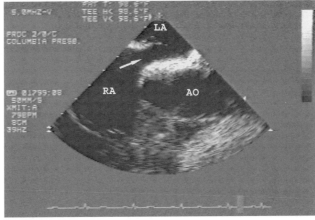

Fig. 8.12 Visualization of patent foramen ovale by transesophageal echocardiography. (A) At baseline, the interatrial septum is visualized without evident opening. (B) During Valsalva maneuver, septal separation becomes visisble (arrow). LA, Left atrium; RA, right atrium; AO, aorta.

(NINDS). In that study [57], the two-year stroke recurrence rate was similar in patients treated with warfarin or aspirin (16.5% vs. 13.2%; hazard ratio 1.29, 95% confidence interval 0.63–2.64, $p = 0.49$), regardless of PFO size and coexistence of an atrial septal aneurysm.

Surgical closure of the PFO has been performed in patients unwilling or unable to be anticoagulated. Stroke or TIA recurrence rates, in relatively small series, have been close to 0% in younger patients [58–60], but up to 18% per year in patients over 45 years of age [58–60]. Percutaneous transcatheter PFO closure has recently been performed using several different devices, with recurrent neurological event rates ranging from

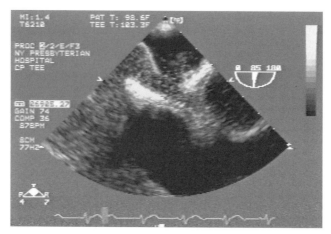

Fig. 8.13 Positive contrast study in patient with a patent foramen ovale. Septal separation is noted, and microbubbles are seen crossing from the right atrium into the left atrium.

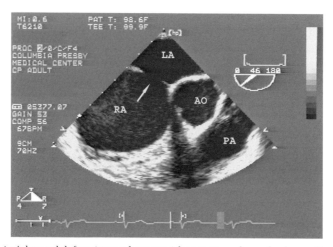

Fig. 8.14 Atrial septal defect (secundum type) by transesophageal echocardiography. An orifice is seen (arrow) at the fossa ovalis level of the interatrial septum. LA, Left atrium; RA, right atrium; AO, aorta; PA, pulmonary artery.

2.2% to 6.3% per year in the most recent series [61–63]. The long-term safety record of these closing devices remains to be established.

Unlike a PFO, which in most cases allows for a right-to-left intracardiac shunt only when the pressure in the right atrium exceeds the pressure in the left atrium, an atrial septal defect (ASD) is an interatrial orifice that remains open at all times (Fig. 8.14), allowing continuous bidirectional blood shunting between the atria. ASD has been much less studied than

PFO as a potential risk factor for stroke/TIA, as a consequence of its much lower frequency in the general population. Right-to-left shunt, and therefore paradoxical embolization, is possible, and becomes more frequent when right ventricular failure develops, predisposing to thrombus formation in the right-sided cardiac chambers. Also, atrial fibrillation is a frequent complication of ASD, greatly adding to its thromboembolic risk. Surgical or transcatheter closure of the ASD before the development of these complications has the potential to decrease markedly the risk of stroke/TIA associated with an ASD.

Atrial septal aneurysm

An atrial septal aneurysm (ASA) is the displacement of more than 10 mm of a portion of the atrial septum into one or both atria during the cardiac cycle. An ASA can occasionally be diagnosed by TTE (Fig. 8.15), but is more often detected by TEE, given the close proximity of the esophagus to the atria (Fig. 8.16). ASA is uncommon in the general population, having been detected in 2.2% of 363 normal subjects undergoing TEE [64], but is three- to four-fold more frequent in patients with cerebral ischemic events [64,65]. In a group of 245 patients with stroke and normal carotid arteries, the prevalence of ASA was reported to be > 25% [66]. When an ASA is present, an associated PFO is found in 54–70% of cases [64,67]. The stroke mechanism associated with an ASA is thought to be mediated through the PFO in most cases [64], but in-situ thrombus formation is also possible, although less frequent. In a series of 195 patients with TEE-detected ASA,

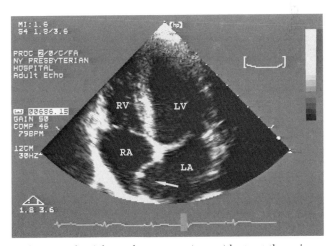

Fig. 8.15 Visualization of atrial septal aneurysm (arrow) by transthoracic echocardiography. Apical four-chamber view. LV, Left ventricle; RV, right ventricle; LA, left atrium; RA, right atrium.

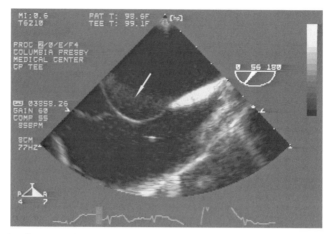

Fig. 8.16 Visualization of atrial septal aneurysm (arrow) by transesophageal echocardiography.

thrombus was visualized in only two cases [67]. However, the association of ASA and PFO seems to carry a greater risk of cerebrovascular events than either condition alone [53,67,68]. PFO characteristics (i.e. larger size of PFOs when associated with ASA), as well as ASA characteristics (thickness, mobility, ability to redirect the blood flow toward the PFO) might play a role in explaining this observation. Increased atrial vulnerability, and therefore predisposition to develop atrial fibrillation, has also been described in patients with atrial septal abnormalities (ASA, PFO, or both) [69].

Antiplatelet agents or systemic anticoagulation with warfarin have been used as secondary prevention of cerebrovascular events in patients with ASA, mostly on an empirical basis. A recently published study of young cryptogenic stroke patients treated with aspirin showed no recurrence of stroke or TIA over 4 years in 10 patients with isolated ASA, a low recurrence rate in 216 patients with isolated PFO (2.3% over 4 years), but a much higher rate in 51 patients with both conditions (15.2% over 4 years) [56]. More data are needed on the comparative efficacy of other preventive approaches.

Valve strands

Filamentous strands are frequently observed by TEE on the mitral and aortic valves (Fig. 8.17), especially in elderly people. Their frequency has varied in the literature, the highest reported frequency in a population undergoing TEE being 40–45% [70]. Valve strands have been shown to be associated with an increased risk of stroke or TIA in several case–control studies [71–73]. However, the prospective follow-up of patients in whom strands were an incidental TEE finding showed a later incidence of 1–2%

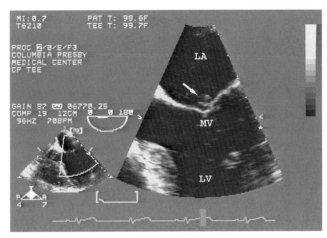

Fig. 8.17 Small filamentous strands (arrow) on the atrial side of the mitral valve (MV). LA, Left atrium; LV, left ventricle.

on an average follow-up of 4 years [70]. In elderly patients with a recent prior stroke, mitral valve strands were not associated with an increased risk of recurrent cerebrovascular events [73]. Therefore, it is not clear whether valve strands represent a risk factor for cerebrovascular events, or a marker of other conditions predisposing to them. The need for preventive treatment in patients with valve strands as an isolated TEE finding is therefore questionable.

TIA and coronary artery disease

It is a matter of debate if the occurrence of a cerebral ischemic event, and especially a transient one such as a TIA, should prompt the search for cardiovascular manifestations of atherosclerosis, and especially coronary artery disease. This issue has been raised by the observation of increased incidence of cardiac ischemic events in patients who had a TIA. In 129 consecutive patients with TIA, 24% mortality from MI over 6 years has been reported, a rate significantly greater than that of patients with minor strokes (6%) [74]. In 390 patients with TIA secondary to atherosclerotic vascular disease, the 5-year cumulative rate of MI or sudden death was only slightly lower than that of fatal and nonfatal cerebral infarction (21.0% vs. 22.7%) [75]. In 132 patients with cerebral ischemia and no prior cardiac history, coronary artery disease was detected in nine (6.8%) [76].

The increased frequency of cardiac events in patients with TIA may be due, at least in part, to an increased frequency in them of cardiovascular risk factors, and especially arterial hypertension [74]. However, in a prospective case–control study on 280 TIA patients and 399 control subjects with comparable cardiovascular risk factor burden, TIA was found to be associated with later incidence of MI even after adjustment for age, race, sex and other pertinent cardiovascular risk factors [77].

From the combined information described above, it appears that an evaluation for coronary artery disease should probably be recommended in patients with TIA secondary to carotid artery disease, or when other manifestations of atherosclerosis, such as the presence of significant aortic arch atheromas, are present. Stress testing, either by exercise or by administration of pharmacological agents such as dobutamine or dipyridamole, coupled with a cardiac imaging technique like transthoracic echocardiography or radionuclide scan, appears as the best option for the non-invasive assessment for coronary artery disease in this group of patients.

Conclusion

The growing awareness of the role of cardioembolism as a mechanism for cerebral ischemic events, and the widespread use of TTE and TEE to search for cardiac and aortic embolic sources, have resulted in recent years in a more rational approach to the prevention of recurrent events. The identification of newer cardioembolic sources, made possible especially by the use of TEE, has led to the reduction of the number of cases considered of unknown origin, and has opened the field to the search of effective therapeutic and preventive strategies.

Acknowledgement

The authors thank Inna Titova BS, and Clarito Dimayuga MD, for their help in the preparation of this chapter.

References

1 Pearson AC, Labovitz AJ, Tatineni S *et al.* Superiority of transesophageal echocardiography in detecting cardiac source of embolism in patients with cerebral ischemia of uncertain etiology. *J Am Coll Cardiol* 1991; 17: 66–72.

2 Cujec B, Polasek P, Voll C *et al.* Transesophageal echocardiography in the detection of potential cardioembolic source of embolism in stroke patients. *Stroke* 1991; 22: 727–33.

3 Flegel KM, Shipley MJ, Rose G. Risk of stroke in nonrheumatic atrial fibrillation. *Lancet* 1987; 1: 526–9.

4 Wolf PA, Abbott RD, Kannel WB. Atrial fibrillation as an independent risk factor for stroke: the Framingham Study. *Stroke* 1991; 22: 983–8.

5 Krahn AD, Manfreda J, Tate RB *et al.* The natural history of atrial fibrillation: incidence, risk factors and prognosis in the Manitoba Follow-Up Study. *Am J Med* 1995; 98: 476–84.

6 Wolf PA, Dawber TR, Thomas HE Jr *et al.* Epidemiologic assessment of atrial fibrillation and risk of stroke: the Framingham Study. *Neurology* 1978; 28: 973–7.

7 Hart RG, Halperin JL. Atrial fibrillation and thromboembolism: a decade of progress in stroke prevention. *Ann Intern Med* 1999; 131: 688–95.

8 Furberg CD, Psaty BM, Manolio TA *et al.* Prevalence of atrial fibrillation in elderly subjects (the Cardiovascular Health Study). *Am J Cardiol* 1994; 74: 236–41.

9 Risk factors for stroke and efficacy of antithrombotic therapy in atrial fibrillation: analysis of pooled data from five randomized controlled trials. *Arch Intern Med* 1994; 154: 1449–57.

10 Kopecky SL, Gersh BJ, McGoon MD *et al.* The natural history of lone atrial fibrillation: a population-based study over three decades. *N Engl J Med* 1987; 317: 669–74.

11 Hart RG, Pearce LA, Rothbart RM *et al.* for the Stroke Prevention in Atrial Fibrillation Investigators. Stroke with intermittent atrial fibrillation: incidence and predictors during aspirin therapy. *J Am Coll Cardiol* 2000; 35: 183–7.

12 Adjusted-dose warfarin versus low-intensity, fixed-dose warfarin plus aspirin for high-risk patients with atrial fibrillation: Stroke Prevention in Atrial Fibrillation III randomised clinical trial. *Lancet* 1996; 348: 633–8.

13 ACC/AHA/ESC guidelines for the management of patients with atrial fibrillation. *J Am Coll Cardiol* 2001; 38: 1231–65.

14 Mooe T, Eriksson P, Stegmayr B. Ischemic stroke after acute myocardial infarction. A population-based study. *Stroke* 1997; 28: 762–7.

15 Bodenheimer MM, Sauer D, Shareef B *et al.* Relation between myocardial infarct location and stroke. *J Am Coll Cardiol* 1994; 24: 61–6.

16 Fifth ACCP Consensus Conference on Antithrombotic Therapy (1998): Summary Recommendations. *Chest* 1998; 114 (Suppl.): 439S–769S.

17 Azar AJ, Koudstaal PJ, Wintzen AR *et al.* Risk of stroke during long-term anticoagulant therapy in patients after myocardial infarction. *Ann Neurol* 1996; 39: 301–7.

18 Loh E, Sutton MS, Wun CC *et al.* Ventricular dysfunction and the risk of stroke after myocardial infarction. *N Engl J Med* 1997; 336: 1916–7.

19 Dries DL, Rosenberg Y, Waclawiw M *et al.* Ejection fraction and risk of thromboembolic events in patients with systolic dysfunction and sinus rhythm: evidence for gender differences in the studies of left ventricular dysfunction trials. *J Am Coll Cardiol* 1997; 29: 80.

20 Koniaris LS, Goldhaber SZ. Anticoagulation in dilated cardiomyopathy. *J Am Coll Cardiol* 1998; 31: 745–8.

21 Mylonakis E, Calderwood SB. Infective endocarditis in adults. *N Engl J Med* 2001; 345: 30.

22 Cabell CH, Pond KK, Peterson GE *et al.* The risk of stroke and death in patients with aortic and mitral valve endocarditis. *Am Heart J* 2001; 142: 75–80.

23 Rohmann S, Erbel R, Gorge G *et al*. Clinical relevance of vegetation localization by transesophageal echocardiography in infective endocarditis. *Eur Heart J* 1992; 13: 446–52.

24 Shapiro SM, Young E, De Guzman S *et al*. Transesophageal echocardiography in diagnosis of infective endocarditis. *Chest* 1994; 105: 377–82.

25 Sanfilippo AJ, Picard MH, Newell JB *et al*. Echocardiographic assessment of patients with infectious endocarditis: prediction of risk for complications. *J Am Coll Cardiol* 1991; 18: 1191–9.

26 Di Salvo G, Habib G, Pergola V *et al*. Echocardiography predicts embolic events in infective endocarditis. *J Am Coll Cardiol* 2001; 15: 1069–76.

27 Aranki SF, Adams DH, Rizzo RJ *et al*. Determinants of early mortality and late survival in mitral valve endocarditis. *Circulation* 1995; 92 (Suppl.): II143–9.

28 Reynan K. Frequency of primary tumors of the heart. *Am J Cardiol* 1996; 77: 107.

29 Reynan K. Cardiac myxomas. *N Engl J Med* 1995; 333: 1610–7.

30 Sastre-Garriga J, Molina C, Montaner J *et al*. Mitral papillary fibroelastoma as a cause of cardiogenic embolic stroke: report of two cases and review of the literature. *Eur J Neurol* 2000; 7: 449–53.

31 Stoddard MF, Dawkins PR, Prince CR *et al*. Left atrial appendage thrombus is not uncommon in patients with acute atrial fibrillation and a recent embolic event: a transesophageal echocardiographic study. *J Am Coll Cardiol* 1995; 25: 452–9.

32 Manning WJ, Silverman DI, Waksmonski CA *et al*. Prevalence of residual left atrial thrombi among patients with acute thromboembolism and newly recognized atrial fibrillation. *Arch Intern Med* 1995; 155: 2193–8.

33 Brickner ME, Friedman DB, Cigarroa CG *et al*. Relation of thrombus in the left atrial appendage by transesophageal echocardiography to clinical risk factors for thrombus formation. *Am J Cardiol* 1994; 74: 391–3.

34 The Stroke Prevention in Atrial Fibrillation Investigators Committee on Echocardiography. Transesophageal echocardiographic correlates of thromboembolism in high-risk patients with nonvalvular atrial fibrillation. *Ann Intern Med* 1998; 128: 639–47.

35 Jaber WA, Prior DL, Thamilarasan M *et al*. Efficacy of anticoagulation in resolving left atrial and left atrial appendage thrombi: a transesophageal echocardiographic study. *Am Heart J* 2000; 140: 150–6.

36 Klein AL, Grimm RA, Murray RD *et al*. Assessment of Cardioversion Using Transesophageal Echocardiography Investigators. Use of transesophageal echocardiography to guide cardioversion in patients with atrial fibrillation. *N Engl J Med* 2001; 344: 1411–20.

37 Leung DY, Black IW, Cranney GB *et al*. Prognostic implications of left atrial spontaneous contrast in nonvalvular atrial fibrillation. *J Am Coll Cardiol* 1994; 24: 755–62.

38 Sadanandan S, Sherrid MV. Clinical and echocardiographic characteristics of left atrial spontaneous echo contrast in sinus rhythm. *J Am Coll Cardiol* 2000; 35: 1932–8.

39 Amarenco P, Duyckaerts C, Tzourio C *et al*. The frequency of ulcerated plaques in the aortic arch in patients with stroke. *N Engl J Med* 1992; 326: 221–5.

40 Amarenco P, Cohen A, Tzourio C *et al*. Atherosclerotic disease of the aortic arch and the risk of ischemic stroke. *N Eng J Med* 1994; 331: 1474–9.

41 Jones EF, Kalman JM, Calafiore P *et al*. Proximal aortic atheroma: an independent risk factor for cerebral ischemia. *Stroke* 1995; 26: 218–24.

42 Di Tullio MR, Sacco RL, Gersony D *et al*. Aortic atheromas and acute ischemic stroke: a transesophageal echocardiographic study in an ethnically mixed population. *Neurology* 1996; 46: 1560–6.

43 Tunick PA, Rosenzweig BP, Katz ES *et al*. High risk for vascular events in patients with protruding aortic atheromas: a prospective study. *J Am Coll Cardiol* 1994; 23: 1085–90.

44 Di Tullio MR, Sacco RL, Savoia MT *et al*. Aortic atheroma morphology and the risk of ischemic stroke in a multiethnic population. *Am Heart J* 2000; 139: 329–36.

45 Ferrari E, Vidal R, Chevalier T *et al*. Atherosclerosis of the thoracic aorta and aortic debris as a marker of poor prognosis: benefit of oral anticoagulants. *J Am Coll Cardiol* 1999; 33: 1317–22.

46 Stern A, Tunick PA, Culliford AT *et al*. Protruding aortic arch atheromas: risk of stroke during heart surgery with and without aortic arch endarterectomy. *Am Heart J* 1999; 138: 746–52.

47 Lechat P, Mas JL, Lascault G *et al*. Prevalence of patent foramen ovale in patients with stroke. *N Engl J Med* 1988; 318: 1148–52.

48 Di Tullio M, Sacco RL, Gopal A *et al*. Patent foramen ovale as a risk factor for ischemic stroke. *Ann Intern Med* 1992; 117: 461–5.

49 Homma S, Di Tullio MR, Sacco RL *et al*. Characteristics of patent foramen ovale associated with cryptogenic stroke: a biplane transesophageal echocardiographic study. *Stroke* 1994; 25: 582–6.

50 Steiner MM, Di Tullio MR, Rundek T *et al*. Patent foramen ovale size and embolic brain imaging findings among patients with ischemic stroke. *Stroke* 1998; 29: 944–8.

51 Stollberger C, Slany J, Schuster I *et al*. The prevalence of deep venous thrombosis in patients with suspected paradoxical embolism. *Ann Intern Med* 1993; 119: 461–5.

52 Di Tullio M, Sacco RL, Venketasubramanian N *et al*. Comparison of diagnostic techniques for the detection of patent foramen ovale in stroke patients. *Stroke* 1993; 24: 1020–4.

53 Mas JL, Zuber M, for the French study group on patent foramen ovale and atrial septal aneurysm. Recurrent cerebral events in patients with patent foramen ovale or atrial septal aneurysm, or both, and cryptogenic stroke. *Am Heart J* 1995; 140: 1083–8.

54 Bogousslavsky J, Garazi S, Jeanrenaud X *et al*. for the Lausanne Stroke with Paradoxical Embolism Study Group. Stroke recurrence in patients with patent foramen ovale: the Lausanne Study. *Neurology* 1996; 46: 1301–5.

55 Cujec B, Mainra R, Johnson DH. Prevention of recurrent cerebral ischemic events in patients with patent foramen ovale and cryptogenic strokes or transient ischemic attacks. *Can J Cardiol* 1999; 15: 57–64.

56 Mas JL, Arquizan C, Lamy C *et al.* for the Patent Foramen Ovale and Atrial Septal Aneurysm Study Group. Recurrent cerebrovascular events associated with patent foramen ovale, atrial septal aneurysm, or both. *N Engl J Med* 2001; 345: 1740–6.

57 Homma S, Sacco RL, Di Tullio MR *et al.*, for the PFO in Cryptogenic Stroke Study (PICSS) Investigators. Effect on medical treatment in stroke patients with patent foramen ovale. *Circulation* 2002; 105: 2625–31.

58 Homma S, Di Tullio MR, Sacco RL *et al.* Surgical closure of patent foramen ovale in cryptogenic stroke patients. *Stroke* 1997; 28: 2376–81.

59 Devuyst G, Bogousslavsky J, Ruchat P *et al.* Prognosis after stroke followed by surgical closure of patent foramen ovale: a prospective follow-up study with brain MRI and simultaneous transesophageal and transcranial Doppler ultrasound. *Neurology* 1996; 47: 1162–6.

60 Dearani JA, Ugurlu BS, Danielson JK *et al.* Surgical patent foramen ovale closure for prevention of paradoxical embolism-related cerebrovascular ischemic events. *Circulation* 1999; 100: 171–5.

61 Sievert H, Babic UU, Hausdorf G *et al.* Transcatheter closure of atrial septal defect and patent foramen ovale with ASDOS device (a multiinstitutional European trial). *Am J Cardiol* 1998; 82: 1405–13.

62 Windecker S, Wahl A, Chatterjee T *et al.* Percutaneous closure of patent foramen ovale in patients with paradoxical embolism: long-term risk of recurrent thromboembolic events. *Circulation* 2000; 101: 893–8.

63 Hung J, Landzberg MJ, Jenkins KJ *et al.* Closure of patent foramen ovale for paradoxical emboli: intermediate-term risk of recurrent neurological events following transcatheter device placement. *J Am Coll Cardiol* 2000; 35: 1311–6.

64 Agmon Y, Khandheria BK, Meissner I *et al.* Frequency of atrial septal aneurysms in patients with cerebral ischemic events. *Circulation* 1999; 99: 1942–4.

65 Pearson AC, Nagelhout D, Castello R *et al.* Atrial septal aneurysm and stroke: a transesophageal echocardiographic study. *J Am Coll Cardiol* 1991; 18: 1223–9.

66 Mattioli AV, Aquilina M, Oldani A *et al.* Atrial septal aneurysm as a cardioembolic source in adult patients with stroke and normal carotid arteries. A multicentre study. *Eur Heart J* 2001; 22: 261–8.

67 Cabanes L, Mas JL, Cohen A *et al.* Atrial septal aneurysm and patent foramen ovale as risk factors for cryptogenic stroke in patients less than 55 years of age. A study using transesophageal echocardiography. *Stroke* 1993; 24: 1865–73.

68 De Castro S, Cartoni D, Fiorelli M *et al.* Morphological and functional characteristics of patent foramen ovale and their embolic implications. *Stroke* 2000; 31: 2407–13.

69 Berthet K, Lavergne T, Cohen A *et al.* Significant association of atrial vulnerability with atrial septal abnormalities in young patients with ischemic stroke of unknown cause. *Stroke* 2000; 31: 398–403.

70 Roldan CA, Shively BK, Crawford MH. Valve excrescences: prevalence, evolution and risk for cardioembolism. *J Am Coll Cardiol* 1997; 30: 1308–14.

71 Freedberg RS, Goodkin GM, Perez JL *et al.* Valve strands are strongly associated with systemic embolization: a transesophageal echocardiographic study. *J Am Coll Cardiol* 1995; 26: 1709–12.

72 Roberts JK, Omarali I, Di Tullio MR *et al.* Valvular strands and cerebral ischemia. Effect of demographics and strands characteristics. *Stroke* 1997; 28: 2185–8.

73 Cohen A, Tzourio C, Chauvel C *et al.* Mitral valve strands and the risk of ischemic stroke in elderly patients. The French Study of Aortic Plaques in Stroke (FAPS) Investigators. *Stroke* 1997; 28: 1574–8.

74 Falke P, Lindgarde F, Stavenow L. Prognostic indicators for mortality in transient ischemic attack and minor stroke. *Acta Neurol Scand* 1994; 90: 78–82.

75 Heyman A, Wilkinson WE, Hurwitz BJ *et al.* Risk of ischemic heart disease in patients with TIA. *Neurology* 1984; 34: 626–30.

76 Gates P, Peppard R, Kempster P *et al.* Clinically unsuspected cardiac disease in patients with cerebral ischemia. *Clin Exp Neurol* 1987; 23: 80.

77 Howard G, Evans GW, Crouse JR 3rd *et al.* A prospective reevaluation of transient ischemic attacks as a risk factor for death and fatal or nonfatal cardiovascular events. *Stroke* 1994; 25: 342–5.

Coagulation Studies

Karen Furie, Peter J. Kelly, J. Philip Kistler

Hypercoagulability and ischemic cerebrovascular disease

Although thrombosis is the fundamental pathological entity in ischemic stroke, the mechanism of coagulation and embolization in ischemic cerebrovascular disease is still being defined. Aberrant regulation of thrombosis and fibrinolysis appears to play a critical role in cardioembolic stroke as well as in the evolution of atherosclerotic plaque from 'stable' to 'vulnerable' [1]. These mechanisms may not be entirely distinct. In addition, although less common, there are primary and secondary hypercoagulable states that may lead to spontaneous thrombosis of intra- or extracranial cerebral vessels [2,3]. In addition to arterial thrombosis, established hypercoagulable disorders predominantly predispose to venous thromboembolism which can result in stroke due to venous sinus occlusion. It has been estimated that 1% of all strokes and 4% of 'stroke in the young' are due to disorders of the coagulation system [4–10]. This is probably an underestimate of the true contribution of coagulation to other stroke mechanisms.

In cases of transient ischemia (TIA) or stroke without a definite mechanism, i.e. nonlacunar symptoms in the absence of large-vessel atherosclerosis or a cardioembolic source, there may be a greater imperative for additional coagulation testing. These 'cryptogenic' embolic cases, which account for up to 40% of all strokes, are most likely to have demonstrable coagulation abnormalities [11,12]. Identification of a prothrombotic tendency can significantly affect therapeutic decision making and long-term prognosis.

Figure 9.1 is a simplified scheme depicting the interplay of intrinsic and extrinsic factors on the coagulation system and the subsequent impact on ischemic stroke risk. In the vast majority of cases, cerebral ischemia is probably the result of a prothrombotic state superimposed on an underlying cardiac anomaly or intrinsic atherosclerotic vascular disease. Less often, thrombus can develop spontaneously in the absence of a structural defect causing *in-situ* thrombosis or embolism. The mechanism of vascular-bed specific hemostasis in cerebral vessels remains poorly understood at

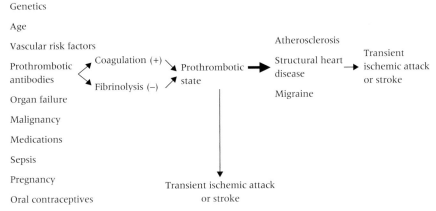

Genetics

Age

Vascular risk factors

Prothrombotic antibodies

Organ failure

Malignancy

Medications

Sepsis

Pregnancy

Oral contraceptives

Fig. 9.1 Coagulation and ischemic stroke.

present [13]. It should be noted that, paradoxically, factors which increase thrombosis will also increase fibrinolysis, although primary hypofunctioning of the fibrinolytic system results in thrombus formation.

Coagulation disorders are often classified as primary or secondary. Genetic polymorphisms or mutations are responsible for primary hypercoagulability. Secondary causes of a prothrombotic state due to increased thrombus formation or reduced fibrinolysis include hepatic failure, nephrotic syndrome, sepsis, malnutrition, malignancy, pregnancy, and oral contraceptives [5,14]. Thrombin generation has also been shown to increase with age [15,16].

Hemostatic markers may also play a prognostic role in patients who have a TIA or risk factors for cerebrovascular disease. In patients with a TIA, F1.2, a marker of thrombin generation, has been predictive of time to ischemic stroke, myocardial infarction, or vascular death [17,18]. Studies have demonstrated that the hemostatic system is activated in conditions associated with an increased stroke risk: hypertension, atrial fibrillation, mitral stenosis, and cardiomyopathy [16,19,20,20–29]. Of those factors related to atherosclerotic disease, fibrinogen has been found most consistently to be an independent predictor of cerebrovascular and cardiovascular events [30–33].

Selecting patients for coagulation testing

Primary coagulation disorders are a relatively uncommon mechanism of TIA and ischemic stroke due to arterial occlusion [4–14]. Routine coagulation testing on all patients would be costly and would not be expected to yield many abnormal or clinically relevant results. In order to maximize the utility of such testing, it is important to select patients with a high

Table 9.1 The hypercoagulable state: clinical features

Absence of conventional stroke risk factors
Family history of venous thromboembolism or early cardiovascular/cerebrovascular
  disease
Thromboembolism involving multiple organs
Livedo reticularis
Hepatic or renal failure
Malignancy
Sepsis

Table 9.2 Suggested coagulation screen

Protein C, protein S, antithrombin III
Immunological assays of total and free protein S
Functional assay for proteins C and S
Activated protein C resistance/factor V Leiden
Fibrinogen
D-dimer
Platelet count
Hematocrit
ELISA for anticardiolipin antibody
Clotting assay for lupus anticoagulant
Homocysteine
Factor VIII
Prothrombin gene G20210A mutation
Thrombin time
Fibrinogen

---

pretest probability of having a disorder of coagulation. Clinical features suggestive of a coagulation derangement are listed in Table 9.1.

It is important to recognize that acute thrombotic events, in which there is active thrombin generation and fibrinolysis, will result in abnormal levels of coagulation factors [34–43]. Coagulation factors are also activated as acute-phase reactants in infection or inflammation. Studies have shown that acute ischemic stroke, particularly stroke due to cardioembolism, is accompanied by higher levels of thrombin–antithrombin complex, D-dimer, and tissue plasminogen activator, reduced functional antithrombin III and plasminogen [34–43]. Therefore, if levels are checked in the acute phase and found to be abnormal, they should be repeated in approximately 12 weeks in order to confirm a sustained derangement. Suggested coagulation studies for screening high-risk patients can be found in Table 9.2.

Hereditary thrombophilias

Although rare, hereditary thrombophilias can manifest with transient cerebral ischemic symptoms, particularly in the young [44,45]. The classic inherited thrombophilias which could potentially be implicated involve factors in the natural anticoagulant system and are transmitted in an autosomal dominant pattern. The natural anticoagulant pathway is activated when thrombin binds to thrombomodulin, activating protein C. Activated protein C inactivates Va and VIIIa, thereby inhibiting thrombosis. Activated protein C resistance can be measured using a clotting assay and then followed up by a genetic test for factor V-Arg506Gln (factor V Leiden). This mutation does not destroy, but rather, slows activated protein C-mediated inactivation and leads to excess thrombin formation [46,47]. Protein S serves as a catalyst for activated protein C.

Protein C is a vitamin K-dependent serine protease expressed by endothelial tissue, which inactivates factors Va and VIIIa, and inhibits tissue plasminogen activator inhibitor-1. In a type I deficiency, the quantity of protein C is diminished, whereas in a type II deficiency, the function is reduced despite normal levels. Protein S is a vitamin K-dependent plasma glycoprotein that acts as a cofactor to protein C, inactivating factors Va and VIIIa. In the circulation, protein S exists in two forms, a biologically active free form and a complex form bound to complement protein C4b [48–52].

There are three forms of congenital protein S deficiency: type I, low levels of free protein S and normal levels of bound protein S; type IIa, low levels of free protein S and low levels of bound protein S; and type IIb, normal levels of free protein S and normal levels of bound protein S [52–56].

Finally, antithrombin is a plasma protein which inhibits virtually all of the coagulation enzymes, primarily factors Xa, IXa, and IIa, but also factors XIIa, XIa and the VIIa–tissue factor complex. As with protein C deficiency, there are two types of antithrombin deficiency, one reduction in quantity (type I), and another related to decreased function (type II) [57–60].

A compelling family history of recurrent venous thromboembolism or ischemic cardiovascular events, particularly at a young age, should alert the clinician to the possibility of a deficiency state [44–60]. Protein C and S deficiencies can cause warfarin-induced skin necrosis. A deficiency in antithrombin III can manifest with heparin 'resistance'. Quantitative and functional assays should be tested in the 'baseline' state, i.e. in the absence of an acute thrombotic event or acute infection in order to prevent confounding. Confirmatory studies should be repeated 2 weeks after a positive screen [14].

Long-term anticoagulation is the mainstay of therapy for patients with a life-threatening thrombotic episode, more than one spontaneous thrombotic episode, thrombosis in an unusual location, i.e. cerebral venous sinus, or a thrombotic episode with a documented genetic defect. Patients with asymptomatic or provoked thrombosis should be prophylaxed with anticoagulation in high-risk situations, i.e. surgery or pregnancy. Warfarin should be initiated with a heparin overlap. Screening of family members should be strongly considered.

Antiphospholipid antibodies

The antiphospholipid antibodies, anticardiolipin antibody and lupus anticoagulant, have been associated with TIAs and cerebral infarctions due to both *in-situ* thrombosis and embolism [61]. These antibodies, lupus anticoagulant which circulates freely and anticardiolipin antibody, bound to β_2-glycoprotein 1, inhibit protein C and protein S, increase platelet aggregation and adhesion, and inhibit vasodilatation. More common in patients with system lupus erythematosus, these antibodies can occur sporadically and appear to play a role predominantly in stroke in the young (age < 50). Medical conditions, i.e. infections and autoimmune disorders, as well as medications such as procainamide, hydralazine, and phenothiazines have been linked to antiphospholipid antibodies [62–65].

Antiphospholipid antibody syndrome, in its fulminant form, Sneddon's syndrome, can present with recurrent venous thromboembolism, TIA or stroke, miscarriage, and livedo reticularis. Although antibodies have been detected in older patients with conventional vascular risk factors, it is unclear whether the presence of antibodies, particularly at low levels, has ramifications for treatment or outcome in this population [66].

Positive ELISA tests should be confirmed through repeat testing in 8–12 weeks. The significance of elevated IgM titers in isolation is unknown. The level of IgG titer does have prognostic significance, with higher titers conveying a greater risk of ischemic events [61,67]. Case series have identified F1.2 as a potential marker of thrombotic potential in patients with antiphospholipid antibodies [68]. Patients who present with antiphospholipid antibodies in the setting of symptoms suggestive of cerebral ischemia should undergo a transthoracic echocardiogram to look for evidence of marantic endocarditis. A platelet count should be checked as immune thrombocytopenic purpura (ITP) has also been found in association with antiphospholipid antibodies [69].

Treatment options are antiplatelet or antithrombotic therapy [70]. The optimal therapy has yet to be definitively determined, but results of the multicentre Antiphospholipid Antibodies in Stroke Study (APASS) will compare aspirin to warfarin [International Normalized Ratio (INR) 1.4–2.8] for the secondary prevention of noncardioembolic stroke [70]. The target INR with warfarin therapy remains controversial, but higher degrees of anticoagulation may be necessary in patients with the fulminant antiphospholipid syndrome [71]. Plasmapheresis has been employed to reduce the burden of circulating antibodies and should be considered if patients continue to have ischemic symptoms despite maximal medical therapy.

Fibrinolysis

Tissue plasminogen activator (tPA) and urokinase convert plasminogen to plasmin in the circulation. This activation is inhibited by plasminogen activator inhibitor-1 (PAI-1). Plasma levels of tPA and PAI-1 are highly correlated and may be elevated as part of an acute-phase reaction. In addition, PAI-1 levels increase in the presence of conventional vascular risk factors, a potential confounder [72]. Cross-sectional studies have found tPA elevated in patients with cerebrovascular disease [72,73,73]. Results from the prospective Physicians Health Study showed that tPA levels in men free of overt cardiovascular disease at baseline but who subsequently suffered a stroke were higher than in controls matched for age and smoking. The age-adjusted relative risk. for thromboembolic stroke in men with baseline tPA > 95th percentile of control values was 3.89 (95% confidence interval 1.83, 8.26) [74].

Homocysteinemia

Recent studies have shown a link between homocysteine (Hcy) levels and activation of coagulation. Levels of tissue factor, tissue factor pathway inhibitor, and thrombin–antithrombin complex correlate with Hcy levels in patients with ischemic heart disease [75]. The prothrombin fragment, F1.2, is a marker of thrombin generation. In patients with coronary artery disease, F1.2 and Hcy levels have been shown to be highly correlated ($r = 0.46$, $P < 0.0001$) with plasma F1+2 levels increasing across quartiles of Hcy [76]. The relationship between the level of Hcy and F1.2 has also been demonstrated in venous thromboembolic disorders [77,78].

Hcy also affects the fibrinolytic system, reducing tissue plasminogen activator binding by as much as 65%, and specifically inhibiting the tPA binding domain of annexin II [79]. Tissue plasminogen activator mass, plasminogen, and PAI-1 levels have been shown to be increased, but tPA activity decreased, in response to methionine loading [80].

A thermolabile variant of methylenetetrahydrofolate reductase (MTHFR) was described in 1988. A single base-pair substitution in the human MTHFR gene results in expression of the thermolabile MTHFR variant and results in hyperhomocysteinemia [81]. Unique because of its low activity at body temperature and drastic reduction in activity after heating, this thermolabile MTHFR variant is highly prevalent in populations with premature vascular disease [82,83]. Thermolabile MTHFR activity has been reported in 17% of premature coronary artery disease patients compared with 5% of controls [84].

Mild hyperhomocysteinemia is more prevalent in individuals homozygous for TT, compared with CT heterozygotes and controls with the CC wild type [85–88]. The relationship between genotype and level of Hcy is contingent upon plasma folate status, as elevated total Hcy occurs primarily in TT homozygotes whose folate concentrations are in the lower half of the reference range [85–88]. There have been conflicting reports with regard to the association between MTHFR genotype and risk of stroke. A study of a patients with early onset (age < 49 years) ischemic stroke found a two-fold independent increased risk of stroke associated with TT genotype [89]. In other international populations, the odds ratios have ranged from 1.6 (Irish, Italian) to 3.4 (Japanese) [90–92].

The potential interaction of hyperhomocysteinemia with other stroke risk factors in different stroke subtypes remains to be clarified. A Swedish study of hyperhomocysteinemic stroke patients found significantly higher total Hcy concentrations in all stroke subtypes (lacunar, large-artery disease, cardioembolic and hemorrhagic) compared with controls, with no difference in mean concentrations between subtypes [93]. In contrast to these results, a more recent Australian study found that hyperhomocysteinemia was associated with large-vessel atherothrombotic and lacunar subtypes, but not cardioembolic strokes [94].

A recent case report demonstrates the thrombotic potential associated with an inherited disorder of Hcy metabolism. A 47-year-old woman presented with symptoms, signs, and a magnetic resonance imaging study consistent with an acute right middle cerebral artery infarction [95]. Carotid duplex ultrasound revealed hypoechoic signal at the internal carotid origin, consistent with intralumenal thrombus. Plasma Hcy was 279 μmol/l (normal < 15 μmol/l). Genotype analysis revealed a cystathionine beta synthase (CBS) I278T heterozygous mutation (with presumed unidentified CBS mutation compound heterozygosity, I278T/?), without the MTHFR 677C→T substitution. Serum folate, B6 and B12 were normal. Following vitamin and anticoagulant treatment, Hcy normalized and carotid thrombus resolved. An asymptomatic sister has severe hyperhomocysteinemia and CBS I278T mutation. Conventional hypercoagulable studies were normal.

Hcy levels should always be drawn in the fasting state since they vary based on the protein content in a meal. Vitamin B12, a cofactor in Hcy metabolism, should routinely be checked, since Hcy levels are expected to be elevated in vitamin B12 deficiency states.

Vitamin therapy with folate, vitamin B6, and when appropriate, vitamin B12, can reduce Hcy levels; however, there have been no studies to date which have demonstrated that vitamin supplementation directly reverses the secondary effects on the hemostatic system or reduces the risk of TIA or stroke.

Von Willebrand factor

Megakaryocytes and endothelial cells synthesize von Willebrand factor (vWF). Activation of vWF at the site of vascular injury leads to binding of fibrin that is then transglutaminated by factor XIII resulting in covalent crosslinking, which stabilizes the clot. The vWF also mediates the incorporation of platelets into thrombus. Elevations in vWF have been associated with an increased risk of ischemic stroke [96–98]. The levels of vWF are elevated in conditions that have a high risk of stroke, such as atrial fibrillation, high-grade carotid stenosis, and hyperhomocysteinemia. Levels of vWF have also been shown to be higher in patients with a greater burden of small vessel/lacunar strokes [96].

The vWF gene, located on chromosome 12, is 180 kb in length and has 52 exons. Single nucleotide polymorphisms (−1793 C/G, −1234 C/T, −1185 A/G, −1051 G/A) in the promoter region of the vWF gene, affecting vWF levels, have been identified [99]. There appears to be an interaction between age and expression of the genotypes. Individuals > 40 years of age with the CC/AA/GG genotypes have the highest mean plasma levels of vWF, with CT/AG/GA being intermediate, and TT/GG/AA lowest [100]. The Thr789Ala polymorphism is associated with coronary artery disease and plasma vWF levels in diabetic patients [101].

Fibrinogen

Fibrinogen is the most consistent hematological marker of stroke risk [30–33]. It is a 340-kDa glycoprotein consisting of three non-identical polypeptides linked by disulfide bonds. Fibrinogen may play a role in atherogenesis by contributing to mechanical vascular wall injury, hyperviscosity and platelet activation. Genetic mutations of fibrinogen may increase the level of fibrinogen or result in fibrinogen more resistant to lysis.

Three genes located on the long arm of chromosome 4 encode fibrinogen's three polypeptides [102]. Data are conflicting regarding the association of specific polymorphisms in the promoter region of fibrinogen and the risk of cerebrovascular disease. The β448 genotype has been associated with cerebrovascular disease in women [103]. The βC/T 148 genotype has been linked to carotid atheroma [104]. Other studies examining the association between fibrinogen, its polymorphisms, and association with cardiovascular disease have failed to demonstrate an association between fibrinogen polymorphisms and cardiovascular disease despite a direct effect on serum fibrinogen levels [105].

Other prothrombotic genes

Several hypercoagulable states under genetic control have been associated with cardiovascular disease and may affect risk of stroke. In a Japanese population, the platelet-activating (PAF) acetylhydrolase polymorphism, which results in a deficiency of the enzyme responsible for inactivating PAF, was found to be a risk factor for stroke [106]. The glycoprotein (GP) receptor IIIa polymorphism P1A2 appears to convey a higher risk of ischemic stroke in Caucasian women with an identifiable cause of stroke [107]. There also appears to be an increased frequency of the GP IIIa P1A2 allele in young patients with atherothrombotic stroke [108].

Despite a role in venous thromboembolism, neither the prothrombin 20210A allele nor factor V Leiden appears to be associated with a higher risk of myocardial infarction [109–116]. The prothrombin G20210A polymorphism, which increases prothrombin levels, has been associated with increased risk of stroke in young female smokers [117,118]. The prothrombin polymorphism increases prothrombin activity by producing greater quantities of thrombin, not by increasing the rate of prothrombin activation (i.e. no increase in F1+2) [119]. Factor V Leiden may be associated with a higher rate of recurrent venous thromboembolism, but the studies are conflicting [120,121]. The presence of multiple prothrombotic genes (i.e. protein S, antithrombin III, prothrombin G20210A, factor V Leiden) appears to convey higher risk than a single polymorphism [113,114].

Trousseau's syndrome

Armand Trousseau first described the syndrome of malignancy-associated hypercoagulability in 1865, and it has since come to be known as Trousseau's syndrome. Most commonly associated with adenocarcinomas, patients with malignancy have a wide range of coagulation abnormalities including increase F1.2, thrombin–antithrombin complex, plasmin–α_2-antiplasmin, and D-dimer (Table 9.3) [120–122].

As in all cases of secondary hypercoagulability, the focus of therapy should be directed at resolving the underlying cause, i.e. excising or treating the malignancy [123]. If patients have documented coagulation abnormalities or meet the criteria for a clinical hypercoagulable state, long-term anticoagulation may be required, although the role of monitoring coagulation in the clinical management of cancer patients has not been

Table 9.3 Coagulation activation markers in malignancy

Elevated fibrinopeptide A (FPA)
Elevated F1.2
Elevated thrombin–antithrombin complex
Elevated D-dimer
Increased fibrinogen
Increased platelet count
Disseminated intravascular coagulation (DIC)
Antiphospholipid antibodies
Activated protein C resistance

fully elucidated [124,125]. It is also important to recognize that patients with malignancy may have other more conventional stroke risk factors which need to be considered [126].

Conclusion

The relationship between disorders of coagulation and venous thromboembolism is well established, but our understanding of their contribution to arterial disease, and cerebrovascular disease in particular, is still emerging. Novel factors in the coagulation system and their genetic determinants will be closely scrutinized in the next decades as they are potential markers of preclinical disease. The potential impact on reducing ischemic stroke risk, particularly stroke of an embolic etiology, may be tremendous with early intervention. At present, we remain relatively naive as to how one or more prothrombotic tendencies interact within a given patient. Existing antithrombotic therapies provide an opportunity to intervene and reduce risk of recurrent thrombosis, and future developments offer the promise of safer and more effective treatments.

Acknowledgement

We acknowledge gratefully the generous support of the Esther U. Sharpe Memorial Fund.

References

1 Reiner AP, Siscovick DS, Rosendaal FR. Hemostatic risk factors and arterial thrombotic disease. *Thromb Haemost* 2001; 85: 584–95.

2 Greaves M. Coagulation abnormalities and cerebral infarction. *J Neurol Neurosurg Psychiatry* 1993; 56: 433–9.

3 Grotta JC, Yatsu FM, Pettigrew LC *et al.* Prediction of carotid stenosis progression by lipid and hematological measurements. *Neurology* 1989; 39: 1325.

4 Mercuri M, Orecchini G, Susta A, Tazza D, Ciuffeti G. Correlation between hemorheologic parameters and carotid atherosclerosis in stroke. *Angiology* 1989; 39: 283.

5 Hart RG, Kanter MC. Haematological disorders and ischemic stroke. A selective review. *Stroke* 1990; 21: 1111–21.

6 Adams HP, Mutler MJ, Biller J, Toffal GJ. Nonhemorrhagic cerebral infarction in young adults. *Arch Neurol* 1986; 43: 793–6.

7 Uchiyama S, Yamazaki M, Hara Y, Iwata M. Alterations of platelet, coagulation, and fibrinolysis markers in patients with ischemic stroke. *Sem Thromb Hemost* 1997; 24: 535–41.

8 Bogousslavsky J, Van Melle G, Regli F. The Lausanne Stroke Registry: Analysis of 1,000 consecutive patients with first stroke. *Stroke* 1988; 19: 1083–92.

9 Adams HP, Mutler MJ, Biller J, Toffal GJ. Non-hemorrhagic cerebral infarction in young adults. *Arch Neurol* 1986; 43: 793–6.

10 Barinagarrementeria F, Cantu-Brito C, De La Pena A, Izaguirre R. Prothrombotic states in young people with idiopathic stroke: a prospective study. *Stroke* 1994; 25: 287–90.

11 Sacco RL, Ellenberg JH, Mohr JP *et al*. Infarcts of undetermined cause: the NINCDS Stroke Data Bank. *Ann Neurol* 1989; 25: 382.

12 Bushnell CD, Siddiqi Z, Goldstein LB. Improving patient selection for coagulopathy testing in the setting of acute ischemic stroke. *Neurology* 2001; 57: 1333–5.

13 Rosenberg RD, Aird WC. Vascular-bed-specific hemostasis and hypercoagulable states. Mechanisms of disease. *N Engl J Med* 1999; 340: 1555.

14 Bushnell CD, Goldsetin LB. Diagnostic testing for coagulopathies in patients with ischemic stroke. *Stroke* 2000; 31: 3067–78.

15 Kistler JP, Bauer KA. The level of activity of the hemostatic system, the rate of embolic stroke and age: is there a correlation? In: Moskowitz MA, Caplan LR, eds. *Cerebrovascular Diseases: 19th Princeton Stroke Conference*. Boston, MA: Butterworth-Heinemann, 1995; 437.

16 Kistler JP, Singer DE, Millenson MM *et al*. for the BAATAF Investigators. Effect of low-intensity warfarin anticoagulation on level of activity of the hemostatic system in patients with atrial fibrillation. *Stroke* 1993; 24: 1360.

17 Cote R, Wolfson C, Solymoss S *et al*. Hemostatic markers in patients at risk of cerebral ischemia. *Stroke* 2000; 31: 1856–62.

18 Feinberg WM, Erickson LP, Bruck D, Kittelson J. Hemostatic markers in acute ischemic stroke: association with stroke type, severity, and outcome. *Stroke* 1996; 27: 1296–300.

19 Junker R, Heinrich J, Schulte H, Erren M, Assman G. Hemostasis in normotensive and hypertensive men: results of the PROCAM study. *J Hypertension* 1998; 16: 917.

20 Gustafsson C, Blomback M, Britton M, Hamsten A, Svensson J. Coagulation factors and the increased risk of stroke in nonvalvular atrial fibrillation. *Stroke* 1990; 21: 47–51.

21 Lip GYH, Lip PL, Zarifis J *et al*. Fibrin D-dimer and beta-thromboglobulin as markers of thrombogenesis and platelet activation in atrial fibrillation. Effects of introducing ultra-low-dose warfarin and aspirin. *Circulation* 1996; 94: 425–31.

22 Lip GYH, Lowe GDO, Metcalfe MJ, Rumley A, Dunn FG. Effects of warfarin therapy on plasma fibrinogen, von Willebrand factor, and fibrin D-dimer in left ventricular dysfunction secondary to coronary artery disease with and without aneurysms. *Am J Cardiol* 1995; 76: 453–8.

23 Li-Saw-Hee F, Blann AD, Goldsmith I, Lip GYH. Indexes of hypercoagulability measured in peripheral blood reflect levels in intracardiac blood in patients with atrial fibrillation secondary to mitral stenosis. *Am J Cardiol* 1999; 83: 1206–9.

24 Li-Saw-Hee FL, Gurney D, Lip GY. Plasma von Willebrand factor, fibrinogen and soluble P-selectin levels in paroxysmal, persistent and permanent atrial fibrillation. Effects of cardioversion and return of left atrial function. *Eur Heart J* 2001; 22: 1635–9.

25 Mitusch R, Slemens HJ, Garbe M, Wagner T, Shelkhzadeh A, Diederich KW. Detection of a hypercoagulable state in nonvalvular atrial fibrillation and the effect of anticoagulant therapy. *Thromb Haemost* 1996; 75: 219–23.

26 Lip GYH, Lowe GDO, Rumley A, Dunn FG. Increased markers of thrombogenesis in chronic atrial fibrillation: effects of warfarin treatment. *Br Heart J* 1995; 73: 527.

27 Soncini M, Casazza F, Mattioli R, Bonfardeci C, Motta A, Cimminiello C. Hypercoagulability and chronic atrial fibrillation: the role of markers of thrombin generation. *Minerva Med* 1997; 88: 501.

28 Yamamoto K, Ikeda U, Furuhashi K, Irokawa M, Nakayama T, Shimada K. The coagulation system is activated in idiopathic cardiomyopathy. *J Am Coll Cardiol* 1995; 25: 1634.

29 Jafri SM, Ozawa T, Mammen E, Levine TB, Johnson C, Goldstein S. Platelet function, thrombin and fibrinolytic activity in patients with heart failure. *Eur Heart J* 1993; 14: 205–12.

30 Lip GYH. Fibrinogen and cardiovascular disorders. *Q J Med* 1995; 88: 155–65.

31 Kannel WB, Wolf PA, Castelli WP, D'Agostino RB. Fibrinogen and risk of cardiovascular disease. The Framingham study. *JAMA* 1987; 258: 1183.

32 Quizilbash N. Fibrinogen and cerebrovascular disease. *Eur Heart J* 1995; 16: 42–5.

33 Qzilbash N, Jones L, Warlow C, Mann J. Fibrinogen and lipid concentrations as risk factors for transient ischemic attacks and minor strokes. *Br Med J* 1991; 303: 605.

34 Wilhelmsen L, Svardsudd K, Korsan-Bengtsen K, Larsson B, Welin L, Tibblin G. Fibrinogen as a risk factor for stroke and myocardial infarction. *N Eng J Med* 1984; 311: 501.

35 Feinberg WM, Erickson LP, Bruck D, Kittelson J. Hemostatic markers in acute ischemic stroke. *Stroke* 1996; 27: 1296.

36 Yamazaki M, Uchiyama S, Maruyama S. Alterations of hemostatic markers in various subtypes and phases of stroke. *Blood Coagul Fibrinolysis* 1993; 4: 707.

37 Altes A, Abellan MT, Mateo J, Avila A, Marti-Vilalta JL, Fontcuberta J. Hemostatic disturbances in acute ischemic stroke: a study of 86 patients. *Acta Haematol* 1995; 94: 10–5.

38 Takano K, Yamaguchi T, Kato H, Omae T. Activation of coagulation in acute cardioembolic stroke. *Stroke* 1991; 22: 12.

39 Takano K, Yamaguchi T, Uchida K. Markers of a hypercoagulable state following acute ischemic stroke. *Stroke* 1992; 23: 194.

40 Kilpatrick TJ, Matkovic Z, Davis SM, McGrath CM, Dauer RJ. Hematologic abnormalities occur in both cortical and lacunar infarction. *Stroke* 1993; 24: 1945.

41 Giroud M, Dutrillaux F, Lemesle M *et al.* Coagulation abnormalities in lacunar and cortical ischemic stroke are quite different. *Neurol Res* 1998; 20: 15.

42 Uchiyama S, Yamazaki M, Hara Y, Iwata M. Alterations in platelet, coagulation, and fibrinolysis markers in patients with acute ischemic stroke. *Sem Thromb Hem* 1997; 23: 535.

43 Lin L, Lin Z, Shen S. Changes of von Willebrand factor and antithrombin III levels in acute stroke: differences between thrombotic and hemorrhagic stroke. *Thromb Res* 1993; 72: 353.

44 Martinez HR, Rangel-Guerra RA, Marfil LJ. Ischemic stroke due to deficiency of coagulation inhibitors: report of 10 young adults. *Stroke* 1993; 24: 19–25.

45 Voetsch B, Damasceno BP, Camargo ECS *et al.* Inherited thrombophilias as a risk factor for the development of ischemic stroke in young adults. *Thromb Haemost* 2000; 83: 229–33.

46 Coller BS, Owen J, Jesty J *et al.* Deficiency of plasma protein S, protein C, or antithrombin III and arterial thrombosis. *Arteriosclerosis* 1987; 7: 456–61.

47 DeLuucia D, d'Alessio D, Pazzella S *et al.* A hypercoagulable state in activated protein C resistant patients with ischemic stroke. *Int J Clin Lab Res* 1998; 28: 74–5.

48 Camerlingo M, Finazzi G, Casto L, Laffranchi C, Barbui T, Mamoli A. Inherited protein C deficiency and nonhemorrhagic arterial stroke in young adults. *Neurology* 1991; 41: 1371.

49 Macko RF, Ameriso SF, Gruber A *et al.* Impairments in the protein C system and fibrinolysis in infection associated stroke. *Stroke* 1996; 27: 2005–11.

50 De Stefano V, Leone G, Teofili L, Ferrelli R, Pollari G, Antonini V. Transient ischemic attack in a patient with nonthrombogenic hereditary protein C deficiency during treatment with stanozolol. *Am J Hematol* 1988; 29: 120–1.

51 D'Angelo A, Landi G, D'Angelo SV *et al.* Protein C in acute stroke. *Stroke* 1988; 19: 579–83.

52 Douay X, Lucas C, Caron C, Goudemand J, Leys D. Antithrombin, protein C, and protein S levels in 127 consecutive young adults with ischemic stroke. *Acta Neurol Scand* 1998; 98: 124–7.

53 Kohler J, Kasper J, Witt I, von Reuten GM. Ischemic stroke due to protein C deficiency. *Stroke* 1990; 50: 361–2.

54 Israels SJ, Seshia SS. Childhood stroke associated with protein C or S deficiency. *J Pediatr* 1987; 111: 562–4.

55 Sacco RL, Owen J, Mohr JP, Tatemichi TK, Grossman BA. Free protein S deficiency: a possible association with cerebrovascular occlusion. *Stroke* 1989; 20: 1657.

56 Mayer SA, Sacco RL, Hurlet-Jensen A, Shi T, Mohr JP. Free protein S deficiency in acute ischemic stroke: a case control study. *Stroke* 1993; 24: 224–7.

57 Ueyama H, Hashimoto Y, Uchino M *et al.* Progressing ischemic stroke in a homozygote with variant antithrombin III. *Stroke* 1989; 20: 815–8.

58 Ernerudh J, Olsson JE, von Schenck H. Antithrombin III deficiency in ischemic stroke. *Stroke* 1990; 21: 967.

59 Shinmyozu K, Ohkatsu Y, Maruyama Y, Osame M, Igate A. A case of congenital antithrombin III deficiency complicated by an internal carotid artery occlusion. *Clin Neurol* 1986; 26: 162–5.

60 Vomberg PP, Breederveld C, Fleury P, Arts WFM. Cerebral thromboembolism due to antithrombin III deficiency in two children. *Neuropediatrics* 1987; 18: 42–4.

61 Verro P, Levine S, Tietjen GE. Cerebrovascular ischemic events with high positive anticardiolipin antibodies. *Stroke* 1998; 29: 2245–53.

62 Levine SR, Kim S, Deegan MJ, Welch KMA. Ischemic stroke associated with anticardiolipin antibodies. *Stroke* 1987; 18: 1101–6.

63 Levine SR, Welch KMA. Cerebrovascular ischemia associated with lupus anticoagulant. *Stroke* 1987; 18: 257–63.

64 Freyssinet JM, Cazenave JP. Lupus-like anticoagulants, modulation of the protein C pathway and thrombosis. *Thromb Haemost* 1987; 58: 679–81.

65 Galli M, Finazzi G, Norbis F, Marziali S, Marchioli R. The risk of thrombosis in patients with lupus anticoagulants is predicted by their specific coagulation profile. *Thromb Haemost* 1999; 81: 695–700.

66 Tanne D, D'Olhaberriague L, Schultz LR, Salowich-Palm L, Sawaya KL, Levine SR. Anticardiolipin antibodies and their associations with cerebrovascular risk factors. *Neurology* 1999; 52: 1368–73.

67 Antiphospholipid Antibodies Stroke Study Group. Anticardiolipin antibodies and the risk of recurrent thrombo-occlusive events and death. *Neurology* 1997; 48: 91–4.

68 Ellis MH, Kesler A, Friedman Z, Drucker I, Radnai Y, Kott E. Value of prothrombin fragment 1.2 in the diagnosis of stroke in young patients with antiphospholipid antibodies. *Clin Appl Thromb Hemost* 2000; 6: 61–4.

69 Macchi L, Rispal P, Clofent-Sanchez G *et al*. Antiplatelet antibodies in patients with systemic lupus erythematosus and the primary antiphospholipid antibody syndrome: their relationship with the observed thrombocytopenia. *Br J Hematol* 1997; 98: 336–41.

70 Levine SR, Brey RL, Tilley BC *et al*. Antiphospholipid antibodies and subseqent thrombo-occlusive events in patients with ischemic stroke. *JAMA* 2004; 291(5): 576–84.

71 Petri M. Treatment of the antiphospholipid antibody syndrome: progress in the last five years? *Curr Rheumatol Rep* 2000; 2: 256–61.

72 Carter AM, Catto AJ, Grant PJ. Determinants of tPA antigen and associations with coronary artery disease and acute cerebrovascular disease. *Thromb Haemost* 1998; 80: 632–6.

73 Margaglione M, Di Minno G, Grandone E *et al*. Abnormally high circulation levels of tissue plasminogen activator and plasminogen activator inhibitor-1 in patients with a history of ischemic stroke. *Arterioscler Thromb* 1994; 14: 1741–5.

74 Ridker PM, Hennekens CH, Stampfer MJ, Manson JE, Vaughan DE. Prospective study of endogenous tissue plasminogen activator and risk of stroke. *Lancet* 1994; 343: 940–3.

75 Marcucci R, Prisco D, Brunelli T *et al*. Tissue factor and homocysteine levels in ischemic heart disease are associated with angiographically documented clinical recurrences after coronary angioplasty. *Thromb Haemost* 2000; 83: 826–32.

76 Al-Obaidi MK, Philippou H, Stubbs PJ *et al*. Relationships between homocysteine, factor VIIa, and thrombin generation in acute coronary syndromes. *Circulation* 2000; 101: 372–7.

77 MacCullum PK, Cooper JA, Martin J, Howarth DJ, Meade TW, Miller GJ. Haemostatic and lipid determinants of prothrombin fragment F1.2 and D-dimer in plasma. *Thromb Haemost* 2000; 83: 421–6.

78 Kyrle PA, Stumpflen A, Hirschl M *et al*. Levels of prothrombin fragment F1+2 in patients with hyperhomocysteinemia and a history of venous thromboembolism. *Thromb Haemost* 1997; 78: 1327.

79 Hajjar KA, Mauri L, Jacovina AT *et al*. Tissue plasminogen activator binding to the annexin II tail domain. Direct modulation by homocysteine. *J Biol Chem* 1998; 273: 9987–93.

80 Kristensen B, Malm J, Nilsson TK *et al*. Hyperhomocysteinemia and hypofibrinolysis in young adults with ischemic stroke. *Stroke* 1999; 30: 974.

81 Frosst P, Blom HJ, Milos R *et al*. A candidate genetic risk factor for vascular disease: a common mutation in methylenetetrahydrofolate reductase. *Nat Genet* 1995; 10: 111.

82 Kang SS, Wong PWK, Zhou J *et al*. Thermolabile methylenetetrahydrofolate reductase in patients with coronary artery disease. *Metabolism* 1988; 37: 611.

83 Kang S-S, Wong PWK, Susmano J, Sora J, Norusis M, Ruggie N. Thermolabile methylenetetrahydrofolate reductase: an inherited risk factor for coronary disease. *Am J Hum Genet* 1991; 48: 536.

84 Jacques PF, Bostom AG, Williams RR *et al*. Relation between folate status, a common mutation in methylenetetrahydrofolate reductase, and plasma homocysteine concentrations. *Circulation* 1996; 93: 7.

85 Rozen R. Molecular genetic aspects of hyperhomocysteinemia and its relation to folic acid. *Clin Invest Med* 1996; 19: 171.

86 Rozen R. Genetic predisposition to hyperhomocysteinemia: deficiency of methylenetetrahydrofolate reductase (MTHFR). *Thromb Haemost* 1997; 78: 523.

87 Harmon DL, Woodside JV, Yarnell JWG *et al*. The common thermolabile variant of methylenetetrahydrofolate reductase is a major determinant of mild hyperhomocysteinemia. *Q J Med* 1996; 89: 571.

88 De Franchis R, Mancini FP, D'Angelo A *et al*. Elevated total plasma homocysteine and 677C T mutation of the 5,10-methylenetetrahydrofolate reductase gene in thrombotic vascular disease. *Am J Hum Genet* 1996; 59: 262.

89 Christensen B, Frosst P, Lussier-Cacan S *et al*. Correlation of a common mutation in the methylenetetrahydrofolate reductase (MTHFR) gene with plasma homocysteine in patients with premature coronary artery disease. *Arterioscler Thromb Vasc Biol* 1997; 17: 569.

90 Harmon DL, Doyle RM, Meleady R *et al.* Genetic analysis of the thermolabile variant of 5, 10-methylenetetrahydrofolate reductase as a risk factor for ischemic stroke. *Arterioscler Thromb Vasc Biol* 1999; 19: 208.

91 Soriente L, Coppola A, Madonna P *et al.* Homozygous C677T mutation of the 5,10 methylenetetrahydrofolate reductase gene and hyperhomocysteinemia in Italian patients with a history of early onset ischemic stroke. *Stroke* 1998; 29: 869.

92 Morita H, Kurihara H, Tsubaki S *et al.* Methylenetetrahydrofolate reductase gene polymorphism and ischemic stroke in Japanese. *Arterioscler Thromb Vasc Biol* 1998; 18: 1465.

93 Brattstrom L, Lindgren A, Israelsson B *et al.* Hyperhomocysteinemia in stroke: prevalence, causes and relationships to type of stroke and stroke risk factors. *Eur J Clin Invest* 1992; 22: 214.

94 Eikelbloom JW, Hankey GJ, Anand SS *et al.* Association between high homocysteine and ischemic stroke due to large and small artery disease but not other etiologic subtypes of ischemic stroke. *Stroke* 2000; 31: 1069.

95 Kelly PJ, Furie KL, Kistler JP, Thornell B, Mandell R, Shih VE. Cystathionine beta-synthase (CBS) mutation causing severe hyperhomocysteinemia, carotid artery thrombosis, and embolic cerebral infarction: a case report and family study. *Ann Neurol* 2000; 48: 424 (Abstract).

96 Kario K, Matsuo T, Kobayashi H, Asada R, Matsuo M. 'Silent' cerebral infarction is associated with hypercoagulability, endothelial cell damage, and high Lp(a) levels in elderly Japanese. *Arterioscler Thromb Vasc Biol* 1996; 16: 734.

97 Catto AJ, Carter AM, Barrett JH, Bamford J, Rice PJ, Grant PJ. von Willebrand factor and factor VIII:C in acute cerebrovascular disease—relationship to stroke subtype and mortality. *Thromb Haemost* 1997; 77: 1104–8.

98 Blann AD, Miller JP, McCollum CN. Von Willebrand factor and soluble E-selectin in the prediction of cardiovascular disease progression in hyperlipidaemia. *Atherosclerosis* 1997; 132: 151–6.

99 Keightly AM, Lam M, Brady JN, Cameron C, Lillicrap D. Variation at the von Wlillebrand factor (vWF) gene locus is associated with plasma vWF:Ag levels: identification of three novel single nucleotide polymorphisms in the vWF gene promoter. *Blood* 1999; 93: 4277.

100 Harvey PJ, Keightly AM, Lam M, Cameron C, Lillicrap D. A single nucleotide polymorphism at nucleotide −1793 in the von Willebrand factor (VWF) regulatory region is associated with plasma VWF:Ag levels. *Br J Hematol* 2000; 109: 349.

101 Lacquemant C, Gaucher C, Delmore C *et al.* Association between high von Willebrand factor levels and the Thr789Ala vWF gene polymorphism but not with nephropathy in type I diabetes. *Kidney Int* 2000; 57: 1437.

102 Kant JA, Furnace AJ, Saxe D, Simon MI, McBride OW, Crabtree GR. Evolution and organization of the fibrinogen locus on chromosome 4: gene duplication accompanied by transcription and inversion. *Proc Natl Acad Sci USA* 1985; 82: 2234.

103 Nishiuma S, Kario K, Yakushijin K *et al.* Genetic variation in the promoter region of the beta-fibrinogen gene is associated with ischemic stroke in a Japanese population. *Blood Coagul Fibrinolysis* 1998; 9: 373.

104 Schmidt H, Schmidt R, Niedkerkorn K *et al.* Beta-fibrinogen gene polymorphism (C148→T) is associated with carotid atherosclerosis. Results of the Austrian stroke prevention study. *Arterioscler Thromb Vasc Biol* 1998; 18: 487.

105 Tyjaerg-Hansen A, Agerholm-Larsen B, Humphries SE, Abildgaard S, Schnohr P, Nordestgaard BG. A common mutation (G455A) in the beta-fibrinogen promoter is an independent predictor of plasma fibrinogen, but not of ischemic heart disease: a study of 9,127 individuals based on the Copenhagen City Heart Study. *J Clin Invest* 1997; 99: 3034.

106 Hiramoto M, Yoshida H, Imaizumi T, Yoshimizu N. A mutation in plasma platelet-activating factor acetylhydrolase (Val 279->Phe) is a genetic risk factor for stroke. *Stroke* 1997; 28: 2417.

107 Wagner KR, Giles WH, Johnson CJ *et al.* Platelet glycoprotein receptor IIIa polymorphism P1A2 and ischemic stroke risk. *Stroke* 1998; 29: 581.

108 Carter AM, Catto AJ, Grant PJ. Platelet GP IIIa PI A and GP Ib variable number tandem repeat polymorphisms and markers of platelet activation in acute stroke. *Arterioscler Thromb Vasc Biol* 1998; 18: 1124.

109 Ridker PM, Hennekens CH, Miletich JP. G20210A mutation in prothrombin gene and risk of myocardial infarction, stroke, and venous thrombosis in a large cohort of US men. *Circulation* 1999; 99: 999.

110 Gardemann A, Arsic T, Katz N *et al.* The factor II G20210A and factor V G1691A gene transitions and coronary artery disease. *Thromb Haemost* 1999; 81: 208–13.

111 Alhenc-Gelas M, Nicaud V, van Gandrille S *et al.* The factor V gene A4070G mutation and risk of venous thromboembolism. *Thromb Haemost* 1999; 81: 193.

112 Emmerich J, Alhenc-Gelas M, Aillaud M *et al.* Clinical features in 36 patients homozygous for the ARG 506→GLN factor V mutation. *Thromb Haemost* 1997; 77: 620–3.

113 de Stefano V, Martinelli I, Mannucci PM *et al.* The risk of recurrent deep venous thrombosis among heterozygous carriers of both factor V Leiden and the G20210A prothrombin mutation. *N Engl J Med* 1999; 341: 801.

114 Lindmarker P, Schulman S, Sten-Linder M *et al.* The risk of recurrent venous thromboembolism in carriers and noncarriers of the G1691A allele in the coagulation factor V gene and the G20210A allele in the prothrombin gene. *Thromb Haemost* 1999; 81: 684.

115 Alhen-Gelas M, Arnaud E, Nicaud V *et al.* Venous thromboembolic disease and the prothrombin, methylenetetrahydrofoalte reductase and factor V genes. *Thromb Haemost* 1999; 81: 506.

116 Tirado I, Mateo J, Oliver A *et al.* Contribution of the prothrombin 20210A allele and the Factor V Leiden as additional genetic risk factors in thrombophilic families with other hemostatic deficiencies. *Thromb Haemost* 1999; (Suppl.) (Abstract).

117 Ridker PM, Glynn RJ, Miletich JP, Goldhaber SZ, Stampfer MJ, Hennekens CH. Age-specific incidence rates of venous thromboembolism among heterozygous carriers of factor V Leiden mutation. *Ann Intern Med* 1997; 126: 528.

118 Rosendaal FR, Siscovick DS, Schwartz SM, Psaty BM, Raghunathan TE, Vos HL. A common prothrombin variant (20210G→A) increases the risk of myocardial infarction in young women. *Blood* 1997; 90: 1747.

119 Arruda VR, Siquiera Chiaparini LC, Coelho OR. Prevalence of the prothrombin gene variant 20210G→A among patients with myocardial infarction. *Cardiovascular Res* 1998; 37: 42.

120 Lopez Y, Paloma MJ, Rifon J, Cuesta B, Paramo JA. Measurement of prothrombotic markers in the assessment of acquired hypercoagulable states. *Thromb Res* 1999; 93: 71–8.

121 Gouin-Thibault I, Achkar A, Samama MM. The thrombophilic state in cancer patients. *Acta Haematol* 2001; 106: 33–42.

122 Gale AJ, Gordon SG. Update on tumor cell procoagulant factors. *Acta Haematol* 2001; 106: 25–32.

123 Falanga A, Rickles FR. Pathophysiology of the thrombophilic state in the cancer patient. *Sem Thromb Hemost* 1999; 25: 173–82.

124 Gouin-Thibault I, Samama MM. Laboratory diagnosis of the thrombophilic state in cancer patients. *Semin Thromb Hemost* 1999; 25: 167–72.

125 Mannucci PM. Markers of hypercoagulability in cancer patients. *Haemostasis* 1997; 27 (Suppl. 1): 25–31.

126 Chaturvedi S, Ansell J, Recht L. Should cerebral ischemic events be considered a manifestation of hypercoagulability? *Stroke* 1994; 25: 1215–8.

PART III

Medical Therapy

Antiplatelet Therapy

Michael J. Schneck

Introduction

Antiplatelet therapy represents the first-line therapy for medical prevention of recurrent stroke following either a stroke or transient ischemia attack (TIA). It is the preferred agent for strokes and TIAs as a result of atherothrombotic disease and is an option for those patients who, by the nature of their cerebrovascular event, would be candidates for anticoagulation but cannot be anticoagulated because of other medical contraindications. Indeed, anticoagulation still plays a role in stroke prevention [1]. Data from the WARSS and SPIRIT studies would suggest, however, that the role of anticoagulation in stroke prevention should be restricted to defined indications such as cardioembolic strokes and hypercoaguable states [1–3]. For all other indications the 'antiplatelet agents' are preferred.

Aspirin remains the paradigm in support of evidence for antiplatelet therapy for stroke prevention following TIAs or ischemic stroke [4]. Over the past decade, however, several new agents have been developed that offer a greater opportunity for efficacy with relatively good side-effect profiles though at a higher expense to the individual. The general indications for these antiplatelet agents are similar with the relative merit of each agent a subject of debate. It should be noted here that many of the clinical trials to evaluate antiplatelet agents in prevention of recurrent cerebral ischemia were performed for patients who had clinically defined stroke. Only a few of the trials included patients with TIAs along with stroke patients or restricted enrollment to patients with transient cerebral ischemia. Nevertheless, it is appropriate to discuss some of these stroke trials for prevention of recurrent cerebral ischemic events in this chapter since the underlying etiology of an incident transient ischemic event or completed stroke are often similar and clinical strategies for prevention should follow the same pattern regardless of whether the ischemic event results in a completed infarct. Currently, there are four antiplatelet drugs available for use in North America for patients with cerebral ischemia: aspirin, ticlopidine, clopidogrel, and sustained-release dipyridamole (DP) (used in combination with low-dose aspirin). Although each of these agents ultimately antagonizes platelet aggregation as their primary mechanism for prevention of thrombus, they have different mechanisms and side-effect profiles.

Aspirin

Aspirin is the common name for acetylsalicylic acid (ASA). It was originally designed as a synthetic pain reliever at the turn of the century because of the recognized properties of its natural analog, salicin, derived from willow bark [4–7]. Aspirin was first suggested, however, as a prophylactic agent for prevention of stroke and myocardial infarction (MI) at mid century but its role in cardiovascular prophylaxis was not widely accepted for another two to three decades when its mechanism became better understood [7,8]. As elucidated, by John Vane, both the anti-inflammatory and antiplatelet activities of aspirin occur because of irreversible inhibition of cyclooxygenase activity [6,9]. Small doses of aspirin (up to 100 mg) can irreversibly block platelet cyclooxygenase with rapid onset of action and maximal peak effect within approximately 20 min. Blockade of cyclooxygenase then results in reduced synthesis of thromboxane A_2 that is necessary for both platelet activation and vasoconstriction. Because platelets cannot synthesize new protein, the resulting inhibition persists through the 7–10-day life span of the affected platelets and though platelet adhesion is not affected, aggregation is impaired clinically manifested as a prolonged bleeding time.

Paradoxically, aspirin at higher doses may actually increase the risk of thrombus formation. Vascular endothelium produces the proaggregant thromboxane A_2. In addition, however, prostaglandin (PGI_2) (prostacyclin) is also produced and this compound inhibits platelet aggregation and vasodilatation. There has been some suggestion, therefore based on animal models and clinical trials, that at higher doses, via an effect on the endothelial wall, aspirin may actually predispose patients to thrombosis [4,10,11].

Many patients cannot tolerate aspirin. The drug is contraindicated for patients with known hypersensitivity or allergic reactions to both salicylates or other nonsteroidal anti-inflammatory drugs (NSAIDs). In particular, some patients with a history of asthma may have associated aspirin hypersensitivity reactions [12]. Up to 20% of patients with asthma may have intolerance to aspirin or NSAIDs. Many patients will experience minor gastrointestinal (GI) discomfort related to aspirin therapy. Coated aspirin or lower dose aspirin may ameliorate the minor GI side-effects but do not eliminate the risk of GI bleeding [13–15]. GI bleeding can be a significant problem for stroke patients receiving aspirin, with an estimated 2–3% rate of bleeding for these patients which represents an approximately two- to three-fold increase in risk [13–16].

There have been many prospective randomized trials testing the efficacy of ASA vs. placebo for patients at high risk of ischemic stroke. In 1977, Fields and colleagues reported on 178 patients with hemispheric TIAs who were not referred for carotid endarterectomy (the selection of patients for surgical or medical treatment was not done on a randomized basis) [17]. Patients were treated with 650 mg ASA twice daily or placebo. They found that the number of unfavorable outcomes (death, cerebral or retinal infarction, or failure to reduce the number of TIAs in a 3-month period) was significantly reduced at 6 months in the ASA-treated group. However, no difference was found in the individual endpoints of ischemic stroke, retinal infarction, or death. Subsequently, in one of many of his landmark trials, Barnett and colleagues demonstrated that, for patients with 'threatened stroke' randomized to aspirin, sulfinpyrazone, a combination of these two drugs, or placebo, men on aspirin had a significant reduction in risk of cerebrovascular events [18]. Sulfinpyrazone conveyed no additional risk reduction. In this Canadian Cooperative Study (CCS) of 585 patients who had a cerebral or retinal TIA, aspirin reduced the risk of recurrent TIA, stroke or death by 19% ($P < 0.05$) and stroke or death by 31% ($P < 0.05$). No benefit was seen in risk reduction for women taking aspirin but, as with most of the early antiplatelet studies, the number of female subjects enrolled was too few to draw any definitive conclusion.

Three other important landmark aspirin trials of patients with TIA that were performed over 15 years ago compared different doses of aspirin. The United Kingdom Transient Ischemic Attack (UK-TIA) trial randomized 2435 patients with minor stroke or TIA in the precomputed tomography era to either 600 mg of aspirin twice daily (high dose), 300 mg of aspirin once daily (medium dose), or placebo [19,20]. Overall, aspirin provided a 15% odds reduction in preventing stroke, MI or vascular death compared with placebo. The authors noted no difference in risk reduction between medium and high-dose aspirin, but there was a significant decrease in GI side-effects. The Swedish Aspirin Low dose Trial (SALT) then demonstrated that low-dose aspirin (75 mg) vs. placebo also conveyed a similar risk reduction of 18% for prevention of stroke or death ($P = 0.02$) in 1360 patients with TIA or minor stroke [21]. The third study, the Dutch TIA trial, compared very low-dose aspirin (30 mg daily) with medium-dose aspirin (283 mg daily) for patients with minor stroke or TIA [10]. The authors commented on the rationale for their trial by observing that the first Antiplatelet Trialists Collaboration (ATC) showed medium to high-dose (300–1500 mg daily) aspirin was effective in reducing the risk of recurrent vascular events [22]. However, low-dose aspirin might be even more effective because of the observation of different effects of low-dose aspirin on inhibition of thromboxane A_2-induced platelet aggregation without affecting the aforementioned endothelial prostacyclin-induced effects [10]. This trial found minimal differences between very low-dose and medium-dose aspirin. Close to 15% of patients on low-dose aspirin had a stroke, MI or death from vascular causes, whereas 15.2% on the medium-dose regimen had a recurrent event. However, there were fewer adverse events on low-dose aspirin including fewer GI side-effects and bleeding complications. The authors concluded that very low-dose aspirin is as effective as medium-dose aspirin for patients with TIA or stroke for prevention of recurrent stroke.

Despite the above data, many North American neurologists had been reluctant to utilize lower doses of aspirin. From *in vitro* studies, Helgason *et al.* had suggested that certain patients responded better to high vs. low-dose aspirin [23]. Data from the Canadian Cooperative Study and a *post hoc* analysis from the North American Symptomatic Carotid Endarterectomy Trial (NASCET) were also very persuasive in supporting the use of higher dose aspirin [14,18,24]. The NASCET trial had suggested that patients had fewer recurrent strokes on higher dose aspirin (650–1300 mg daily) vs. low or medium-dose aspirin (81–350 mg daily). A subsequent randomized trial of low vs. high-dose aspirin following carotid endarterectomy failed to support the NASCET *post hoc* analysis, however. In fact, the opposite was the case, as the Aspirin and Carotid Endarterectomy (ACE) trial found that low-dose aspirin was associated with fewer postoperative vascular events [25]. The ACE trial has been frequently used as a justification for low-dose aspirin in stroke prevention. There are caveats about this trial that need to be raised, however. Among these are that the low-dose regimen in the ACE trial should really be considered as a justification for 'medium-dose' aspirin. Also, the extrapolation of data from a short-term postendarterectomy trial to long-term cerebrovascular prophylaxis following an incident TIA must be viewed with caution.

The most recent trial incorporating patients with minor stroke or TIA is the European Stroke Prevention Study 2 (ESPS2) [26]. This trial is discussed in further detail in the dipyridamole section below and is a large multicentre randomized comparison of sustained-release DP or low-dose aspirin (50 mg daily) singly or in combination vs. placebo. For the patients on aspirin only, the relative risk reduction was 18% for nonfatal stroke or death. This finding is in line with prior aspirin TIA trials using both a high or low-dose regimen.

In general, the benefits of aspirin reported in all of the above-described trials are consistent with the large meta-analyses presented in the Aspirin Trialists' Collaboration [22,27]. By the 1994 ATC report, 145 trials of antiplatelet therapy vs. control, in approximately 70 000 high-risk and 30 000 low-risk patients, were analyzed. Eighteen of the trials enrolled stroke or TIA patients for a total of close to 12 000 subjects with a mean of approximately 650 patients per study. By comparison, most of the 'modern' individual cerebrovascular trials have enrolled between five and 10 times the number of subjects. The results of the 1994 ATC suggest an overall odds reduction of approximately 20–25% in stroke/TIA or other vascular events. For patients with an incident stroke or TIA, there was a 23% odds reduction in nonfatal stroke but there was no significant reduction in fatal stroke risk.

Subsequent meta-analyses encompassing the modern trials have confirmed the findings of the ATC and have reported a significant odds reduction of approximately 15% for the prevention of stroke as well as prevention of a composite vascular disease endpoint compared with placebo [4,28–31]. There appeared to be no differences in risk reduction between low, medium or high-dose aspirin regimens in any of the meta-analyses.

Thienopyridine derivatives

As thienopyridine derivatives, both ticlopidine and clopidogrel have a similar mechanism of action [4,9,11,32]. The two agents are chemically very similar, with clopidogrel differing only by the addition of an acetate moiety on the benzyl ring of ticlopidine. These agents inhibit platelet aggregation through ADP-induced modification of the GPII/IIIa glycoprotein receptor on the platelet membrane that is critical in binding platelets to fibrinogen during platelet activation. Both agents require metabolism in the liver for their antiaggregant activity and then irreversibly inhibit platelet aggregation. Ticlopidine inhibits platelet function within 24–48 h of administration that peaks at 3–7 days. The standard daily dose is 250 mg twice daily, though some patients who experience GI side-effects may be tried on 250 mg once daily. Compared with ticlopidine, clopidogrel displays dose-related inhibition of platelet aggregation with the recommended 75-mg once-daily dose being equivalent to 250 mg twice daily of ticlopidine. For clopidogrel the onset of action is more rapid at about 2 h, although peak inhibition occurs with a similar time-course to ticlopidine.

The major limitation of ticlopidine is its side-effect profile [29,32–35]. GI side-effects of diarrhea, dyspepsia and nausea are fairly common and are frequent reasons for discontinuation of ticlopidine. Rash is also a common side-effect. In addition, ticlopidine has two serious adverse hematological effects. These are neutropenia and thrombotic thrombocytopenic purpura (TTP). Serious, though reversible, neutropenia occurs in 0.9% of all patients on ticlopidine. TTP, though less common, is estimated to occur in one of every 5000 ticlopidine users [36]. Because of the risk of these serious adverse events, complete blood count monitoring is required every 2 weeks for the first 3 months of ticlopidine use with annual blood counts thereafter. Thus, as a result of these side-effects, ticlopidine is no longer considered a 'first-line antiplatelet agent' [29].

Overall, clopidogrel is a much safer drug than ticlopidine, with a safety profile similar to that of aspirin [4,11,29,32]. GI side-effects are, in fact, relatively uncommon and neutropenia does not appear to be an issue with this agent. Athough it is rare and much less common than with ticlopidine, there is some concern, however, about TTP with this agent [37]. Interestingly, the clopidogrel-associated TTP appears to occur early in the course of therapy, whereas ticlopidine-induced TTP can occur later in the course of therapy [37]. No routine blood monitoring is needed with clopidogrel, although the clinician should keep the possibility of TTP in mind if there are suggestive symptoms.

The rationale for the use of the thienopyridines in either stroke or TIA was established at the beginning of the last decade. At that time, the Canadian American Ticlopidine Study (CATS) and the Ticlopidine Aspirin Stroke Study (TASS) were published [33,38,39]. The CATS study compared ticlopidine with placebo in 1053 patients with completed ischemic stroke with mean follow-up of 2 years and showed significant relative risk reduction (RRR) of 23% ($P = 0.02$) in the combined endpoint of stroke, MI or vascular death (RRR 23%, $P = 0.02$) [38]. Of greater relevance to this discussion, the TASS study looked at 3069 patients enrolled within 3 months of a TIA or minor stroke with mean follow-up of 3.4 years with endpoints of stroke and stroke or death compared with high-dose aspirin (1300 mg/daily) [33]. The TASS study found a RRR of 21% ($P = 0.024$) in favor of ticlopidine for nonfatal stroke and 12% RRR ($P = 0.048$) in favor of ticlopidine for stroke or death. Because of the previously mentioned predominantly GI side-effects, there was a significant drop-out rate in TASS. A subgroup efficacy analysis, however, suggested that for those patients who were able to stay in the trial until the end of the study or until a stroke endpoint was reached, there was an even greater RRR of 27% in favor of ticlopidine ($P = 0.011$). Additional *post hoc* analyses had suggested that non-whites, women, patients with vertebrobasilar symptoms, patients whose initial event occurred on other antithrombotic agents such as aspirin, and patients without high-grade carotid stenosis were thought possibly to derive greater risk reduction with ticlopidine [40]. In particular, African-Americans were thought to derive particular benefit with ticlopidine in the TASS study with a more favorable safety profile as well [41]. Therefore in 1995, the African American Antiplatelet Stroke Prevention Study (AAASPS) was initiated and enrollment was recently completed [42]. Though a study of patients with completed stroke rather than TIA, this study of ticlopidine vs. moderate-dose aspirin may cause resurgence in the use of ticlopidine if a favorable risk–benefit profile is demonstrable.

Clopidogrel was actually designed as a specific replacement for ticlopidine because of the latter agent's adverse safety profile. There are, however, limited data about the use of clopidogrel for patients who have sustained a TIA. The use of clopidogrel in this population must be extrapolated from the Clopidogrel vs. ASA in Patients at Risk of Ischemic Events (CAPRIE) [43]. This was a large multicenter randomized trial of patients with atherosclerotic vascular disease who were randomized to either clopidogrel or medium dose (325 mg) of aspirin. A total of 19 185 patients with MIs, peripheral vascular disease or stroke were enrolled up to 6 months after the initial event. There were 6431 patients with ischemic strokes and 40% of these strokes were described as lacunar infarcts. For the CAPRIE study, primary endpoint being reduction of stroke, MI, or vascular death, there was an absolute risk reduction of 0.5% per year with a RRR of 8.7% ($P = 0.043$) in favor of clopidogrel for all subjects enrolled. When a secondary analysis was performed restricted only to the 6431 stroke patients enrolled in CAPRIE, there was an absolute risk reduction of 0.6% per year for the primary endpoint with a RRR of 7.3% that was not, however, statistically significant [28,34]. The absolute risk reduction of stroke alone for these stroke patients was also not significant at 0.5% annually. Paradoxically, only the patients entering the study with peripheral arterial disease sustained a large benefit from clopidogrel compared with aspirin. However, an important caveat of all these subgroup analyses was that the study was designed with power to discover a difference only for the primary endpoint for all patients enrolled rather than for the individual cerebrovascular, cardiac, or peripheral vascular subgroups.

Though currently there are no other supporting data regarding the use of clopidogrel in patients with either stroke or TIA, there is some corroborating information from a series of trials in patients with coronary heart disease, some of which have been recently published [44,45]. These trials (CLASSICS, CURE, CREDO and COMMIT) would suggest that the combination of clopidogrel and aspirin is more effective than aspirin alone in patients following placement of coronary stents, patients with unstable angina, or MI. Based on these cardiovascular trials, the current trend is toward combination antiplatelet therapy with the thienopyridines. The CURE (Clopidogrel in Unstable Angina to Prevent Recurrent Events) study in patients with unstable angina or non-Q wave MI reported that the combination of clopidogrel and aspirin provided a 20% RRR in fatal and nonfatal cardiovascular events (including stroke and MI) compared with aspirin alone ($P = 0.001$) with an absolute risk reduction of 2.1% [46]. Given the 38% relative excess rate of bleeding complications seen with combination therapy in CURE, some have argued, however, that the CURE results may not be applicable to patients with cerebrovascular disease [47]. The MATCH (Management of Atherothrombosis with Clopidogrel in High-risk Patients with Recent Transient Ischaemic Attack or Ischaemic Stroke) study will provide similar data in over 7000 patients with cerebrovascular disease on combination therapy vs. clopidogrel alone and may give a better perspective about the appropriate role for clopidogrel and for combination therapy in patients with TIAs [44]. Another study, the Prevention of Small Subcortical Strokes study, is planned to begin in 2003 and this trial will evaluate aspirin vs. aspirin and clopidogrel in patients with lacunar stroke, as well as testing two different blood pressure regimens.

Dipyridamole

Antithrombotic effects of DP are mediated through multiple pathways by increases in platelet cyclic AMP levels and blockade of adenosine uptake, as well as direct potentiation of prostacyclin synthesis in both the platelets and vascular endothelium with potentiation of prostacyclin-induced antiplatelet aggregation [11,48]. This results in a reversible inhibition of platelet thrombus aggregants, though there is no effect on bleeding times or *in vitro* platelet aggregation. Immediate-release DP has a rapid onset of action, with peak concentrations developing within approximately 1 h, but a trough below which therapeutic action is detected occurs within 4–6 h of the first dose. As a result, immediate-release DP requires four to six times a day dosing. The development of a sustained-release preparation has allowed for twice daily dosing with maintenance of adequate trough levels for optimal antiplatelet effect. The sustained-release preparation is available in Europe singly or in combination with aspirin. In the USA, only the combination agent of aspirin (25 mg) and sustained-release DP (200 mg) is Food and Drug Administration (FDA) approved as a twice-daily regimen for prevention of stroke for patients with stroke or TIA.

The side-effect profile of this combination therapy reflects the individual components, with no significant increase in side-effects due to combination therapy above and beyond those attributable to either aspirin or DP alone [49]. Headache is probably the largest barrier to use of this agent and relates to the vasodilatator effects of DP. There was an excess of 15.3% of subjects complaining of headache ($P < 0.001$) who received sustained-release DP alone or in combination in the second European Stroke Prevention Study (ESPS2) with a drop-out rate of 6% attributable to headache on DP in this study. Headache seemed to occur in the early phase of treatment and subjects reported that headache appeared to wear off over time. Diarrhea ($P < 0.001$) and vomiting ($P = 0.046$) were the other side-effects attributable to DP. The incidence of GI or other bleeding complications was, however, mainly reflective of the aspirin treatment and 65% of the subjects with some form of bleeding complication had been on aspirin combination or monotherapy. Only 14% of the bleeding complications in ESPS2 were deemed to be severe or fatal and close to 80% of those subjects had been on aspirin (singly or in combination).

The use of DP in stroke prevention actually dates back, similar to aspirin, over 30 years. When the data for all vascular events were pooled in the Antiplatelet Trialists meta-analyses, DP had a 23% odds reduction for stroke, MI, or vascular death compared with placebo in 10 reported trials [22,27]. There was also a 28% odds reduction for this combined endpoint of stroke, MI, and vascular death in the 34 trials comparing a combination of DP and aspirin with placebo. The AICLA and Toulouse TIA studies were two early studies of cerebrovascular disease that demonstrated a benefit of immediate release DP and aspirin vs. placebo for stroke prevention [26,30,48,50]. The largest of these studies was ESPS-1, published in 1987, that suggested a combination of high-dose aspirin and DP could provide a significant stroke risk reduction of 38% in patients with TIA or minor stroke [51]. Several small stroke or TIA studies in the 1970s and 1980s failed to show definitive efficacy for immediate-release DP (in combination with aspirin) vs. aspirin alone, however. High withdrawal rates and small sample sizes limited these early trials. Thus, the question of whether DP, alone or in combination with aspirin, had any real benefit remained unresolved until the second European Stroke Prevention Study (ESPS2).

ESPS2 was a double-blind placebo-controlled randomized trial with a factorial design comparing low-dose ASA alone (25 mg twice daily), DP alone (200 mg twice daily), a combination of ASA plus DP, or placebo with primary endpoints of stroke and death and secondary endpoints of stroke, MI, or vascular death in over 6600 patients [26,49,52,53]. Approximately one-quarter of the patients enrolled in this study had an atherothrombotic TIA. In ESPS2, the risk of stroke was reduced by 18% for ASA alone ($P = 0.013$), 16% for DP alone ($P = 0.039$) and 37% for the combination ($P < 0.001$) compared with placebo. There was a RRR for stroke of 23% favoring the combination compared with ASA alone ($P = 0.006$). The risk of stroke and/or death was reduced by 13.2% for ASA alone ($P = 0.016$), 15.4% for DP alone ($P = 0.015$) and 24.4% for the combination ($P < 0.001$).

The composite endpoint of stroke, MI, or sudden death was a prespecified secondary endpoint [53]. The risk reduction for this composite endpoint was 32.6% ($P < 0.001$) for combination therapy compared with placebo. Combination therapy was also more effective than aspirin alone with a RRR of 21.9% ($P = 0.003$) or DP alone with a RRR of 23.3% ($P = 0.01$), though much of the benefit seemed to be driven by the number of recurrent stroke events.

TIA and stroke or TIA were also prespecified secondary endpoints [26,53]. Stroke or TIA occurred in 1526 subjects and TIA only in 824 subjects and the combination therapy provided a 36% risk reduction that was highly significant ($P < 0.001$) compared with placebo and was equally significant compared with aspirin or DP monotherapy.

The conclusions of ESPS2 were therefore that combination of ASA plus ER-DP has the advantage of being more effective than ASA in preventing stroke in high-risk patients. When these results were pooled with the other DP/aspirin trials in cerebral vascular disease, a 25% reduction in the odds of nonfatal stroke and 18% reduction in the odds of all vascular events were reported [29]. The ESPS2 results were driven by the nonfatal stroke endpoints. As such, whether the benefits of this combination are applicable to patients at high risk of cardiac events and vascular death is unproven. Additionally, though the odds ratios described for the low-dose aspirin arm in ESPS2 are compatible with similar data for stroke patients reported by the Aspirin Trialists Collaboration, some concern remains, however, in the USA about whether the 50-mg daily dose of aspirin used in this trial is sufficient for patients with previous ischemic heart disease.

Comparative discussion of antiplatelet treatment options

There are no available trials that directly compare ticlopidine, clopidogrel, or sustained-release DP with each other. The relative benefits of any of these agents in prevention of recurrent stroke are typically a matter of 'expert opinion'. As noted earlier, even the dose of aspirin remains controversial. Traditionally, Europeans have used lower doses of aspirin than North American vascular neurologists, with many of the European vascular neurologists recommending aspirin doses as low as 30 mg/day [54]. Prior to the updated United States FDA recommendations, many North American vascular neurologists (including this author) would prescribe up to 1300 mg of aspirin per day with the typical approach being medium-dose aspirin (325 mg daily). As a result of the theoretical arguments that higher dose aspirin may actually promote thrombogenesis, the lack of clinical trial data to support the use of higher doses of aspirin despite the *in vitro* observation of 'aspirin nonresponders' at lower doses, and the increase in minor GI side-effects at higher doses, the aspirin wars must be declared in favor of the low-dose camp. With the current FDA prescribing guidelines for aspirin in prevention of recurrent stroke now in a lower range (50–325 mg daily), there is a greater acceptance of low-dose aspirin (typically 81 mg in the USA) [55]. However, an interesting paradox has seemingly arisen. Anecdotally, cardiologists in the past had prescribed 81 mg of aspirin daily for MI prevention but have recently shifted to 325 mg alone or in combination with other agents. Thus, from the cardiology perspective, where stroke neurologists had previously 'overdosed' their patients on aspirin, currently some stroke specialists are underdosing their patients.

This dilemma in part reflects this lack of direct comparison between varying doses of the different antiplatelet agents. As a result, there are attempts to make indirect comparisons based on interpretations from studies with different sample sizes, inclusion criteria and choice of endpoints that compared aspirin (with or without placebo) against the newer antiplatelet agents.

Advocates of the thienopyridines point out that atherosclerosis is a systemic vascular disease and the cause of death in most stroke patients is a cardiac event. They therefore argue that antiplatelet agents should reduce the risk of both stroke and MI [45]. The counter argument is that the rate of MI in the first 2 years post stroke is low [56]. Therefore, the most critical issue for patients with TIA or stroke is prevention of recurrent cerebrovascular disease, especially because of patient concerns about post-stroke disability [56,57]. This school of thought argues that prevention of coronary heart disease, while relevant, is most appropriately regarded as a secondary endpoint when attempting to make comparisons of clinical efficacy between drugs.

Tables 10.1, 10.2 and 10.3 illustrate the relative merits of each of the available antiplatelet agents in the USA. Based on the ACCP guidelines (January 2001), aspirin, clopidogrel and the combination of sustained-release DP are all acceptable first-line agents for stroke prevention [29]. The merits of aspirin rest primarily with its cost. Since aspirin is very inexpensive, many physicians will first use aspirin for patients who have experienced a TIA due to atherothrombotic disease or who have experienced a cardioembolic event but are not candidates for warfarin, if the patient has never been on any prior antiplatelet agent. Compared with

Table 10.1 List of available antiplatelet agents with cost and side-effect comparisons

	Mechanism	Side-effect profiles	Cost per month*
Aspirin	Inhibits cyclooxygenase	GI side-effects predominate	< $3 (< £1.70)
Ticlopidine	Inhibits platelet ADP receptor	Diarrhea, nausea, anorexia, neutropenia, TTP	$130.64 (£74.63)
Clopidogrel	Inhibits platelet ADP receptor	Similar to aspirin with less GI side-effects. Possible TTP	$96.44 (£55.09)
Aspirin and sustained-release dipyridamole	Mixed action (see text)	Headache, GI side-effects	$88.50 (£50.56)

*Based on figures from PriceProbe, 2000. GI, Gastrointestinal; TTP, thrombotic thrombocytic purpura.

Table 10.2 Relative comparisons of efficacy of thienopyridines and dipyridamole vs. aspirin for the endpoint of recurrent stroke in cerebrovascular disease patients

	Relative risk reduction	Absolute risk reduction	Numbers needed to treat
Ticlopidine* 500 mg/daily	21%	2.5	1 : 40
Clopidogrel† 75 mg/daily	8%	0.8	1 : 125
Aspirin and sustained release dipyridamole‡ 50/400 mg daily	23%	3.0	1 : 33

Data are derived from the TASS*, CAPRIE†, and ESPS2‡ trials.

Table 10.3 Relative comparisons of efficacy of thienopyridines and dipyridamole vs. aspirin for the endpoint of stroke, myocardial infarction or vascular death for patients with cerebrovascular disease

	Relative risk reduction	Absolute risk reduction	Numbers needed to treat
Ticlopidine* (500 mg daily)	9%	2.3	1 : 43
Clopidogrel (75 mg daily)	7.3%	1.0	1 : 100
Aspirin and sustained-release dipyridamole* (50/400 mg daily)	22%	3.6	1 : 28

*A secondary endpoint of the TASS and ESPS2 trials, respectively.

placebo, however, the RRR is only 15% for prevention of recurrent stroke. Furthermore, though the risk of significant GI bleeding is only about 1–2%, minor GI irritation is a frequent patient complaint. Therefore, clopidogrel and sustained-release DP are worthy of consideration even for patients with TIAs who have not previously been on aspirin.

The major advantage of clopidogrel compared with aspirin is the side-effect profile. There are significantly fewer GI side-effects and a somewhat lower risk of GI bleeding. This agent is particularly useful in those patients who are aspirin allergic or aspirin intolerant, as there does not seem to be any allergic cross-reactivity, and it is therefore the drug of choice in aspirin-intolerant patients. The dilemma for those who prescribe clopidogrel is that the RRR for stroke, MI or vascular death compared with aspirin was only about 7% for the over 6000 patients enrolled in the CAPRIE study who had a stroke as their initial entry event into that study, and this finding of itself was not statistically significant. Still, despite its significant expense and relatively lower benefit, overall this has been the most popular of the prescription antiplatelet agents (possibly because of its dual use for cardiac disease). In the year 2000, it was among the top 50 brand-name drugs by retail sales and top 100 drugs by number of prescriptions in the USA. In fact, there were more prescriptions for clopidogrel than prescription enteric-coated aspirin (which, however, is also available over the counter in the USA) [58]. Combination therapy using clopidogrel and either 81 mg or 325 mg of aspirin is also increasingly popular. Though there is no direct evidence to support this approach in patients with cerebrovascular disease, this author favors using clopidogrel in combination with aspirin as opposed to clopidogrel monotherapy because of the indirect evidence in extrapolation from the coronary disease trials and the ESPS2 observations that combination antiplatelet therapy is more effective than antiplatelet monotherapy. When clopidogrel is used in combination with aspirin, the 81-mg dose of aspirin is probably preferable to minimize bleeding complications.

Although ticlopidine was shown to have significant RRR compared with high-dose aspirin, its significantly greater side-effect profile including the high-risk complications of neutropenia and TTP and also the high cost of even the generic form of ticlopidine and the added cost and inconvenience of required blood testing, precluded its inclusion as a first-line antiplatelet agent in the ACCP guidelines. In addition to the potential hematological side-effects, the almost two-fold increased frequency of the so-called minor GI side-effects of diarrhea, nausea and anorexia as well as the risk of rash are real barriers to compliance with the use of ticlopidine. Starting at 250 mg once daily for the first week can minimize some of these side-effects, but they are still relatively frequent. The recent finding that ticlopidine was not superior to aspirin in the African American Antiplatelet Stroke Prevention Study also dampens enthusiasm for ticlopidine [59].

The last of the FDA-approved antiplatelet agents, sustained-released DP in combination with low-dose aspirin, is possibly the most effective of the antiplatelet therapies in stroke prevention according to the ACCP guidelines [29]. Furthermore, it is considered to have a side-effect profile deemed equally favorable with aspirin or clopidogrel, though this is based on indirect comparison of the clinical trials. Indeed, the risk of significant bleeding complications was no greater than low-dose aspirin in the ESPS2 trial. The major barriers to its widespread use are an increased risk of headache, the continued hesitancy of North American physicians toward low-dose aspirin, and cost to the individual patient. The headache, in particular, can be a significant limiting factor in the use of this agent, and though this side-effect often resolves within a few weeks of initiation of therapy, the symptom can be of such severity as to mandate immediate discontinuation. Prophylactic treatment with acetaminophen or starting with one capsule at bedtime can decrease the frequency of headache. Drug-related headache can be a significant concern for those patients with premorbid symptoms of migraine-type headache or who had their TIA or stroke onset accompanied by headache. However, based on a need-to-treat analysis, the combination of sustained-release DP and low-dose aspirin is highly cost-effective compared with aspirin for managed-care and other preferred formulary lists [60]. Using a need-to-treat ratio of 1 : 33 [with the annual cost of this drug per patient of approximately $1060 (£605)] for the prevention of recurrent cerebrovascular events and an assumed annual direct and indirect cost of stroke of approximately $50 000 (£28 550), there is a net gain in terms of cost per stroke averted. Therefore, for moderate to high-risk patients who have sustained a TIA, the sustained-release DP/aspirin combination is appropriate even if the patient has not previously been on aspirin alone.

Sustained-release DP without aspirin is not available for use in the USA and so patients who are aspirin intolerant cannot receive the sustained-release DP/aspirin drug. Immediate-release DP might be considered an option for those aspirin-intolerant patients. However, this preparation is not approved for stroke prevention in the USA and, in order to achieve an adequate therapeutic level, frequent multiple high daily doses would be necessary. In aspirin-intolerant patients, a thienopyridine is therefore indicated.

Conclusion

An antiplatelet regimen is the preferred medical therapy for patients with atherothrombotic cerebrovascular disease or for patients with cardioembolic stroke or TIA for whom anticoagulation is contraindicated. There are now a number of different options available and the choice of a specific drug depends on relative efficacy for cerebrovascular or cardiovascular prophylaxis vs. cost and potential for side-effects and tolerability by the individual patient.

Although data regarding therapy for patients who had a transient ischemic TIA are not available for clopidogrel, it is appropriate to extrapolate from the stroke data. There is no theoretical argument against the use of this agent in patients with TIAs, and in the future more information will be forthcoming about the role of clopidogrel in patients with TIA and the benefit of combination therapies that include clopidogrel. A direct head-to-head trial comparing aspirin and extended release dipyridamole vs. clopidogrel began in 2003 (PROFESS Trial).

Based on the available evidence, the ACCP guidelines suggesting a possible greater benefit for combination therapy with sustained-release dipyridamole and low-dose aspirin appear reasonable and some vascular neurologists would argue that this agent should represent the first-line medical therapy for patients who have sustained an atherothrombotic stroke assuming cost to the individual patient is not an issue. Other vascular neurologists would favor clopidogrel as first-line therapy, if cost to the patient is not an issue, considering its dual cerebrovascular and cardiac benefits. Otherwise, even though aspirin is possibly less effective than the prescription antiplatelet agents, its low retail cost and proven efficacy for different vascular beds still make it an appropriate first-line agent for cerebrovascular risk reduction.

References

1 Schneck MJ. Anticoagulation for stroke prevention. In: Gorelick PB, Alter M, eds. *The Prevention of Stroke.* New York: Parthenon Publishing Group, 2002: 208–22.
2 Mohr JP, Thompson. JL, Lazar RM. Warfarin-Aspirin Recurrent Stroke Study Group, a comparison of warfarin and aspirin for the prevention of recurrent ischemic stroke. *N Engl J Med* 2001; 345: 1444–51.

3 Anonymous. A randomized trial of anticoagulants versus aspirin after cerebral ischemia of presumed arterial origin. *Ann Neurol* 1997; 42: 857–65.

4 Patrono C, Coller. B, Dalen JE *et al*. Platelet-active drugs: the relationships among dose, effectiveness and side-effects. *Chest* 2001; 119 (Suppl. 1): 39S–63S.

5 Roth GH, Calverley. DC. Aspirin, platelets and thrombosis: theory and practice. *Blood* 1994; 83: 885–98.

6 Patrono C. Aspirin as an antiplatelet drug. *N Engl J Med* 1994; 330: 1287–94.

7 Stassen JM, Nystrom A. A historical overview of hemostasis, thrombosis, and antithrombotic therapy. *Ann Plast Surg* 1997; 38: 317–29.

8 Millikan C, Futrell. N. The strange story of aspirin and the prevention of stroke. *J Stroke Cerebrovasc Dis* 1995; 5: 248–54.

9 Schafer A. Antiplatelet therapy. *Am J Med* 1996; 101: 199–209.

10 Dutch TIA Study Group. A comparison of two doses of aspirin (30 mg vs. 283 mg a day) in patients after a transient ischemic attack or minor ischemic stroke. *N Engl J Med* 1991; 325: 1261–6.

11 Pettigrew LC. Antithrombotic drugs for secondary stroke prophylaxis. *Pharmacotherapy* 2001; 21: 452–63.

12 Babu KS, Salvi SS. Aspirin and asthma. *Chest* 2000; 118: 1470–6.

13 Hart RG, Harrison. MJG. Aspirin wars: the optimal dose of aspirin to prevent stroke. *Stroke* 1996; 27: 585–7.

14 Barnett HJM, Kaste M, Meldrum H, Eliasziw M. Aspirin dose in stroke prevention: beautiful hypotheses slain by ugly facts. *Stroke* 1996; 27: 588–92.

15 Savon JJ, Allen ML, DiMarino AJ *et al*. Gastrointestinal blood loss with low dose (325 mg) plain and enteric-coated aspirin administration. *Am J Gastroenterol* 1995; 90: 581–5.

16 Roderick J, Wilkes HC, Mead TW. The gastrointestinal toxicity of aspirin: aAn overview of randomized controlled trials. *J Clin Pharmacol* 1993; 35: 219–26.

17 Fields W, Lemak NA, Frankowski RF, Hardy RJ. Controlled trial of aspirin in cerebral ischemia. *Stroke* 1977; 8: 301–6.

18 Canadian Cooperative Study Group. A randomized trial of aspirin and sulfinpyrazone in threatened stroke. *N Engl J Med* 1978; 299: 53–9.

19 UK-TIA Study Group. United Kingdom transient ischaemic attack (UK-TIA) aspirin trial: interim results. *Br Med J* 1988; 296: 316–20.

20 UK-TIA Study Group. United Kingdom Transient Ischemic Attack (UK-TIA.) aspirin trial: final results. *J Neurol Neurosurg Psychiatry* 1991; 54: 1044–54.

21 SALT Collaborative Group. Swedish Aspirin Low dose Trial (SALT) of 75 mg aspirin as secondary prophylaxis after cerebral ischemic events. *Lancet* 1991; 338: 1345–9.

22 Antiplatelet Trialists Collaboration. Secondary prevention of vascular disease by prolonged antiplatelet treatment. *Br Med J* 1988; 296: 320–31.

23 Helgason CM, Tortorice KL, Winker SR *et al*. Aspirin response and failure in cerebral infarction. *Stroke* 1993; 24: 345–50.

24 Barnett HJM, Eliasziw M, Meldrum HE. Drugs and surgery in the prevention of ischemic stroke. *N Engl J Med* 1995; 332: 238–48.

25 Taylor WD, Barnett HJM, Haynes RB *et al.* (ACE Collaborators). Low-dose and high-dose acetylsalicylic acid for patients undergoing carotid endarterectomy: a randomized controlled trial. *Lancet* 1999; 353: 2179–84.

26 Diener HC, Cunha L, Forbes C *et al.* European Stroke Prevention Study 2. Dipyridamole and acetylsalicylic acid in the secondary prevention of stroke. *J Neurol Sci* 1996; 143: 1–13.

27 Antiplatelet Trialists Collaboration. Collaborative overview of randomised trials of antiplatelet therapy I. Prevention of death, myocardial infarction, and stroke by prolonged antiplatelet therapy in various categories of patients. *Br Med J* 1994; 308: 81–106.

28 Albers GW, Tijssen JG. Antiplatelet therapy: new foundations for optimal treatment decisions. *Neurology* 1999; 53 (Suppl. 4): S25–S31.

29 Albers GW, Amarenco P, Easton JD *et al.* Antithrombotic and thrombolytic therapy for ischemic stroke. *Chest* 2001; 119 (Suppl. 1): 300S–320S.

30 Gelmers H, Tijssen JG. Platelet antiaggregants in secondary prevention after stroke: does dipyridamole add to the effect of aspirin? *J Stroke Cerebrovasc Dis* 1993; 3: 115–20.

31 Johnson ES, Lanes SF, Wentworth CE *et al.* A metaregression analysis of the dose–response effect of aspirin on stroke. *Arch Intern Med* 1999; 159: 1248–53.

32 Quinn MJ, Fitzgerald. DJ. Ticlopidine and clopidogrel. *Circulation* 1999; 100: 1667–72.

33 Haas WK, Easton JD, Adams HP Jr. *et al.* A randomized trial comparing ticlopidine hydrochloride with aspirin for the prevention of stroke in high-risk patients: Ticlopidine Aspirin Stroke Study Group. *N Engl J Med* 1989; 321: 501–7.

34 Hankey GJ, Sudlow CLM, Dunbabin DW. Thienopyridines or aspirin to prevent stroke and other serious vascular events in patients at high risk of vascular disease? A systemic review of the evidence from randomized trials. *Stroke* 2000; 31: 1779–84.

35 Ticlopidine Aspirin Stroke Study Group. Ticlopidine versus aspirin for stroke prevention: on-treatment results from Ticlopidine Aspirin Stroke Study. *J Stroke Cerebrovasc Dis* 1993; 3: 168–76.

36 Bennet CL, Weinberg. PD, Rozenberg-Ben-Dor K *et al.* Thrombotic thrombocytopenic purpura associated with ticlopidine. A review of 60 cases. *Ann Intern Med* 1998; 128: 541–4.

37 Bennet CL, Connors JM, Carwile JM *et al.* Thrombotic thrombocytopenic purpura associated with clopidogrel. *N Engl J Med* 2000; 342: 1773–7.

38 Gent M, Blakely JA, Easton JD *et al.* The Canadian American Ticlopidine Study (CATS) in thromboembolic stroke. *Lancet* 1989; 1: 1215–20.

39 Harbison JW, Ticlopidine Aspirin Stroke Study Group. Ticlopidine versus aspirin for the prevention of recurrent stroke: analysis of patients with minor stroke from the Ticlopidine Aspirin Stroke Study. *Stroke* 1992; 23: 1723–7.

40 Grotta JC, Norris JW, Kamen B. Prevention of stroke with ticlopidine: who benefits most? TASS baseline and angiographic data subgroup. *Neurology* 1992; 42: 111–5.

41 Weisberg LA, Ticlopidine Aspirin Stroke Study Group. The efficacy and safety of ticlopidine and aspirin in nonwhites: analysis of a patient subgroup from the Ticlopidine Aspirin Stroke Study. *Neurology* 1993; 43: 27–31.

42 Gorelick PB, Leurgans S, Richardson D *et al.* African-American Antiplatelet Stroke Prevention Study (AAASPS): clinical trial design. *J Stroke Cerebrovasc Dis* 1998; 7: 426–34.

43 CAPRIE Steering Committee. A randomized blinded trial of clopidogrel versus aspirin in patients at risk of ischaemic events (CAPRIE). *Lancet* 1996; 348: 1329–39.

44 Easton JD. Future perspectives for optimizing oral antiplatelet therapy. *Cerebrovasc Dis* 2001; 11 (Suppl. 2): 23–8.

45 Hacke W. From CURE to MATCH: ADP receptor antagonists as the treatment of choice for high-risk atherothrombotic patients. *Cerebrovasc Dis* 2002; 13 (Suppl. 1): 22–6.

46 Yusuf S, Zhao F, Mehta SR *et al.* Effects of clopidogrel in addition to aspirin in patients with acute coronary syndromes without ST-segment elevation. *N Eng J Med* 2001; 345: 494–502.

47 Albers GW, Amarenco P. Combination therapy with clopidogrel and aspirin: can the CURE results be extrapolated to cerebrovascular patients. *Stroke* 2001; 32: 2948–9.

48 Wilterdink JL, Easton JD. Dipyridamole plus aspirin in cerebrovascular disease. *Arch Neurol* 1999; 56: 1087–92.

49 ESPS2 Study Group. Safety. European Stroke Prevention Study 2. *J Neurol Sci* 1997; 151: S41–51.

50 Bousser MG, Eschwege E, Haguenau M *et al.* 'AICLA' controlled trial of aspirin and dipyridamole in the secondary prevention of athero-thrombotic cerebral cerebral ischemia. *Stroke* 1983; 14: 5–14.

51 European Stroke Prevention Study Group. European Stroke Prevention Study. *Stroke* 1990; 21: 1122–30.

52 ESPS2 Study Group. Primary endpoints: European Stroke Prevention Study 2. *J Neurol Sci* 1997; 151 (Suppl.): S13–26.

53 ESPS2 Study Group. Secondary Endpoints: European Stroke Prevention Study 2. *J Neurol Sci* 1997; 151: S27–S37.

54 Masuhr F, Busch M, Einhäupl KM. Differences in medical and surgical therapy for stroke prevention between leading experts in North America and Western Europe. *Stroke* 1998; 29: 339–45.

55 Anonymous. Internalanalgesic antipyretic, and antirheumatic drug products for over-the-counter human use; final rule for professional labeling of aspirin, buffered aspirin, and aspirin in combination with antacid drug products. *Federal Register* 1999; 64: 49652–5.

56 Albers GW. Choice of endpoints in antiplatelet trials: which outcomes are most relevant to stroke patients? *Neurology* 2000; 54: 1022–8.

57 Samsa GP, Matchar DB, Goldstein LB *et al.* Utilities for major stroke: results from a survey of preferences among persons at increased risk for stroke. *Am Heart J* 1998; 136: 703–13.

58 Scott-Levin Associates. *Prescription Audit Calendar Year 2000.* 2000.

59 Gorelick PB, Richardson D, Kelly M *et al.* Aspirin and ticlopidine for prevention of recurrent stroke in black patients. *JAMA* 2003; 289: 2947–57.

60 Sarasin F, Gaspoz J-M, Bounameaux H. Cost-effectiveness of new antiplatelet regimens used as secondary prevention of stroke or transient ischemic attack. *Arch Intern Med* 2000; 160: 2773–8.

CHAPTER 11

Role of Oral Anticoagulants

Richard K.T. Chan, Seemant Chaturvedi, Patrick Pullicino

There is uncertainty as to whether anticoagulation is beneficial or harmful for patients with transient ischemic attacks (TIAs). There are very few clinical trials that address the management of TIAs, and of these, none has sufficient statistical power to provide unequivocal evidence to support or refute the use of anticoagulation. The current chapter will discuss the rationale for the use of anticoagulation in specific clinical situations.

General considerations

The main pathogenic mechanisms of TIAs appear to be embolism, *in-situ* thrombosis or hypoperfusion. Penetrating artery spasm is another potential cause [1]. Anticoagulants are used to prevent the formation of thrombus along diseased endothelial surfaces, thus reducing the potential for embolism in the arterial system and preventing intralumenal thrombosis that may compromise cerebral blood flow. By inhibiting the prothrombotic arm of the coagulation/fibrinolysis homeostatic mechanisms, anticoagulants also allow spontaneous thrombolysis in patients who already have intralumenal or intracardiac thrombus.

Anticoagulants can be divided into two main groups. Unfractionated heparin, low-molecular-weight heparins and heparinoids exert their effect by inhibiting the activity of factor IIa (thrombin), Xa and XIa through their action on antithrombin III. Warfarin and other associated oral anticoagulants prevent carboxylation (that is dependent on vitamin K) of key coagulant factors, thereby rendering coagulation ineffective. Heparin and related agents are discussed in a separate chapter. Oral anticoagulants are the preferred agents for long-term anticoagulation and will be the focus of this chapter.

The most common, and potentially serious, adverse effect of anticoagulants is hemorrhage. Thus, anticoagulation should be avoided in the following situations:
• patients with a bleeding diathesis (hemophiliacs, thrombocytopenia);
• patients with a bleeding tendency (e.g. peptic ulcers, recent major surgery, cerebral amyloid angiopathy);

• patients in whom hemorrhage could be potentially fatal (e.g. enlarging aortic aneurysm, intracranial aneurysm);
• patients with high risk of intracranial hemorrhage (e.g. poorly controlled hypertension, previous intracerebral hemorrhage).

Any potential benefits from anticoagulation could be offset by the associated hemorrhagic side-effects. In the case of patients with definite stroke, the risk of hemorrhagic transformation of the infarction often equals or exceeds the risk of recurrent stroke. However, the risk of intracerebral hemorrhage among patients with TIA is probably low, since the volume of infarcted brain tissue is small, if any. If anticoagulation is contemplated, a computed tomography scan of the head is mandatory since patients with chronic subdural hematoma may present with TIA-like episodes [2].

Early studies of oral anticoagulation in TIAs

Perkin reviewed the studies of anticoagulation for TIA prior to 1980 [3]. There have been four randomized [4–7] and six nonrandomized studies [8–13]. The randomized trials included relatively small numbers of patients and showed no difference between warfarin and placebo. Three studies compared warfarin with aspirin with or without dipyridamole [5–7] and these showed no difference in stroke rates between patient groups. Eriksson [14] compared aspirin and dipyridamole with heparin for early treatment of TIA, followed by warfarin in both groups. Although there was no difference in stroke or death between the treatment groups, recurrent TIA was more frequent in the antiplatelet agent group. None of these studies supported anticoagulation for TIAs.

Recent studies of anticoagulation in patients with TIA/stroke

In general, one can consider the use of oral anticoagulants for either broad groups of TIA/stroke patients or for specific pathophysiological conditions. Two recent studies have examined the use of warfarin for broad groups of patients. These will be reviewed first and specific conditions will be discussed thereafter.

The first large study which was planned for patients with noncardioembolic stroke was the Stroke Prevention in Reversible Ischemia Trial (SPIRIT) [15]. This trial compared aspirin and warfarin with an International Normalized Ratio (INR) of 3.0–4.5. The study was terminated early due to an excess of major bleeding events in the warfarin group. There were 36 major bleeding episodes in the warfarin group compared with only five in the aspirin group. The excess bleeding risk was probably due to the high level of anticoagulation targeted in this study.

Another study which compared warfarin and aspirin in a broad group of patients did reach the completion stage. This was the Warfarin Aspirin Recurrent Stroke Study (WARSS) [16]. The WARSS trial was a multicenter study in the USA between 1993 and 2001 which enrolled 2206 patients with noncardioembolic stroke. Patients with severe carotid stenosis and scheduled carotid endarterectomy were also excluded. The trial population consisted primarily of patients with lacunar stroke (56.1%), large-vessel atherosclerosis (11.8%), or cryptogenic stroke (26.1%).

The WARSS treatment regimens were either aspirin 325 mg per day or warfarin with a target INR of 1.4–2.8. Over a follow-up period of 2 years, 17.8% of warfarin patients experienced either death or recurrent stroke, whereas 16.0% of the aspirin patients reached this outcome (hazard ratio of 1.13 for warfarin compared with aspirin, $P = 0.25$). When stroke subtypes were analyzed, there was no convincing evidence that any of the subtypes (cryptogenic, large-artery atherosclerosis, etc.) derived benefit from treatment with warfarin. With the mean daily INR of 2.1 in the study, there was no increase in the number of major hemorrhages with warfarin in this study.

The 'bottom line' of this study was that in a broad group of patients with diverse stroke mechanisms, there was no advantage seen with an oral anticoagulant. Thus, clinicians must consider if warfarin is advantageous for more specific conditions.

Anticoagulation for specific disease states

There are some situations in which anticoagulation is either preferred over antiplatelet agents for TIAs or where anticoagulants are still being investigated for stroke prevention. They include conditions that are associated with a high risk of conversion to stroke or that have the potential to lead to severe or fatal stroke. The following conditions deserve special mention.

TIA associated with intralumenal or intracardiac thrombus [17]

Patients who have an intralumenal thrombus in the arteries supplying the brain or intracardiac thrombus are probably at higher risk of developing stroke following an episode of TIA. The thrombus may fragment, causing ongoing embolization. In the case of intralumenal thrombus, further growth of the thrombus may lead to significant stenosis or occlusion, precipitating a further cerebral ischemic event. Anticoagulation may delay the growth of the thrombus and, in the case of on-going embolization, anticoagulation may prevent thrombus propagation from the site of embolic occlusion. Although there are no data to prove that anticoagulants are beneficial in these instances, many vascular neurologists would recommend anticoagulation for patients with left ventricular thrombi or intralumenal thrombi of the major cervical vessels. In the latter circumstance, follow-up imaging with either ultrasound or angiography is recommended, since there may be a severe stenosis underlying the lumenal thrombus and it may be warranted to remove the stenotic lesion via endarterectomy.

'Crescendo TIAs'

'Crescendo TIAs' is a clinical syndrome characterized by recurrent, usually stereotyped episodes of transient neurological dysfunction from a presumed vascular cause, occurring within a short period of time. Most authorities believe that crescendo TIAs represent either recurrent embolism to the affected brain tissue from an unstable, thrombogenic, atheromatous plaque or intralumenal thrombus, or marginal perfusion of brain tissue distal to a critical stenosis of the cerebral arteries. Heparin or warfarin had no effect on outcome in seven patients with the capsular warning syndrome (pure motor crescendo TIAs) compared with controls [18]. Anticoagulation may help to prevent embolism from a critical arterial stenosis but definitive proof of efficacy is lacking.

TIA associated with critical extracranial carotid artery stenosis

Some clinicians believe that patients with critical (99%) stenosis of the extracranial internal carotid artery or common carotid artery may benefit from anticoagulation prior to carotid endarterectomy. Anticoagulation in this setting may reduce thrombus formation at or near the site of maximum stenosis, thereby preventing embolization and maintaining adequate cerebral perfusion. The efficacy of this approach is not proven and there is no indication that patients with severe carotid stenosis who are awaiting carotid endarterectomy will fare any better with anticoagulation compared with aspirin or another antiplatelet strategy. As mentioned above, in the WARSS trial there was a nonsignificant benefit favoring aspirin for patients with large-artery stenosis or occlusion [16]. Thus, in general, warfarin for extracranial stenosis is not recommended.

Short-term anticoagulation for stroke prevention

In some conditions, patients are considered for short-term anticoagulation (3–12 months) depending on clinical status. These conditions include postmyocardial infarction and in the setting of arterial dissection.

Myocardial infarction

Patients who experience TIA or minor stroke after myocardial infarction (MI) may be considered for short-term anticoagulation and even some high-risk patients may receive anticoagulation as part of a primary prevention strategy. Cerebral ischemia is thought to be caused by embolism from a mural thrombus forming on the damaged endocardial surface. Short-term anticoagulation reduces the risk of development of an intracardiac thrombus and subsequent embolization [19].

The National Stroke Association commentary on prevention of a first stroke recommends warfarin treatment following a MI if other conditions are present such as persistent atrial fibrillation, decreased left ventricular function (ejection fraction < 28%), or if left ventricular thrombi are detected in the first few months following MI [20].

The recent Warfarin Aspirin Reinfarction Study (WARIS II) found that patients receiving either warfarin alone (INR 2.8–4.2) or warfarin (INR 2.0–2.5) and aspirin 75 mg per day following MI had a reduced rate of cardiovascular events, including embolic stroke, compared with aspirin alone (160 mg per day) [21]. For stroke, the aspirin group had 32 events, compared with 17 in each of the two warfarin groups ($P < 0.03$). There was a significantly higher rate of bleeding in the warfarin groups and therefore, whether an increased use of warfarin following MI is embraced by cardiologists remains to be seen.

Arterial dissection

Arterial dissections are an important cause of stroke or TIA in young adults. They can involve either the extracranial or intracranial portions of major vessels such as the carotid artery or vertebral artery. Although there have not been any randomized trials to evaluate the treatment of these patients in terms of differential efficacy of antiplatelet agents vs. anticoagulation, many vascular neurologists favor the use of intravenous heparin followed by oral anticoagulation with warfarin (INR 2–3) for these patients [22]. One rationale for this treatment selection is that most ischemic events following dissection are believed to be thromboembolic in nature.

The vast majority of patients with dissection will need only short-term anticoagulation since many dissections heal spontaneously [23]. It is recommended that patients be followed with either angiography or a noninvasive imaging study at 3–6-month intervals and anticoagulation is typically discontinued when severe stenosis resolves or when only minor lumenal irregularities are present.

Long-term anticoagulation for stroke prevention

The major proven indication for long-term anticoagulation for secondary stroke prevention is for patients with atrial fibrillation [24]. The European Atrial Fibrillation Trial (EAFT) investigated the use of warfarin, aspirin, or placebo for patients with nonvalvular atrial fibrillation and a prior TIA or minor stroke. The warfarin group had a substantial reduction in the annual stroke rate with a INR target of 2.0–3.9. The annual stroke rate was 12% with placebo, approximately 10% with aspirin, and 4% with warfarin. Therefore, it is clear that if the patient is a safe anticoagulation candidate, warfarin is preferred for atrial fibrillation patients with a previous central nervous system (CNS) embolic event.

TIA associated with intracranial arterial stenosis

Stenosis of the intracranial vertebral, intracranial internal carotid, middle cerebral, and basilar arteries is a recognized cause of TIA/stroke. The stenosis disturbs blood flow and, if severe, produces hypoperfusion distally. Thrombus formation and subsequent embolization are promoted by the irregular surface of the arterial internal surface and by slow flow distal to the stenosis. While logical, it is not known if the risk of stroke can be significantly reduced by anticoagulation. Any potential benefit may also be offset by the hemorrhagic complications associated with anticoagulation.

Chimowitz *et al.* conducted a retrospective, nonrandomized analysis of patients treated with intracranial atherosclerotic disease [25]. In this study, the intracranial disease was angiographically verified as being between 50 and 99% stenosis. Treatment with aspirin or warfarin was at the discretion of the local physician. One hundred and fifty-one patients were identified and stroke was recorded in 59% of patients, with TIA being the qualifying event in 41%. The degree of narrowing of the symptomatic vessel was 50–69% in 41% and 70–99% in 59% of patients. There was an almost equal distribution of anterior circulation and posterior circulation lesions.

In the subsequent follow-up, 88 patients were treated with warfarin and 63 patients with aspirin. The median follow-up time averaged 14.7 months for the warfarin group and 19.3 months for the aspirin group. It was found that treatment with warfarin resulted in fewer strokes and total ischemic events. Major cardiovascular events (stroke, MI, or vascular death) occurred in 26 aspirin patients during 143 patient years and 14 warfarin patients during 166 patient years ($P < 0.01$, log rank test). Patients with higher degrees of stenosis (70–99%) and those with posterior circulation disease had higher stroke rates.

One should interpret these data with caution, however, since there have been several instances in which retrospective, nonrandomized data have not been confirmed in prospective fashion [26]. The current optimal antithrombotic regimen for intracranial atherosclerosis is not known. The Warfarin Aspirin Symptomatic Intracranial Disease (WASID) study is an on-going clinical trial aimed at conclusively determining the best stroke prevention strategy in this condition [27]. The preliminary results of the prospective WASID trial did not show benefit of warfarin compared to aspirin in this population.

TIA associated with low cardiac output state

Reduced cardiac output, regardless of the presence or absence of congestive heart failure, is associated with a 1–2% annual risk of systemic embolization, including TIA and stroke [28,29]. There are two main reasons for cerebral ischemia in patients with low cardiac output state. Low ejection fraction promotes intracardiac thrombus formation due to stasis within the ventricles, leading to systemic (including cerebral) embolization. The low output state may also cause a reduction in cerebral blood flow and systemic hypoperfusion, leading to regional or global cerebral hypoperfusion. As is the case in intracranial arterial stenosis, the benefit of warfarin remains unproven. The Warfarin vs. Aspirin in Reduced Cardiac Ejection Fraction (WARCEF) Study [30] is a randomized study of patients with ejection fraction of < 30% in which patients are assigned to warfarin (INR 2.5–3.0) or aspirin 325 mg per day. This study includes both patients with prior TIA/stroke and those patients without prior CNS embolism. The trial is currently in an early stage and results will probaby not be available for at least 5 years.

TIA associated with hypercoagulable state

Venous thrombosis is common among patients with deficient intrinsic fibrinolytic factors (protein C, protein S, antithrombin III), but TIAs and stroke are quite unusual. If no other cause of TIA is detected, clinicians may consider employing long-term anticoagulation for secondary stroke prevention.

Patients with antiphospholipid antibody syndrome represent another potential cause of TIA or stroke. The exact pathogenesis leading to TIA or stroke in this condition is poorly understood, but it is believed that the antibodies causes endothelial damage, thus promoting thrombus formation.

Although one previous retrospective study suggested that high-intensity (INR ≥ 3.0) anticoagulation should be considered in preventing strokes or other systemic thrombotic event, many vascular neurologists were skeptical about this finding [31].

The Antiphospholipid Antibodies and Stroke Study (APASS) was a component of the previously mentioned WARSS trial. In the APASS analysis, there was no significant difference in the number of arterial or venous thrombotic events in patients with an antiphospholipid antibody or lupus anticoagulant according to whether they received treatment with warfarin or aspirin [32]. Therefore, unless the patient has multiple features of the so-called primary antiphospholipid antibody syndrome (previous spontaneous abortions, venous and/or arterial thromboses, thrombocytopenia), the role of anticoagulation is unclear. For patients with low-titer anticardiolipin antibodies especially, antiplatelet therapy is preferred.

TIA associated with paradoxical embolism

Occasionally, TIA may be due to emboli from the venous system that enter the cerebral circulation through a right-to-left shunt in the pulmonary vasculature, an atrial septal defect [including a patent foramen ovale (PFO)] or ventricular septal defect. Warfarin has been shown to reduce the risk of deep venous thrombosis and pulmonary embolism in high-risk individuals, but its efficacy in preventing stroke from paradoxical embolism is not proven. A recent multicenter study from France found that the rate of recurrent stroke in patients with an isolated PFO was low even with aspirin (300 mg per day) treatment [33]. In this study, 581 patients between ages 18 and 55 years were recruited following a crypto-genic stroke. With aspirin treatment, the stroke rate at 4 years was 2.3%. The stroke rate increased with an associated atrial septal aneurysm (ASA) to 15.2% at 4 years.

Another multicenter study was conducted in concert with the WARSS trial. The Patent Foramen Ovale in Cryptogenic Stroke Study (PICSS) analyzed the outcomes in patients with a PFO who received either aspirin 325 mg per day or warfarin (INR 1.4–2.8) [34]. A PFO was identified in 203 patients and during 2 years' follow-up, there was a nonsignificant trend favoring aspirin in prevention of either recurrent stroke or death. The event rates were 13.2% in the aspirin group and 16.5% in the war-farin group ($P = 0.49$). In contrast to the French study, there was no increase in the event rate among those patients with both a PFO and ASA.

The conclusion of recent studies is that either antiplatelet or anticoagu-lation treatment can be justified for patients with a TIA/stroke and PFO. The decision between these treatments should take into account, at a min-imum, the presence of hypercoagulable states, the age of the patient, and the bleeding risk of the patient [35].

Conclusion

The role of anticoagulation in the management of patients with TIA has been insufficiently studied. To a large extent, the role of anticoagulation in the setting of TIA depends on the putative cause of the TIA and the balance of the expected benefit (stroke risk reduction) and the associated risk (hemorrhage). Given that the risk of stroke may be different for patients with TIA alone and patients with frank cerebral infarction, future second-ary stroke prevention studies need to include sufficient numbers of patients with TIA so that the role of anticoagulants can be clearly established. The major indication at present for anticoagulation in TIA patients is in the setting of atrial fibrillation and other high-risk sources of cardioembolism.

For many of the conditions mentioned above, the role of anticoagula-tion is controversial. With current clinical trials, the appropriateness of oral anticoagulation will be clarified in the next decade for important conditions such as intracranial atherosclerosis and reduced cardiac ejection fraction. In the interim, clinicians are advised to use oral anticoagulants in a judicious and cautious manner.

References

1 Friberg L, Olsen TS. Cerebrovascular instability in a subset of patients with stroke and transient ischemic attack. *Arch Neurol* 1991; 48: 1026–31.

2 Moster ML, Johnston DE, Reinmuth OM. Chronic subdural hematoma with transient neurological deficits: a review of 15 cases. *Ann Neurol* 1983; 14: 539–42.

3 Perkin GD. Anticoagulants in transient ischemic attacks. In: Greenhalgh RM, Rose FC, eds. *Progress in Stroke Research*. Bath: Pitman Medical, 1980: 181–203.

4 Veterans Adminstration Cooperative Study of Atherosclerosis Neurology Section. An evaluation of anticoagulant therapy in the treatment of cerebrovascular disease. *Neurology* 1961; 11: 132–8.

5 Olson JE, Brechter C, Backlund H *et al.* Anticoagulant vs antiplatelet therapy as prophylactic against cerebral infarction in transient ischemic attacks. *Stroke* 1980; 11: 4–119.

6 Buren A, Ygge J. Treatment program and comparison between anticoagulants and platelet aggregation inhibitors after transient ischemic attack. *Stroke* 1981; 12: 578–80.

7 Garde A, Samuelsson K, Fahlgren H, Hedberg E, Hjerne LG, Ostman J. Treatment after transient ischemic attacks: a comparison between anticoagulant drug and inhibition of platelet aggregation. *Stroke* 1983; 14: 677–81.

8 Fisher CM. The use of anticoagulants in cerebral thrombosis. *Neurology* 1958; 8: 311–32.

9 Sekert RG, Whisnant JP, Millikan CH. Surgical and anticoagulant therapy of occlusive cerebrovascular disease. *Ann Intern Med* 1963; 58: 637–41.

10 Fazekas JF, Alman RW, Sullivan JF. Vertebral-basilar insufficiency. *Arch Neurol* 1963; 8: 215–20.

11 Friedman GD, Wilson S, Mosier JM, Colandrea MA, Inchaman MZ. Transient ischemic attacks in a community. *JAMA* 1969; 210: 1428–34.

12 Toole JF, Janeway R, Choi K *et al.* Transient ischemic attacks due to atherosclerosis: a prospective study of 160 patients. *Arch Neurol* 1975; 32: 5–12.

13 Olsson JE, Muller R, Berneli S. Long-term anticoagulant therapy for TIAs and minor stroke with minimum residuum. *Stroke* 1976; 7: 444–51.

14 Eriksson SE. Enteric-coated acetylsalicylic acid plus dipyridamole compared with anticoagulants in the prevention of ischemic events in patients with transient ischemic attacks. *Acta Neurol Scand* 1985; 71: 485–93.

15 The Stroke Prevention in Reversible Ischemia Trial (SPIRIT) Study Group. A random trial of anticoagulants versus aspirin after cerebral ischemia of presumed arterial origin. *Ann Neurol* 1997; 42: 857–65.

16 Mohr JP, Thompson JLP, Lazar RM *et al.* A comparison of warfarin and aspirin for the prevention of recurrent ischemic stroke. *N Engl J Med* 2001; 345: 1444–51.

17 Cerebral Embolism Task Force. Cardiogenic brain embolism. *Arch Neurol* 1989; 46: 727–43.

18 Donnan GA, O'Malley HM, Quang L, Hurley S. The capsular warning syndrome: the high risk of early stroke. *Cerebrovasc Dis* 1996; 6: 202–7.

19 Collins R, MacMahon S, Flather M *et al.* Clinical effects of anticoagulant therapy in suspected acute myocardial infarction: systematic overview of randomized trials. *Br Med J* 1996; 313: 652–9.

20 Gorelick PB, Sacco RL, Smith DB *et al.* Prevention of a first stroke. A review of guidelines and a multidisciplinary consensus statement from the National Stroke Association. *JAMA* 1999; 281: 1112–20.

21 Hurlen M, Abdelnoor M, Smith P, Erikssen J, Arnesen H. Warfarin, aspirin, or both after myocardial infarction. *N Engl J Med* 2002; 347: 969–74.

22 Schievink WI. Spontaneous dissection of the carotid and vertebral arteries. *N Engl J Med* 2001; 344: 898–906.

23 Kasner SE, Hankins LL, Bratina P, Morgenstern LB. Magnetic resonance angiography demonstrates vascular healing of carotid and vertebral artery dissections. *Stroke* 1997; 28: 1993–7.

24 EAFT Study Group. Secondary prevention in nonrheumatic atrial fibrillation after transient ischemic attack or minor stroke. *Lancet* 1993; 342: 1255–62.

25 Chimowitz MI, Kokkinos J, Strong J *et al.* The Warfarin Aspirin Symptomatic Intracranial Disease Study. *Neurology* 1995; 45: 1488–93.

26 Taylor DW, Barnett HJM, Haynes RB *et al.* Low dose and high dose acetylsalicylic acid for patients undergoing carotid endarterectomy: a randomized controlled trial. *Lancet* 1999; 353: 2179–84.

27 Benesch CG, Chimowitz MI. Best treatment for intracranial arterial stenosis? 50 years of uncertainty. *Neurology* 2000; 55: 465–6.

28 Katz SD, Marantz PR, Biasucci L *et al.* Low incidence of stroke in ambulatory patients with heart failure: a prospective study. *Am Heart J* 1993; 126: 141–6.

29 Cioffi G, Pozzoli M, Forni G *et al.* Systemic thromboembolism in chronic heart failure. A prospective study in 406 patients. *Eur Heart J* 1996; 17: 1381–9.

30 Pullicino PM, Halperin JL, Thompson JL. Stroke in patients with heart failure and reduced left ventricular ejection fraction. *Neurology* 2000; 54: 288–94.

31 Cuadrado MJ, Khamashta MA. The anti-phospholipid antibody syndrome (Hughes syndrome): therapeutic aspects. *Baillieres Best Pract Res Clin Rheumatol* 2000; 14: 151–63.

32 The APASS Investigators. Antiphospholipid antibodies and subsequent thrombo-occlusive events in patients with ischemic stroke. *JAMA* 2004; 291: 576–84.

33 Mas JL, Arquizan C, Lamy C *et al.* Recurrent cerebrovascular events associated with patent foramen ovale, atrial septal aneurysm, or both. *N Engl J Med* 2001; 345: 1740–6.

34 Homma S, Sacco RL, DiTullio M, Sciacca RR, Mohr JP, for the PFO in Cryptogenic Stroke Study (PICSS) Investigators. Effect of medical treatment in stroke patients with patent foramen ovale. *Circulation* 2002; 105: 2625–31.

35 Chaturvedi S. Coagulation abnormalities in adults with cryptogenic stroke and patent foramen ovale. *J Neurol Sci* 1998; 160: 158–60.

CHAPTER 12

Heparin and Related Compounds

James F. Meschia

Introduction

Physicians have only recently had reliable evidence to guide decisions about the use of heparin and related compounds in patients with acute ischemic stroke. Use of these agents in patients who experience a transient ischemic attack (TIA) remains a relative blindspot of evidence-based medicine. The unfortunate, but predictable, result is excessive variability in clinical practice [1]. Randomized clinical trials in acute ischemic stroke may give important insights into the potential risks and benefits of giving heparin to patients with TIA, but patients who present with a TIA may respond differently to treatments with these agents. Future trials may provide additional evidence that applies more directly to patients with TIA. At present, the decision to use heparin in patients with TIA is based on extrapolation from a wealth of stroke trial data and a paucity of TIA trial data.

Pharmacology of heparins and heparinoids

Heparin is a glycosaminoglycan derived from bovine, caprine, ovine, or porcine intestine. The mean molecular weight of unfractionated (UF) heparin is 15 000 Da and ranges from 5000 to 30 000 Da. One-third of the molecules in UF heparin contain a pentasaccharide sequence that exhibits high-affinity binding to antithrombin. Molecules with this pentasaccharide sequence and a total of 18 or more saccharide units are capable of forming a trimolecular complex consisting of heparin, antithrombin, and thrombin (also known as factor IIA). Formation of this trimolecular complex catalyzes inactivation of thrombin by antithrombin. Heparin molecules with fewer than 18 saccharides cannot simultaneously bind thrombin and antithrombin and are incapable of neutralizing thrombin. However, the smaller heparin molecules retain the ability of the larger heparin molecules to neutralize factor Xa via antithrombin (Fig. 12.1) [2].

Low-molecular-weight (LMW) heparins are produced by the enzymatic or chemical depolymerization of UF heparin. The mean molecular weights

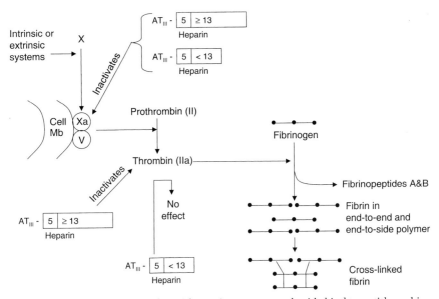

Fig. 12.1 Only heparin molecules with a unique pentasaccharide bind to antithrombin III (ATIII). All ATIII-heparin species inhibit factor Xa, but ATIII–heparin can inhibit thrombin only if the heparin has at least 13 saccharides in addition to the ATIII-binding pentasaccharide. Low-molecular-weight heparin preparations have a greater ATIII-to-thrombin binding ratio than unfractionated heparin.

Table 12.1 A comparison of Anti-Xa/IIa activity in heparin preparations

Drug	Anti-Xa/IIa activity
Unfractionated heparin	1 : 1
Dalteparin	2.7 : 1
Nadoparin	3.6 : 1
Enoxaparin	3.8 :1

of the various LMW heparin preparations range from 4000 to 6000 Da. LMW heparins have a greater percentage of molecules with less than 18 saccharides than UF heparin. The antifactor Xa : antifactor IIa activity ratio is higher in LMW than in UF heparins, which is 1.0 by definition. The anti-Xa : anti-IIa ratio is a convenient means of comparing various commercially available LMW heparin preparations (Table 12.1).

LMW heparins have distinct pharmacokinetic advantages over UF heparin. The half-life of anti-Xa activity of LMW heparins after subcutaneous administration is about 4 h, permitting continuous anticoagulation with daily or twice-daily subcutaneous injections. Because LMW heparins have a lower affinity for plasma and matrix proteins than their UF counterpart, a more predictable anticoagulant response can be achieved with a fixed dose. LMW heparin preparations have improved bioavailability after subcutaneous administration compared with UF heparin. Heparinoids like danaparoid are a mixture of semisynthetic or natural sulfated glycosaminoglycans derived from animal sources [3]. For further details regarding anticoagulation with heparin and related compounds, readers are encouraged to refer to the exhaustive review by Hirsh and colleagues [4].

Randomized clinical trials of heparin for acute ischemic stroke

There are now several completed trials of heparin and related compounds in acute ischemic stroke. In a trial performed by the Cerebral Embolism Study Group, 45 patients with acute cardioembolic stroke presenting within 48 h of onset of symptoms randomly received either early or delayed treatment [5]. In the early-treatment group, patients received an intravenous (i.v.) bolus of 5000–10 000 U of UF heparin followed by a continuous infusion of heparin for at least 96 h before being treated with warfarin. Patients in the delayed-treatment group were not treated with heparin but instead were treated with platelet antiaggregants or warfarin beginning 10 days after stroke. None of the 24 heparin recipients had a recurrent stroke or hemorrhage within the 96-h treatment period. Of the 21 patients who received delayed treatment, two had early recurrent ischemic strokes, one had a deep venous thrombosis, two had hemorrhagic transformations of their infarct, and three died. Enrollment was terminated because of an insignificant trend toward fewer thromboembolic events in the early-treatment group. The study did not address whether early anticoagulation reduced neurological impairment or disability.

A randomized trial by Duke and colleagues evaluated UF heparin compared with placebo in 225 patients with noncardioembolic stroke [6]. Patients with a neurological deficit that worsened during the first hour of observation were excluded from the study because of the prevailing belief at the time that patients with so-called stroke-in-evolution should immediately receive anticoagulation. The study excluded patients with recent myocardial infarction or valvular heart disease. Five patients with atrial fibrillation were randomized in the first year of patient recruitment, but atrial fibrillation subsequently became an exclusion criterion. No difference was seen in stroke progression or death at 7 days.

In the International Stroke Trial (IST) 19 435 patients were randomized in a 3×2 factorial design to medium-dose subcutaneous UF heparin (12 500 IU twice daily), low-dose subcutaneous heparin (5000 IU twice daily), or no heparin and aspirin (300 mg daily) or no aspirin [7]. Patients and treating physicians were not blinded to treatment allocation. Functional outcome was stratified into four groups based on responses to three questions: 'Is the patient alive?', 'Do you/they require help from another person for everyday activities?', and 'Do you feel that you/they have made a complete recovery from your/their stroke?'. The median time interval from stroke onset to randomization was 19 h. Sixty-seven percent of patients had head computed tomography (CT) before randomization. Four percent of the patients never had head CT during the course of the trial. There was no significant difference at 14 days between the heparin and no-heparin groups in the combined endpoint of death or nonfatal stroke recurrence. Patients allocated to the heparin group had significantly fewer recurrent ischemic strokes within 14 days (2.9% vs. 3.8%, $P = 0.005$). When the medium- and low-dose groups were analyzed separately, the low-dose heparin group had a significant reduction in the combined endpoint of death or nonfatal stroke recurrence within 14 days (10.8% vs. 12.0%, $P = 0.03$). There was no difference in the heparin and no-heparin groups in the percentage of patients who were either dead or dependent at 6 months.

Subgroup analysis of the 3169 patients with atrial fibrillation at baseline showed that the proportion of patients with atrial fibrillation with fatal or nonfatal recurrent ischemic stroke within 14 days allocated to UF heparin 12 500 IU BID, UFH 5000 IU BID, and no heparin were: 2.3%, 3.4%, 4.9% ($P = 0.001$) [8]. The proportion with symptomatic intracerebral hemorrhage allocated to UFH 12 500 IU BID, UFH 5000 IU BID, and no heparin were: 2.8%, 1.3%, and 0.4% ($P < 0.0001$). There was no effect on the proportion of patients who were dead or dependent at 6 months.

In the Fraxiparine for Ischemic Stroke Study (FISS), 312 patients with a motor deficit due to an acute ischemic stroke were randomized within 48 h of onset of symptoms to one of three treatment groups: nadroparin calcium at 4100 IU antifactor Xa subcutaneously either once or twice daily or placebo [9]. After 10 days of the experimental treatment, patients received aspirin (100 mg/day). CT evidence of hemorrhage, age > 80 years, and sustained hypertension were among the exclusion criteria. The primary endpoint was poor outcome, defined as mortality or dependence on others for performing activities of daily living in the 6 months after randomization. There was a significant dose-dependent reduction in the rate of poor outcome in favor of patients treated with nadroparin calcium twice daily at 6 months but not at 3 months. Results of this trial could not be replicated, however.

A total of 1281 patients were enrolled in the Trial of ORG10172 in Acute Stroke Treatment (TOAST), a randomized double-blind placebo-controlled trial of danaparoid (also known as ORG10172) given by continuous i.v. infusion to maintain the anti-Xa activity at 0.6–0.8 IU/ml [10]. Patients were required to have symptoms lasting > 1 h but < 24 h. Cranial

CT evidence of blood or mass effect, abnormal coagulation studies, thrombolytic therapy within the previous 24 h, and mean arterial blood pressure
> 130 mmHg were among the initial exclusion criteria. In the entire trial,
80 patients with a National Institutes of Health Stroke Scale Score (NIHSS)
> 15 (severe stroke) received danaparoid and 80 patients received placebo.
Eleven patients who had a baseline NIHSS > 15 had serious bleeding within
10 days; 10 (91%) of these patients had received danaparoid ($P = 0.01$).
Because of this safety concern, NIHSS > 15 was added as an exclusion
criterion early in the trial. Favorable outcomes, defined as a Glasgow Outcome Scale (GOS) of 1 or 2 and a Barthel Index (BI) > 12, were achieved in
59.2% given danaparoid and 54.3% given placebo ($P = 0.07$) at 7 days.
Very favorable outcomes, defined as GOS of 1 and BI of 19 or 20, were
achieved in 33.9% given danaparoid and 27.8% given placebo ($P = 0.01$).
At 3 months, there were no significant differences between the treatment
groups either for favorable or for very favorable outcomes. A subgroup
analysis suggested that danaparoid improved favorable (68.1% vs. 54.7%;
$P = 0.04$) and very favorable (43.4% vs. 29.1%; $P = 0.02$) outcomes in
patients with large-artery atherothrombotic stroke at 3 months. There
was no demonstrable benefit, however, for patients with cardioembolic,
lacunar, or cryptogenic stroke.

Tinzaparin in Acute Ischemic Stroke (TAIST) was a three-arm, double-
blind, double-dummy, aspirin-controlled trial of two doses of subcutaneous tinzaparin (100 IU/kg anti-Xa daily for 10 days vs. 175 IU/kg anti-Xa
daily for 10 days) [11]. Aspirin was given at 300 mg/day. A total of 1486
patients were randomized. The main entry criterion was an acute ischemic
stroke that could be treated within 48 h of onset. Major clinical exclusion
criteria were age > 90 years, coma, mild stroke, or bleeding tendency. Major
CT exclusion criteria were intracranial hemorrhage or ≥ 5 mm midline shift
of intracranial contents. Follow-up was both clinical and radiographic,
with a protocol-mandated second head CT obtained 10 days after enrollment. The primary endpoint was independence (modified Rankin scale
of ≤ 2) at 6 months. The rates of independence did not differ among
the treatment groups. Anticoagulation had the expected effects on deep
vein thrombosis and symptomatic intracerebral hemorrhage. None of 486
patients randomized to tinzaparin experienced deep vein thrombosis
compared with nine (1.8%) of 491 patients randomized to aspirin. Seven
(1.4%) of 486 patients in the high-dose tinzaparin group experienced
symptomatic intracerebral hemorrhage compared with one (0.2%) of 491
patients in the aspirin group [odds ratio (OR) 7.15; 95% confidence interval (CI) 1.10, 163]. The effect of tinzaparin on the primary outcome was
not contingent upon clinical subtype of stroke (i.e. whether the patient
had a cardioembolic stroke).

Heparin and Acute Embolic Stroke Trial (HAEST) was a randomized, double-blind, double-dummy trial of the LMW heparin compound

known as dalteparin (100 IU/kg subcutaneously twice a day) vs. aspirin (160 mg/day) for the treatment of acute ischemic stroke in patients with atrial fibrillation [12]. A total of 449 patients were randomized within 30 h of stroke onset. All patients had electrocardiographic documentation of atrial fibrillation either on admission or within 24 h before the stroke. The median age was 80 years. At 14 days postrandomization, 19 patients (8.5%) who received dalteparin had a recurrent ischemic stroke compared with 17 patients (7.5%) who received aspirin. The difference was not significant. Head CTs were done before randomization and repeated after 7 days and on clinical deterioration. The rate of symptomatic and asymptomatic cerebral hemorrhages detected on CT was 11.6% on dalteparin vs. 14.2% on aspirin (OR 0.79, CI 0.44, 1.43). A combined endpoint including recurrent ischemic stroke, cerebral hemorrhage, progression of symptoms, or death favored aspirin. This raises the question of whether heparin can be bypassed in patients with atrial fibrillation and stroke. Patients could potentially receive aspirin initially, followed by direct initiation of warfarin on day 2 or 3 if a follow-up imaging study does not show hemorrhagic transformation.

At the end of all these randomized clinical trials, one is left to conclude that the use of heparin and related compounds in patients with recent ischemic stroke provides no net benefit. IST suggests that the modest reduction in recurrent stroke brought about by subcutaneous heparin is offset by an increase in the rate of intracerebral hemorrhage. HAEST and subgroup analyses of IST and TOAST suggest that heparin and related compounds have no obvious role in the acute management of cardioembolic stroke. A subgroup analysis in TOAST suggests that danaparoid may be of benefit to patients with stroke due to large-vessel atherosclerosis, but prospective confirmation of this finding is lacking.

Can results of stroke trials be applied to TIAs?

There is a new push to treat stroke as a medical emergency, in part because tissue plasminogen activator is approved for the treatment of stroke within 3 h of onset of symptoms. Exploratory analyses of the NINDS rt-PA (recombinant tissue plasminogen activator) stroke study suggest that even within this 3-h therapeutic time window, earlier drug delivery leads to better outcome [13]. The Brain Attack Coalition recommended that the key elements of a primary stroke center include acute stroke teams, units, written care protocols, and an integrated emergency response system [14]. Many centers already have well-developed stroke pathways and teams expediting evaluation of acute ischemic stroke in the emergency department [15]. Some centers have emergency physicians who, with specialty consultation as required, identify patients with acute ischemic stroke and deliver rt-PA [16]. Other centres are developing mechanisms for remote

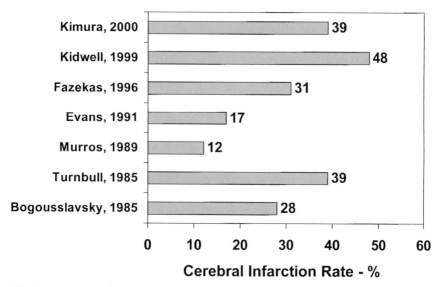

Fig. 12.2 Bar graph showing the proportion of patients who had evidence of cerebral infarction detected by head computed tomography or magnetic resonance imaging at the time of presentation with transient ischemic attack [18–24].

cerebrovascular specialty consultations through teleconferencing [17]. The result of all these efforts is that patients are being identified and evaluated in emergency departments at many centers with greater efficiency, and treatment decisions can be made within 1 h of presentation.

Communities are being advised to activate the emergency medical service as soon as a person experiences the symptoms of a stroke. One consequence of treating stroke as a medical emergency is that TIA is now considered an acute illness. Many patients with TIA will be free of symptoms by the time they arrive in the emergency room, while others will have rapidly improving symptoms. It is not entirely clear how heparin trials in acute ischemic stroke apply to patients presenting in the emergency room with recent symptoms of stroke that have either already resolved or are rapidly on the way to resolution within 24 h. The justification for heparin in these patients would be stroke prevention rather than reduction of neurological deficit.

Randomized clinical trials in acute ischemic stroke show that intracranial hemorrhage is the major risk of giving heparin. It is likely that acute anticoagulation of patients with TIA carries a lower risk of intracranial hemorrhage. However, hemorrhagic transformation of an infarct may remain an important clinical concern when acutely anticoagulating patients with TIA. Many patients who present with TIA have radiographic evidence of infarction (Fig. 12.2). Several radiographic case series of patients presenting with TIA show detection rates for cerebral infarction ranging from 12 to 48% [18–24]. These percentages should be taken as a rough estimate because of the potential for referral bias, but it is fair to say that many patients who present with TIA are not entirely free of the risk of hemorrhagic transformation of an infarct. Even though roughly 20% of patients with TIA will have radiographic evidence of infarction, the lesions tend to be small [25]. Some of these lesions will be cerebral infarcts with transient symptoms, while others will be chronic infarcts in so-called silent areas of the brain. The results of the TOAST study suggest that larger infarcts are more likely to undergo hemorrhagic transformation.

Case series clearly show that heparin is not universally effective in preventing cerebral infarction. In a series of 74 patients treated at the University of Iowa, heparin given by continuous infusion to maintain an activated partial thromboplastin time (APTT) of 1.5–2.5 times control was not able to prevent 12 patients (16.2%) from having recurrent TIAs and five (6.8%) from having cerebral infarction [26]. The clinically meaningful question is whether heparin is superior to aspirin or similar antiplatelet agents for preventing stroke. This question can only be answered by a properly controlled clinical trial.

There is very little evidence from randomized clinical trials to guide the decision to use heparin in patients presenting with a recent TIA. Biller and colleagues conducted a pilot randomized clinical trial comparing aspirin with i.v. adjusted-dose heparin in hospitalized patients with recent TIA [27]. To be eligible, patients had to have at least one TIA within 7 days before admission. Patients were excluded if they had focal neurological deficits for more than 24 h, evidence on baseline CT of an intracranial aneurysm or hemorrhage, or laboratory evidence of a coagulopathy. Patients in the heparin group received an i.v. bolus injection of 5000 IU of UF heparin followed by a continuous infusion. The maintenance infusion of heparin was started at 1000 IU/h and was adjusted to maintain a partial thromboplastin time of 1.5–2.0 times the baseline value. The heparin was continued for a minimum of 3 days and a maximum of 9 days. Heparin was discontinued at the time of cerebrovascular surgery or when maintenance therapy was begun. During short-term follow-up, cerebral infarction occurred in one (3.7%) patient assigned to heparin and four (14%) patients assigned to aspirin. The difference was not significant, but there were no hemorrhagic complications noted during the course of the study.

SPIRIT [28] and WARSS [29] suggest that many patients with stroke derive no added benefit from warfarin vs. chronic antiplatelet therapy. However, in the restricted subgroup of patients who are best served with long-term anticoagulation, such as patients who have a mechanical heart valve or atrial fibrillation, the question is not whether to anticoagulate the patient but when. The European Atrial Fibrillation Trial provides compelling evidence that patients with atrial fibrillation and TIA or minor stroke

Table 12.2 Heparin preparations for which there is a published experience in patients presenting with transient ischemic attack

Generic name	Trade name	Dose
Unfractionated heparin	—	Continuous intravenous infusion with dose adjusted to an activated partial thromboplastin time of 1.5–2.5 times control [26]
Enoxaparin	Lovenox	1 mg/kg subcutaneously every 12 h [63]
Nadoparin	Fraxiparine	4100 IU anti-Xa subcutaneously every 12 h [36]

should receive long-term anticoagulation [30]. A total of 669 patients with nonrheumatic atrial fibrillation and a history of TIA or minor ischemic stroke within the preceding 3 months were randomized to anticoagulation, aspirin or placebo. Physicians were free in their choice of oral anticoagulation (most choosing Coumadin derivatives) but treatment was adjusted to obtain an International Normalized Ratio (INR) of 2.5–4.0 (target value 3.0). The combined endpoint was death from vascular disease, any stroke, myocardial infarction, or systemic embolism. During a mean follow-up of 2.3 years, the annual rate of outcome events was 8% in patients treated with anticoagulants vs. 17% in patients treated with placebo (hazard ratio 0.53; 95% CI 0.36, 0.79). Anticoagulation was also found to be superior to aspirin.

In patients with TIA and no evidence of cerebral infarction on head imaging who have a clear indication for long-term anticoagulation, it may be advisable to initiate anticoagulation as soon as possible with either UF or LMW heparin. To date, there have been no adequately powered, randomized trials of bridging therapy with heparin vs. bridging therapy with aspirin or similar antiplatelet agent. The absolute reduction in stroke risk for acute bridging anticoagulation is likely to be low. Table 12.2 shows the heparin preparations that have a published track record as treatment for TIA, although not with proven efficacy.

Use of heparin in patients with crescendo TIAs

Crescendo TIAs are recurrent transient cerebral or retinal ischemia of increasing frequency, duration, or severity [31]. Crescendo TIAs often involve the same vascular territory. For example, a patient with crescendo TIAs might present to medical attention after sequentially experiencing transient blindness in the right eye, transient left facial droop, and transient left facial droop with left upper extremity paresis. Crescendo TIAs are commonly associated with large-vessel atherosclerosis. In a series of 47 consecutive patients with crescendo TIAs seen at University of California San Diego Medical Center, 26 (55%) had anatomically significant disease

[32]. Many investigators have stressed the importance of expeditious endarterectomy in patients with crescendo TIAs and symptomatic carotid stenosis [31,33–35]. A common recommendation is to give heparin to patients with crescendo TIAs as a bridge to surgery or long-term antiplatelet or anticoagulant therapy [36,37]. The American Heart Association considers i.v. heparin adjusted to an APTT of 1.5–2.0 times control to be a Grade C recommendation [38]. There has not been a randomized trial of heparin vs. aspirin which specifically focused on patients with crescendo TIAs. The use of heparin is likely to be of relatively minor clinical importance compared with prompt carotid endarterectomy where indicated.

Use of heparin in patients with endocarditis

TIAs can rarely occur in the setting of bacterial endocarditis. A review of the Cleveland Clinic experience over a 12-year period identified 175 patients with neurological complications of bacterial endocarditis [39]. Two (1.1%) had TIA, and in both cases the TIA heralded stroke. A review of 20 cases of late prosthetic valve endocarditis with neurological complications at the University of Iowa yielded one (5%) case of TIA [40]. There has been additional anecdotal report of TIA as the presenting feature of bacterial endocarditis [41]. Controversy surrounds the use of heparin to prevent stroke in bacterial endocarditis. As is common when addressing rare clinical events, there is no randomized trial upon which to base firm recommendations for treatment. Just as intracranial hemorrhage is the most feared complication of heparin when used to treat patients with TIA unrelated to endocarditis, so too is intracranial hemorrhage the most feared complication of heparin when used to treat patients with TIA in the setting of endocarditis. However, in endocarditis there is not only the routine concern of hemorrhagic transformation of an infarct, but also the risk of intracranial hemorrhage caused by an erosive arteritis or rupture of a mycotic aneurysm [42]. In 51 patients who had head imaging for neurological complications of endocarditis in one series, two (4%) had hemorrhagic infarction and three (6%) had intracerebral hematoma [39].

Anticoagulation should probably not be used routinely for native valve endocarditis, but some have recommended that patients with prosthetic valve endocarditis continue to receive appropriate anticoagulant therapy [43]. Not everyone considers it is safe to anticoagulate patients with prosthetic valve endocarditis. The US Army Collaborative Group found intracranial hemorrhage to be the principal cause of death in their series of patients with prosthetic valve endocarditis, most of whom received anticoagulation [44]. After reviewing cases of prosthetic valve endocarditis at eight university-affiliated hospitals, Davenport and Hart found no obvious protective effect from anticoagulation therapy with warfarin [45].

Patients with mechanical prosthetic valve endocarditis who are maintained on anticoagulation should have intensive monitoring of coagulation and neurological status. Brain hemorrhage can occur in about 3% of cases [46]. In patients who develop intracranial hemorrhage, heparin should be stopped immediately, and patients should be transfused to correct the coagulopathy. In one retrospective study, temporary interruption of anticoagulation could be done safely for 1–2 weeks after intracranial hemorrhage in patients with mechanical heart valves [47].

Management of TIAs in pregnant women with high-risk cardioembolic source

Fortunately, pregnant women rarely experience TIAs. Medical management of this group of patients is challenging. A small case-control study of 12 previously healthy pregnant women and 24 healthy women matched for age, ethnicity, and smoking status demonstrated that transient cerebrovascular ischemic events during pregnancy were associated with a high rate of inherited thrombophilias [48]. In addition, women in the first trimester of pregnancy who present with TIA may have a comorbid high-risk source of cardioembolism such as a mechanical heart valve. Warfarin cannot be used because of its teratogenic effects. Warfarin embryopathy is associated with hypoplasia of the nose, stippling of bone (chondrodysplasia punctata), optic atrophy, mental retardation, and possibly the Dandy-Walker malformation [49,50]. Behavioral outcome in school-age children can also be affected adversely by *in-utero* exposure to warfarin [51]. Skeletal development in children may not be affected if warfarin exposure is avoided during the first trimester [52]. There can be little doubt that vitamin K deficiency brings about skeletal and neurological problems in embryos. A rat model can reproduce some of the skeletal abnormalities associated with warfarin embryopathy [53]. Epoxide reductase deficiency can bring about the so-called pseudowarfarin embryopathy syndrome, and maternal vitamin K malabsorption can lead to punctate calcifications, nasal hypoplasia, and abnormalities of the spine, along with the Dandy-Walker malformation [54].

Because of concerns of warfarin embryopathy, pregnant women who require anticoagulation are often placed on UF or LMW heparin. Because UF heparin is associated with practical disadvantages, including the risk of heparin-induced thrombocytopenia and osteoporosis with long-term use, some physicians have advocated use of LMW heparins [55]. Rowan and colleagues treated 11 women with mechanical heart valves with enoxaparin (1 mg/kg twice daily) and aspirin (100–150 mg daily) during the course of 14 pregnancies [56]. There were nine live births, three miscarriages, and two terminations. In the 48 months of enoxaparin treatment, one woman who had a documented valve thrombosis when she presented at 8 weeks' gestation had persistent valve thrombosis at 20 weeks' gestation. It was concluded that successful pregnancy may be achieved with therapeutic enoxaparin but that further studies were required before its use could be recommended for pregnant women with mechanical heart valves. While there are certain advantages of LMW heparins in pregnancy, the medications contraindicate the use of regional anesthesia, and it has been recommended that a switch to i.v. UF heparin before delivering may allow greater flexibility in the use of regional anesthesia [57]. Pregnant women who present with TIA and who are found to have a high-risk potential source of cardioembolism represent a therapeutic challenge and are best served by a multidisciplinary approach with expertise in the areas of high-risk obstetrics, hematology, cardiology, and neurology.

Practice patterns

Despite the plethora of negative trials discussed above, some vascular neurologists still feel that heparin may be useful when used selectively in patients. Caplan recommends that heparins should be considered in patients with large-artery occlusions and severe stenosis as well as cardiogenic embolism conditions with a high acute recurrence risk [58].

Previous surveys have shown that practising neurologists continue to use i.v. heparin in certain scenarios, although heparin use may have declined over the past decade. Anderson conducted a survey of neurologists in Minneapolis in 1991 and found that the vast majority of neurologists would use heparin for patients with atrial fibrillation-related stroke (92%) and stroke in evolution (94%) [59]. For patients with vertebrobasilar stroke, the figure was 74% and for carotid distribution stroke, it was 53%.

A more recent survey conducted in 2001, after the publication of six major multicenter studies mentioned above, found that i.v. heparin was still popular among US and Canadian neurologists for patients with atrial fibrillation-related stroke (88% and 84%, respectively) [60]. For other conditions such as stroke in evolution, vertebrobasilar stroke, or carotid territory stroke, US neurologists were more inclined to use i.v. heparin compared with their Canadian counterparts (US 51%, 30%, and 31% vs. Canadian 33%, 8%, and 4%, respectively; $P < 0.001$). For a patient with two TIAs in a 48-h period, US neurologists were also more likely to prescribe i.v. heparin compared with Canadian neurologists (47% vs. 9%, $P < 0.001$). Medicolegal concerns may partly explain this disparity in treatment patterns [60].

Guidelines

In 2002 a joint committee from the American Academy of Neurology and the American Stroke Association published their report on early use of anticoagulants and antiplatelet agents in ischemic stroke [61]. The report commented that 'dose-adjusted, unfractionated heparin is not recommended for reducing morbidity, mortality, or early recurrent stroke because the evidence indicates it is not efficacious and may be associated with increased bleeding complications'. Furthermore, 'i.v., unfractionated heparin or high dose LMW heparin/heparinoids are not recommended for any specific subgroup of patients with acute ischemic stroke that is based on any presumed stroke mechanism or location (e.g. cardioembolic, large vessel atherosclerotic)'.

A slightly different conclusion was articulated in the American College of Chest Physicians Antithrombotic supplement [62]. With regard to heparin, it was commented that 'clinical trials evaluating i.v. heparin for stroke treatment are inconclusive with heterogeneous results. Clinicians may consider early anticoagulation for treatment of acute cardioembolic and large-artery ischemic strokes and for progressing stroke where the suspected mechanism is ongoing thromboembolism'.

Conclusion

Recent randomized clinical trials show that acute ischemic stroke in general and acute cardioembolic stroke in particular are not indications for acute anticoagulation with heparin, LMW heparins or heparinoids. Any reduction in early recurrent cerebral infarction appears to be offset by an increase in intracranial hemorrhage. However, the risk of intracranial hemorrhage is likely lower for TIA than for stroke. Heparin has not been shown to be superior to aspirin as a bridge to long-term oral anticoagulation in patients with TIA and a high-risk source of cardioembolism. Neither has heparin been shown to be superior to aspirin as a bridge to carotid endarterectomy in patients with crescendo TIAs. Additional controlled clinical trial data are needed. Proving the superiority of a short course of heparin over aspirin will be challenging, since the risk of stroke in the first week following a TIA is relatively low. At this point heparin cannot be recommended for routine use in patients with TIAs.

References

1 Johnston SC, Smith WS. Practice variability in management of transient ischemic attacks. *Eur Neurol* 1999; 42: 105–8.
2 Hirsh J, Raschke R, Warkentin TE *et al*. Heparin: mechanism of action, pharmacokinetics, dosing considerations, monitoring, efficacy, and safety. *Chest* 1995; 108 (suppl.): 258S–275S.
3 Meuleman DG, Hobbelen PM, van Dedem G *et al*. A novel antithrombotic heparinoid (Org 10172) devoid of bleeding inducing capacity: a survey of its

pharmacological properties in experimental animal models. *Thromb Res* 1982; 27: 353–63.

4 Hirsh J, Anand SS, Halperin JL *et al.* Guide to anticoagulant therapy: Heparin: a statement for healthcare professionals from the American Heart Association. *Circulation* 2001; 103: 2994–3018.

5 Cerebral Embolism Study Group. Immediate anticoagulation of embolic stroke: a randomized trial. *Stroke* 1983; 14: 668–76.

6 Duke RJ, Bloch RF, Turpie AG *et al.* Intravenous heparin for the prevention of stroke progression in acute partial stable stroke. *Ann Intern Med* 1986; 105: 825–8.

7 International Stroke Trial Collaborative Group. The International Stroke Trial (IST): a randomised trial of aspirin, subcutaneous heparin, both, or neither among 19 435 patients with acute ischaemic stroke. *Lancet* 1997; 349: 1569–81.

8 Saxena R, Lewis S, Berge E *et al.* Risk of early death and recurrent stroke and effect of heparin in 3169 patients with acute ischemic stroke and atrial fibrillation in the International Stroke Trial. *Stroke* 2001; 32: 2333–7.

9 Kay R, Wong KS, Yu YL *et al.* Low-molecular-weight heparin for the treatment of acute ischemic stroke. *N Engl J Med* 1995; 333: 1588–93.

10 The Publications Committee for the Trial of ORG 10172 in Acute Stroke Treatment (TOAST) Investigators. Low molecular weight heparinoid, ORG 10172 (danaparoid), and outcome after acute ischemic stroke: a randomized controlled trial. *JAMA* 1998; 279: 1265–72.

11 Bath PM, Lindenstrom E, Boysen G *et al.* Tinzaparin in acute ischaemic stroke (TAIST): a randomised aspirin-controlled trial. *Lancet* 2001; 358: 702–10.

12 Berge E, Abdelnoor M, Nakstad PH *et al.* Low molecular-weight heparin versus aspirin in patients with acute ischaemic stroke and atrial fibrillation: a double-blind randomised study. HAEST Study Group. Heparin in Acute Embolic Stroke Trial. *Lancet* 2000; 355: 1205–10.

13 Marler JR, Tilley BC, Lu M *et al.* Early stroke treatment associated with better outcome: the NINDS rt-PA stroke study. *Neurology* 2000; 55: 1649–55.

14 Alberts MJ, Hademenos G, Latchaw RE *et al.* Recommendations for the establishment of primary stroke centers. Brain Attack Coalition. *JAMA* 2000; 283: 3102–9.

15 Bonnono C, Criddle LM, Lutsep H *et al.* Emergi-paths and stroke teams: an emergency department approach to acute ischemic stroke. *J Neurosci Nurs* 2000; 32: 298–305.

16 Smith RW, Scott PA, Grant RJ *et al.* Emergency physician treatment of acute stroke with recombinant tissue plasminogen activator: a retrospective analysis. *Acad Emerg Med* 1999; 6: 618–25.

17 Levine SR, Gorman M. 'Telestroke': the application of telemedicine for stroke. *Stroke* 1999; 30: 464–9.

18 Kimura K, Minematsu K, Wada K *et al*. Lesions visualized by contrast-enhanced magnetic resonance imaging in transient ischemic attacks. *J Neurol Sci* 2000; 173: 103–8.

19 Kidwell CS, Alger JR, Di Salle F *et al*. Diffusion MRI in patients with transient ischemic attacks. *Stroke* 1999; 30: 1174–80.

20 Fazekas F, Fazekas G, Schmidt R *et al*. Magnetic resonance imaging correlates of transient cerebral ischemic attacks. *Stroke* 1996; 27: 607–11.

21 Evans GW, Howard G, Murros KE *et al*. Cerebral infarction verified by cranial computed tomography and prognosis for survival following transient ischemic attack. *Stroke* 1991; 22: 431–6.

22 Murros KE, Evans GW, Toole JF *et al*. Cerebral infarction in patients with transient ischemic attacks. *J Neurol* 1989; 236: 182–4.

23 Turnbull IW, Bannister CM. CT observations on the natural history of asymptomatic cerebral infarction following transient ischaemic attacks. *Neurol Res* 1985; 7: 190–3.

24 Bogousslavsky J, Regli F. Cerebral infarct in apparent transient ischemic attack. *Neurology* 1985; 35: 1501–3.

25 Koudstaal PJ, van Gijn J, Lodder J *et al*. Transient ischemic attacks with and without a relevant infarct on computed tomographic scans cannot be distinguished clinically. Dutch Transient Ischemic Attack Study Group. *Arch Neurol* 1991; 48: 916–20.

26 Putman SF, Adams HP Jr. Usefulness of heparin in initial management of patients with recent transient ischemic attacks. *Arch Neurol* 1985; 42: 960–2.

27 Biller J, Bruno A, Adams HP Jr *et al*. A randomized trial of aspirin or heparin in hospitalized patients with recent transient ischemic attacks. A pilot study. *Stroke* 1989; 20: 441–7.

28 The Stroke Prevention in Reversible Ischemia Trial (SPIRIT) Study Group. A randomized trial of anticoagulants versus aspirin after cerebral ischemia of presumed arterial origin. *Ann Neurol* 1997; 42: 857–65.

29 Mohr JP, Thompson JLP, Lazar RM *et al*. A comparison of warfarin and aspirin for the prevention of recurrent ischemic stroke. *N Engl J Med* 2001; 345: 1444–51.

30 EAFT (European Atrial Fibrillation Trial) Study Group. Secondary prevention in nonrheumatic atrial fibrillation after transient ischaemic attack or minor stroke. *Lancet* 1993; 342: 1255–62.

31 Wilson SE, Mayberg MR, Yatsu F *et al*. Crescendo transient ischemic attacks: a surgical imperative. Veterans Affairs trialists. *J Vasc Surg* 1993; 17: 249–55; discussion 255–46.

32 Rothrock JF, Lyden PD, Yee J *et al*. 'Crescendo' transient ischemic attacks: clinical and angiographic correlations. *Neurology* 1988; 38: 198–201.

33 Schneider C, Johansen K, Konigstein R *et al*. Emergency carotid thromboendarterectomy: safe and effective. *World J Surg* 1999; 23: 1163–7.

34 Mentzer RM Jr, Finkelmeier BA, Crosby IK *et al*. Emergency carotid endarterectomy for fluctuating neurologic deficits. *Surgery* 1981; 89: 60–6.

35 Eckstein HH, Schumacher H, Klemm K *et al*. Emergency carotid endarterectomy. *Cerebrovasc Dis* 1999; 9: 270–81.

36 Venketasubramanian N, Chua HC. Subcutaneous low molecular weight heparin in place of heparin infusion during warfarin dose optimisation in cerebral ischaemia. *Clin Neurol Neurosurg* 1998; 100: 193–5.

37 Paterson HM, Holdsworth RJ. Extracranial arterial aneurysms: a cause of crescendo transient ischaemic attacks. *Int J Clin Pract* 2000; 54: 675–6.

38 Feinberg WM, Albers GW, Barnett HJ *et al*. Guidelines for the management of transient ischemic attacks. From the Ad Hoc Committee on Guidelines for the Management of Transient Ischemic Attacks of the Stroke Council of the American Heart Association. *Circulation* 1994; 89: 2950–65.

39 Salgado AV, Furlan AJ, Keys TF *et al*. Neurologic complications of endocarditis: a 12-year experience. *Neurology* 1989; 39: 173–8.

40 Keyser DL, Biller J, Coffman TT *et al*. Neurologic complications of late prosthetic valve endocarditis. *Stroke* 1990; 21: 472–5.

41 Stalenhoef AF, Timmermans J, van der Meer JW. Transient bilateral cortical blindness as a presenting symptom of infective endocarditis. *Neth J Med* 1996; 48: 163–4.

42 Hart RG, Kagan-Hallet K, Joerns SE. Mechanisms of intracranial hemorrhage in infective endocarditis. *Stroke* 1987; 18: 1048–56.

43 Tunkel AR, Kaye D. Neurologic complications of infective endocarditis. *Neurol Clin* 1993; 11: 419–40.

44 Carpenter JL, McAllister CK. Anticoagulation in prosthetic valve endocarditis. *South Med J* 1983; 76: 1372–5.

45 Davenport J, Hart RG. Prosthetic valve endocarditis 1976–1987. Antibiotics, anticoagulation, and stroke. *Stroke* 1990; 21: 993–9.

46 Delahaye JP, Poncet P, Malquarti V *et al*. Cerebrovascular accidents in infective endocarditis: role of anticoagulation. *Eur Heart J* 1990; 11: 1074–8.

47 Wijdicks EF, Schievink WI, Brown RD *et al*. The dilemma of discontinuation of anticoagulation therapy for patients with intracranial hemorrhage and mechanical heart valves. *Neurosurgery* 1998; 42: 769–73.

48 Kupferminc MJ, Yair D, Bornstein NM *et al*. Transient focal neurological deficits during pregnancy in carriers of inherited thrombophilia. *Stroke* 2000; 31: 892–5.

49 Zakzouk MS. The congenital warfarin syndrome. *J Laryngol Otol* 1986; 100: 215–9.

50 Kaplan LC. Congenital Dandy Walker malformation associated with first trimester warfarin: a case report and literature review. *Teratology* 1985; 32: 333–7.

51 Wesseling J, Van Driel D, Heymans HS *et al*. Behavioral outcome of school-age children after prenatal exposure to coumarins. *Early Hum Dev* 2000; 58: 213–24.

52 Van Driel D, Wesseling J, Rosendaal FR *et al*. Growth until puberty after *in utero* exposure to coumarins. *Am J Med Genet* 2000; 95: 438–43.

53 Howe AM, Webster WS. The warfarin embryopathy: a rat model showing maxillonasal hypoplasia and other skeletal disturbances. *Teratology* 1992; 46: 379–90.

54 Menger H, Lin AE, Toriello HV *et al.* Vitamin K deficiency embryopathy: a phenocopy of the warfarin embryopathy due to a disorder of embryonic vitamin K metabolism. *Am J Med Genet* 1997; 72: 129–34.

55 Eldor A. Thrombophilia and its treatment in pregnancy. *J Thromb Thrombolysis* 2001; 12: 23–30.

56 Rowan JA, McCowan LM, Raudkivi PJ *et al.* Enoxaparin treatment in women with mechanical heart valves during pregnancy. *Am J Obstet Gynecol* 2001; 185: 633–7.

57 Hague WM, North RA, Gallus AS *et al.* Anticoagulation in pregnancy and the puerperium. *Med J Aust* 2001; 175: 258–63.

58 Caplan LR. Resolved: heparin may be useful in selected patients with brain ischemia. *Stroke* 2003; 34: 230–1.

59 Anderson DC. How Twin Cities neurologists treat ischemic stroke. *Arch Neurol* 1993; 50: 1098–103.

60 Al-Sadat A, Sunbulli M, Chaturvedi S. Use of intravenous heparin by North American neurologists: do the data matter? *Stroke* 2002; 33: 1574–7.

61 Coull BM, Williams LS, Goldstein LB *et al.* Anticoagulants and antiplatelet agents in acute ischemic stroke. *Neurology* 2002; 59: 13–22.

62 Albers GW, Amarenco P, Easton JD, Sacco RL, Teal P. Antithrombotic and thrombolytic therapy for ischemic stroke. *Chest* 2001; 119: 300S–320S.

63 Kalafut MA, Gandhi R, Kidwell CS *et al.* Safety and cost of low-molecular-weight heparin as bridging anticoagulant therapy in subacute cerebral ischemia. *Stroke* 2000; 31: 2563–8.

CHAPTER 13

Diabetes Mellitus Treatment

George Grunberger, Fadi Al-Khayer

Diabetes mellitus represents several syndromes of abnormal carbohydrate metabolism that are characterized by hyperglycemia. It is associated with an absolute (Type 1) or relative (Type 2) impairment in insulin secretion, along with varying degrees of peripheral resistance to the action of insulin.

Epidemiological data demonstrate an increased risk of stroke among patients with diabetes [1,2]. The Copenhagen Stroke Study found that a stroke patient with diabetes was 3.2 years younger than a stroke patient without diabetes. The incidence of stroke was 2.5 times higher in diabetic men and 3.6 times higher in diabetic women when compared with persons without diabetes and the presence of diabetes independently increased the relative death risk from a stroke by 80% [3].

Diabetes is the leading cause of blindness among working-age people, of end-stage renal disease (ESRD), and of nontraumatic limb amputations [4]. In 1997, the direct cost of diabetes (cost of medical care) and its indirect cost (cost of short-term disability, permanent disability, and premature death) was $44.1 (£24.9) billion and $54.1 (£30.6) billion, respectively [5], or one in every seven healthcare dollars spent in the country (about 15% of all US healthcare expenditure).

Epidemiology

In the United States, approximately 16 million persons have diabetes [6] or approximately one in 16 people. The vast majority of these (> 90%) have Type 2 diabetes. Depending on the region and ethnicity, anywhere between 10 and 20% of North Americans have impaired glucose tolerance. This group has a very high risk of developing Type 2 diabetes (about 7% conversion rate per year) [7].

While nearly 800 000 Americans develop diabetes every year, or approximately 2200 every day, individuals with Type 2 diabetes may have it and remain undiagnosed for over 10 years.

Table 13.1 The classification of diabetes mellitus

Type 1 diabetes	A. Immune-mediated
	B. Idiopathic
Type 2 diabetes	
Other specific types of diabetes	Genetic defects of β-cell function (previously MODY), genetic defects in insulin action, diseases of the exocrine pancreas, endocrinopathies, drug- or chemical-induced, infections, etc.
Gestational diabetes mellitus	

MODY, Maturity-onset diabetes of the young.

Worldwide, an estimated 135 million people had diabetes in 1995. By 2025, the number of people with diabetes is expected to rise to about 300 million [8].

Classification

The American Diabetes Association (ADA) issued new recommendations in 1997 [9]. There is no distinction between primary and secondary causes of diabetes. The terms 'Type 1' and 'Type 2' are to be used instead of 'insulin-dependent (IDDM)' and 'non-insulin-dependent (NIDDM)', respectively. Table 13.1 illustrates the classification of diabetes mellitus.

Type 1 diabetes

Type 1 diabetes is characterized by destruction of the pancreatic β-cells, leading to absolute insulin deficiency. This is usually due to autoimmune destruction of the pancreatic β-cells (Type 1A), but some patients have no evidence of autoimmunity and have no other known cause for β-cell destruction (Type 1B, idiopathic).

Type 2 diabetes

Type 2 diabetes is by far the most common type of diabetes, and is characterized by variable degrees of insulin resistance (with its attendant increased glucose production and peripheral glucose under-utilization), combined with impaired insulin secretion.

Symptoms

Type 1 diabetes mellitus usually presents with symptomatic hyperglycemia or diabetic ketoacidosis (DKA). Type 2 diabetes may present with

Table 13.2 Criteria for the diagnosis of diabetes mellitus

	Plasma glucose level
Normal	Fasting < 110 mg/dl (6.1 mmol/l)
Impaired fasting glucose	Fasting plasma glucose between 110 and 125 mg/dl (6.1–6.9 mmol/l)
Impaired glucose tolerance	Two-hour plasma glucose 140–199 mg/dl (7.8 and 11.1 mmol/l) during an oral glucose tolerance test*
Diabetes mellitus	Fasting plasma glucose ≥ 126 mg/dl (7.0 mmol/l) Symptoms of diabetes† plus random‡ plasma glucose concentration ≥ 200 mg/dl (11.1 mmol/l) Two-hour plasma glucose = 200 mg/dl (11.1 mmol/l) during an oral glucose tolerance test‡

*The test should be performed using a glucose load containing the equivalent of 75 g anhydrous glucose dissolved in water. It is not recommended for routine clinical use.
†Polyuria, polydipsia, and unexplained weight loss.
‡Random is defined as any time of the day without regard to the time since last meal.

symptomatic hyperglycemia or hyperosmolar hyperglycemic state (HHS) (Table 13.4), but is frequently diagnosed in asymptomatic patients during a routine medical examination or when patients present with clinical manifestations of a late complication.

The symptoms of uncontrolled hyperglycemia are polyuria (elevated plasma glucose levels cause marked glucosuria and osmotic diuresis), polydipsia, and weight loss. Hyperglycemia may also lead to blurred vision, nausea, and fatigue. In Type 2 diabetes, these symptoms may persist for weeks or longer before medical attention is sought.

Diagnosis

A new criterion for diagnosing diabetes mellitus has been issued by the ADA in 1997 [9]. It strongly suggests that the diagnosis of diabetes be made on the basis of fasting plasma glucose (FPG). If patients are asymptomatic, the diagnosis needs to be confirmed by a repeated test on a different day. Table 13.2 shows the definitions that have been suggested along with the criteria for the diagnosis of diabetes mellitus [9,10].

Screening

As mentioned above, the majority of patients with Type 1 diabetes present with an acute decompensated metabolic state (DKA) and are therefore diagnosed after symptoms develop. The clinical testing of asymptomatic

Table 13.3 Risk factors for Type 2 diabetes

Obesity (ideal body weight 120% or body mass index 27 kg/m²)

Family history of diabetes mellitus in a first-degree relative

Habitual physical inactivity

Belonging to a high-risk ethnic or racial group (African-American, Hispanic American, Native American, Asian American, or Pacific Islander)

History of delivering a baby weighing > 4.1 kg (9 lb) or of gestational diabetes mellitus

Hypertension (blood pressure 140/90 mmHg)

Dyslipidemia defined as a serum high-density lipoprotein cholesterol concentration < 35 mg/dl (0.9 mmol/l) and/or a serum triglyceride concentration > 250 mg/dl (2.8 mmol/l)

Previously identified impaired glucose tolerance or impaired fasting glucose

Polycystic ovary syndrome

---

individuals for the presence of autoantibodies related to Type 1 diabetes is not currently recommended to identify persons at risk.

On the other hand, in Type 2 diabetes, a long asymptomatic period exists. The early detection and prompt treatment of the disease may reduce its burden and complications. The ADA recommends starting measuring fasting blood glucose in individuals who do not have risk factors for Type 2 diabetes at age 45 years. It should be performed every 3 years if normal [11,12]. Screening of high-risk subjects should be started before the age of 45 years and be done annually. The American College of Endocrinology (ACE) recommends screening for such individuals at age 30 years [13].

Table 13.3 shows the risk factors for Type 2 diabetes [12] (refer to Table 13.1 for normal and abnormal plasma blood glucose values).

Complications

There are acute and chronic complications of diabetes.

Acute complications

Diabetic ketoacidosis and hyperosmolar hyperglycemic state are acute complications of diabetes. The former is usually seen in Type 1 diabetes and was reported to be responsible for more than 160 000 hospital admissions per year in the USA [14]. The latter is seen in Type 2 diabetes, especially in the elderly. Both conditions are potentially life threatening if not treated promptly. They are both associated with absolute or relative insulin deficiency, volume depletion, and hyperglycemia.

Table 13.4 summarizes the above two conditions.

Table 13.4 Comparison between diabetic ketoacidosis (DKA) and hyperosmolar hyperglycemic state (HHS)

	DKA	HHS
Type of diabetes	Usually type 1	Usually type 2
Precipitating factors	Inadequate insulin administration; infection; infarction (cerebral, coronary, mesenteric, peripheral); drugs (cocaine)	Myocardial infarction; stroke; sepsis; pneumonia; urinary tract infection; other serious infections; medications (thiazide diuretics, glucocorticoids, phenytoin)
Symptoms	Nausea/vomiting; thirst/polyuria; abdominal pain; altered mental function; shortness of breath	Polyuria; weight loss; altered mental status; lethargy; obtundation; seizure; coma. Notably absent are symptoms of nausea, vomiting, and abdominal pain
Physical findings	Dehydration; hypotension; tachycardia; tachypnea/ Kussmaul respiration (rapid, deep breathing); acetone odour on the patient's breath; abdominal tenderness; fever; lethargy; obtundation	Profound dehydration; hypotension; tachycardia; altered mental status. Notably absent is Kussmaul respirations and acetone odour on the patient's breath
Glucose	300–600 mg/dl	600–1200 mg/dl
Plasma ketones	+++	+/–
Serum bicarbonate	< 15 meq/l	Normal to slightly low
Potassium	Normal to high	Normal
Phosphate	Low	Normal
Serum osmolality	300–320 mOsm/ml	330–380 mOsm/ml
Arterial pH	6.8–7.3	> 7.3
Anion gap*	High	Normal to slightly high
Treatment	Replace fluids i.v. Give insulin i.v. Replace potassium and other minerals. Treat precipitating factor	Replace fluids i.v. Give insulin i.v. Monitor electrolytes. Treat precipitating factor

*[Na – (Cl + HCO$_3$)], meq/l.

Table 13.5 Chronic complications of diabetes mellitus

Microvascular complications	Retinopathy: nonproliferative and proliferative Nephropathy Neuropathy: distal symmetrical polyneuropathy; mononeuropathies; autonomic neuropathy; and thoracic and lumbar nerve root disease (polyradiculopathy)
Macrovascular complications	Coronary artery disease Peripheral vascular disease Cerebrovascular disease

Chronic complications

The chronic complications of diabetes are responsible for the majority of morbidity and mortality associated with this disease. They are divided into microvascular and macrovascular complications.

Table 13.5 illustrates the chronic complications of diabetes mellitus.

Microvascular complications

The microvascular complications probably represent a distinctive feature of diabetes that result from chronic hyperglycemia. As will be mentioned below, randomized, prospective clinical trials involving large numbers of patients with Type 1 and Type 2 diabetes have conclusively demonstrated that a reduction in chronic hyperglycemia prevents or reduces retinopathy, nephropathy, and neuropathy. However, a genetic predisposition to these complications may be implicated in their development in some patients with diabetes [15].

Retinopathy
Diabetic retinopathy is the leading cause of new blindness among middle-aged Americans, accounting for 12% of all new cases in the USA each year [16]. The presence of severe retinopathy may be a risk factor for death due to ischemic heart disease [17].

Diabetic retinopathy is divided into two categories: nonproliferative and proliferative.

Nonproliferative diabetic retinopathy is characterized by abnormalities of the retinal circulation, including microaneurysms, intraretinal hemorrhages, cotton-wool spots, retinal edema and exudates, and intraretinal microvascular abnormalities. Proliferative diabetic retinopathy is characterized by the proliferation of newly formed blood vessels from the optic disc, retina or iris as the result of widespread retinal ischemia. Panretinal laser photocoagulation performed in patients with high-risk proliferative diabetic retinopathy reduced the risk of severe vision loss by more than 50% [18,19].

Nephropathy
Diabetic nephropathy is the most common cause of ESRD in most of the developed world and is responsible for 43% of all new patients requiring renal replacement therapy in the USA [20]. In contrast to what was thought in the past, there are no substantial differences in the occurrence of diabetic nephropathy between Type 1 and Type 2 diabetes [21]. The peak onset of nephropathy in diabetes is between 10 and 15 years after the onset of the disease. Microalbuminuria (defined as 30–300 mg/day of albumin in a 24-h urine collection) is the earliest clinical finding of diabetic nephropathy [22,23]. ACE inhibitors lower protein excretion and may preserve renal function in diabetics with microalbuminuria [24,25]. The sixth report of the Joint National Committee on Prevention, Detection, Evaluation, and Treatment of High Blood Pressure (JNC VI) recommends a blood pressure of ≤ 125/75 in any patient with renal disease [26].

Neuropathy
Diabetic polyneuropathy is the most common neuropathy in the Western world [27]. Approximately 50% of patients with diabetes will eventually develop neuropathy [28]. The high rate of diabetic neuropathy results in substantial morbidity, including recurrent lower extremity infections, ulcerations, and subsequent amputations. The most frequently encountered neuropathies include the following.

Distal symmetrical polyneuropathy This is the most common form. It most frequently presents with distal sensory loss. Classic 'stocking-glove' sensory loss is typical in this disorder. Motor involvement with frank weakness can occur but usually later and in more severe cases.

Mononeuropathy Mononeuropathy is less common than distal symmetrical polyneuropathy and presents with pain and motor weakness in the distribution of a single nerve. It can affect the cranial nerves (especially the third nerve) or the peripheral nerves (especially the median nerve at the wrist causing carpal tunnel syndrome).

Polyradiculopathy Polyradiculopathy is characterized by severe disabling pain in the distribution of one or more nerve roots. It can affect the lumbar plexus causing pain in the thigh or hip and may be associated with muscle weakness in the hip muscles (diabetic amyotrophy); or the thoracic roots causing severe abdominal pain.

Autonomic neuropathy This is a common complication of diabetes and can affect multiple systems causing resting tachycardia, orthostatic hypotension, gastroparesis, enteropathy, bladder dysfunction, retrograde ejaculation, erectile impotence, hyperhidrosis, and anhidrosis.

Does tight glycemic control prevent microvascular complications?
The prospective Diabetes Control and Complications Trial (DCCT) provided conclusive evidence that strict glycemic control in relatively young patients with Type 1 diabetes can both delay the onset of microvascular complications (primary prevention) and slow the rate of progression of already established complications (secondary prevention) [29].

The DCCT was initiated in 1983 to test whether treatment of individuals with Type 1 diabetes to maintain blood glucose as close to normal as possible would reduce the microvascular complications of diabetes when compared with conventional treatment. It was conducted at 29 clinical centres in the USA and Canada and followed 1441 subjects—726 with no retinopathy at baseline (the primary-prevention cohort) and 715 with mild retinopathy (the secondary-intervention cohort)—for a mean of 6.5 years. Intensive therapy consisted of intensive education in self-management, with frequent contact from support staff, three or more insulin injections per day or an insulin pump, and frequent blood monitoring. Conventional therapy was to achieve the goal of clinical self-being; patients received up to two daily insulin injections and a standard schedule of monitoring. The appearance and progression of retinopathy and other complications were assessed regularly. The mean hemoglobin A_{1c} (HbA$_{1c}$) values during the study were 7.2% with intensive therapy as opposed to 9.1% with conventional therapy; the respective mean blood glucose concentrations were 155 mg/dl (8.6 mmol/l) and 235 mg/dl (12.8 mmol/l).

Highlights of DCCT results include:
• In the primary-prevention cohort, intensive therapy reduced the adjusted mean risk for the development of retinopathy by 76% compared with conventional therapy.
• In the secondary-intervention cohort, intensive therapy slowed the progression of retinopathy by 54% and reduced the development of proliferative or severe nonproliferative retinopathy by 47%.
• Intensive therapy reduced the occurrence of microalbuminuria by 39%, and macroalbuminuria (urinary albumin excretion of > 300 mg per 24 h) by 54%.
• Intensive therapy reduced clinical neuropathy by 60%.

The Stockholm Diabetes Intervention Study (SDIS) has shown similar results [30]. Forty-three patients with Type 1 diabetes were randomized to intensified treatment and 48 patients were randomized to standard treatment. The patients were followed up for 10 years. The HbA$_{1c}$ was reduced to ~ 7% in the intensive group, and ~ 8.3% in the conventionally managed group.

Highlights of SDIS results include:

• A lower incidence of the development of serious retinopathy was seen in the intensive group (33% vs. 63% in the conventional group).

• A lower incidence of the development of nephropathy in the intensive group (7% vs. 26% in the conventional group).

• A lower incidence of the development of symptoms of neuropathy in the intensive group (14% vs. 32% in the conventional group).

The United Kingdom Prospective Diabetes Study (UKPDS) and the Kumamoto study in Japan confirmed the above findings in patients with Type 2 diabetes. The UKPDS was designed to compare the efficacy of different treatment regimens on glycemic control and the complications of diabetes in patients with Type 2 diabetes [31]. It recruited 5102 patients with newly diagnosed Type 2 diabetes in 23 centres within the UK between 1977 and 1991. The patients were randomly assigned to intensive treatment with a sulfonylurea (metformin was added to the sulfonylurea if optimal control was not achieved with the latter alone) or with insulin, or conventional treatment with diet. The target fasting blood glucose concentration was 108 mg/dl (6 mmol/l) or less in the intensive group. In the conventional group, the aim was the best achievable FPG with diet alone; drugs were added only if there were hyperglycemic symptoms or FPG > 270 mg/dl (15 mmol/l). Over 10 years, HbA_{1c} was 7.0% in the intensive group compared with 7.9% in the conventional group.

The UKPDS found a 25% reduction in risk of microvascular complications in the intensive group:

• The incidence of retinopathy was 17% in the intensive group vs. 21% in the conventional group.

• The incidence of nephropathy was 24% in the intensive group vs. 33% in the conventional group.

A few years before publishing the results of UKPDS, the Kumamoto trial, a trial of 110 patients with Type 2 diabetes on insulin from Japan, found similar results [32]. A group of 55 patients without evidence of microvascular complications (the primary prevention cohort) was randomly assigned to receive multiple doses of insulin or less intensive insulin treatment. The other 55 patients with evidence of simple retinopathy and urinary albumin excretion > 30 mg/day (the secondary intervention cohort) were randomly assigned to the same treatment regimens. The patients were followed for 6 years. The goal of therapy in the multiple-dose insulin groups was to reduce the HbA_{1c} value below 7.0%. The following benefits were noted in the multidose insulin group:

• A lower incidence of the development or progression of retinopathy after 6 years (7.7% vs. 32% in the primary prevention cohort, and 19.2% vs. 44% in the secondary intervention cohort).

- A lower incidence of the development or progression of nephropathy after 6 years (7.7% vs. 28% in the primary prevention cohort, and 11.5% vs. 32% in the secondary intervention cohort).

In the Kumamoto trial, the investigators concluded that the glycemic threshold to prevent the onset and the progression of diabetic micro-angiopathy was HbA_{1c} 6.5%, fasting blood glucose < 110 mg/dl, and 2-h postprandial blood glucose concentration < 180 mg/dl.

A 10-year follow-up on the Kumamoto trial further supported the above findings [33].

Macrovascular complications

The macrovascular complications are not specifically a result of hyper-glycemia. These clinical conditions also occur in the general population. However, in persons with diabetes they present at earlier age, more fre-quently, and in a more severe fashion, as illustrated below.

Coronary artery disease (CAD)

Cardiovascular complications are the most frequent cause of mortality in Type 2 diabetes mellitus [34]. The risk of a first myocardial infarction in patients with diabetes is higher or equal to that in nondiabetic individuals who have already suffered such an event [35]. The Framingham Study found that the incidence of cardiovascular disease among diabetic men was twice that among nondiabetic men, and among diabetic women the incid-ence of cardiovascular disease was three times that among nondiabetic women [36]. The decline in heart disease mortality noted in recent years in the USA was less in diabetic persons than in nondiabetic persons, and mortality even increased in women with diabetes [37]. Compared with nondiabetics, the diabetic patients had a greater incidence of multivessel disease and a greater number of diseased vessels [38]. In addition to the in-creased frequency of symptomatic CAD, another important clinical finding in diabetes is silent ischemia or even silent infarction [39]. Controlling blood pressure, treating dyslipidemia, and avoiding smoking are mandatory thera-peutic modalities to reduce CAD mortality among patients with diabetes.

Peripheral vascular disease (PVD)

PVD in the lower extremities is an important reason for disabling pain and amputations in patients with and without diabetes. However, presence of diabetes increases the incidence of PVD. The Framingham heart study of 381 men and women who were followed for 38 years revealed that the odds ratio for developing intermittent claudication was 2.6 for diabetes mellitus [40]. In patients with peripheral arterial disease, diabetic patients have worse arterial disease and a poorer outcome than nondiabetic patients [41]. Patients with PVD, regardless of the etiology, have a high risk of death from cardiovascular disease [42].

Cerebrovascular disease

Diabetic patients tend to have dyslipidemia, hypertension, CAD, physical inactivity, and obesity. These factors increase the likelihood of developing large-vessel cerebral atherosclerosis.

Cohort studies have demonstrated an independent effect of diabetes on stroke risk after controlling for other risk factors, with relative risks ranging from 1.5 to 3.0 [43,44]. As was stated before, the Copenhagen Stroke Study found that the diabetic stroke patient was 3.2 years younger than the nondiabetic stroke patient, the incidence of stroke was 2.5 times higher in diabetic men and 3.6 times higher in diabetic women when compared with persons without diabetes, and diabetes independently increased the relative death risk from a stroke by 80% [3]. A Swedish study showed a six-fold rise in the risk of stroke in men with diabetes compared with a 13-fold rise in women [45]. The main source of thromboembolic strokes in patients with diabetes is the internal carotid artery [46].

Although 'traditional' risk factors are important contributors to coronary heart disease and stroke also in persons with diabetes, they do not fully explain the excess risk of macrovascular disease produced by diabetes. There is currently strong interest in 'nontraditional' risk factors for coronary heart disease. The Atherosclerosis Risk in Communities (ARIC) Study showed that levels of albumin, fibrinogen, von Willebrand factor, factor VIII activity, and leukocyte count were predictors of coronary heart disease among persons with diabetes. These associations may reflect (i) the underlying inflammatory reaction or microvascular injury related to atherosclerosis and a tendency toward thrombosis, or (ii) common antecedents for both diabetes and coronary heart disease [47]. Epidemiological studies have demonstrated that hyperinsulinemia, a marker for insulin resistance, is an independent risk factor for cardiovascular disease [48]. Elevated plasma levels of plasminogen activator inhibitor type 1 (PAI-1) are associated with cardiovascular disease. Levels of PAI-1, the primary inhibitor of endogenous-type fibrinolysis, are elevated in persons with diabetes and in obese nondiabetic persons with insulin resistance. Impaired fibrinolytic function in diabetes correlates with the severity of vascular disease in diabetes [49]. Peroxisome proliferator-activated receptor-γ (PPAR-γ), a nuclear receptor that has a regulatory role in differentiation of cells, is present in human endothelial cells, vascular smooth-muscle cells, monocytes and macrophages, and human arterial lesions, all of which play important pathogenic roles in atherosclerosis. Thiazolidinediones, such as pioglitazone (Actos®) and rosiglitazone (Avandia®), bind and activate PPAR-γ. These drugs are currently used for treatment of hyperglycemia in patients with Type 2 diabetes. Thiazolidinediones may also target various aspects of the insulin resistance syndrome in addition to hyperglycemia (a decrease in plasma insulin and triglyceride levels, an increase in HDL-cholesterol level, a decrease in lipid oxidation, favorable redistribution of body fat, a decrease in vascular resistance, and improvement in endothelial function) [50]. Thus, therapy with these drugs might reduce the risk of cardiovascular disease.

To support the importance of the nontraditional risk factors in atherosclerosis, a new report about the use of HMG-CoA reductase inhibitors (statins) showed that these drugs in patients with atherosclerosis might result in more marked reduction of morbidity and mortality than expected from trials using conventional cholesterol-lowering therapies that looked at only decreasing the cholesterol. The mechanism was by stimulation of angiogenesis, improvement of endothelial function, plaque stabilization, inhibition of coagulation and/or thrombocyte aggregation and inhibition of the inflammatory response associated with atherosclerosis [51].

Does tight glycemic control prevent macrovascular complications?
As mentioned above, tight glycemic control reduces the risk of microvascular complications in patients with diabetes mellitus. However, there is much more limited information on the effect of glycemic control on the macrovascular complications of diabetes. The DCCT in patients with Type 1 diabetes found a nonsignificant trend toward fewer cardiovascular events with intensive therapy [29]. It was suggested that the relatively short duration of diabetes mellitus and the young age of these individuals might have masked the true benefit of glycemic control.

In the primary analysis of the UKPDS, there was no difference in macrovascular disease in the intensive and conventional therapy groups [31]. However, a subanalysis of the UKPDS found that, in patients with diabetes, glucose control plus tight blood pressure control could reduce the macrovascular complications of diabetes, including stroke and death [52]. Importantly, the UKPDS showed that treatment with insulin and the sulfonylureas did not appear to increase the risk of cardiovascular disease in individuals with Type 2 diabetes, proving prior claims about the atherogenic potential of these agents to be wrong.

Treatment of diabetes mellitus

Therapy of diabetes mellitus involves daily self-management by the patient and a host of lifestyle adaptations.

Treatment of Type 1 diabetes

Patients with Type 1 diabetes generally have absolute insulin deficiency. The clinical goals of treatment include (i) decreasing plasma glucose to prevent the symptoms of hyperglycemia, (ii) preventing ketosis and the risk of DKA, (iii) avoiding hypoglycemia as possible, (iv) a balanced diet that maintains lean body mass and minimizes the risk of symptomatic

Table 13.6 The American Diabetes Association (ADA) standards for glycemic control in diabetes mellitus

Parameter	Normal	Goal	Additional action suggested
Fasting or preprandial glucose (capillary whole blood)	< 110	80–120	< 80 or > 140 mg/dl
Bedtime glucose (capillary whole blood)	< 120	100–140	< 100 or > 160 mg/dl
Hemoglobin A_{1c} (%)	< 6%	< 7%	> 8%

Table 13.7 The American College of Endocrinology targets for glycemic control

	Target
Fasting glucose (capillary whole blood)	< 110 mg/dl
Postprandial glucose (capillary whole blood)	< 140 mg/dl
Hemoglobin A_{1c}	< 6.5%

hyperglycemia and/or hypoglycemia at the same time, (v) and tight control of plasma glucose to prevent late complications. The ADA revised their standards of care after the publication of the DCCT.

Table 13.6 summarizes the ADA standards for glycemic control in diabetes (both Type 1 and Type 2) [53]. Table 13.7 summarizes the ACE guidelines [13].

Blood glucose monitoring

The current glucose meters are inexpensive, small, simple, accurate, and use less blood. Ideally, testing at home should to be done four to seven times daily (premeals and/or 2 h after meals). Blood glucose monitoring allows daily glycemic control to be assessed and guides insulin treatment. An important supplement to home blood glucose testing is monitoring of plasma levels of HbA_{1c} so that chronic level of glucose control can be estimated.

Nutrition

Nutrition is essential in the management of Type 1 diabetes. A meal plan based on the individual patient's lifestyle, food preferences, and eating habits should be used as a basis for integrating insulin therapy into lifestyle. To facilitate the matching of insulin doses to meals and to prevent hypoglycemia, patients with Type 1 diabetes should eat consistent regular meals comprising about 50% carbohydrate calories, ~ 10–20% protein calories, < 30% total fat calories, and < 300 mg cholesterol a day [54]. A dietitian should be part of the diabetes care team.

Exercise

Exercise is an important component of diabetes care. It is helpful to avoid weight gain frequently induced by increased insulin administration [55]. Patients must be instructed how to adjust their meals, their insulin doses and timing to prevent hypoglycemia during, immediately after, or even 6–12 h after exercise, as moderately intensive exercise may deplete glycogen stores, resulting in sustained food requirement to replace the glycogen. Absorbed carbohydrate should be available during activity in case of hypoglycemia.

Insulin

The basic principle of insulin replacement treatment is (i) to maintain a fairly constant basal level of insulin in the serum by administering one or two daily injections of intermediate or long-acting insulin (NPH, lente, ultralente, glargine), or by a continuous subcutaneous insulin infusion (insulin pump); (ii) and to superimpose short-acting insulin on this basal level via premeal bolus doses (the dose of this insulin can be adjusted according to the premeal blood glucose or the size of the meal to be eaten, and the anticipated activity following the meal). Table 13.8 summarizes the different insulin preparations currently available in the USA.

It is important to recognize that there is considerable variability in the pharmacokinetic characteristics of these insulins both from individual to individual and within the same individual from day to day.

The most commonly used multiple-dose regimen consists of basal and prandial component. The general rule is that basal insulin and mealtime

Table 13.8 Different insulin preparations currently available in the USA

Insulin type	Onset (h)	Duration (h)	Peak (h)
Short acting (regular insulin, R)	0.5–1.0	6–8	2–3
Rapid acting			
Lispro (Humalog®)	0.05–0.15	3–5	1–2
Aspart (NovoLog®)	0.05–0.15	3–5	1–2
Intermediate acting			
NPH	1–3	13–18	5–7
Lente	1–3	13–20	4–8
Long acting			
Ultralente	2–4	18–30	10–14
Glargine (Lantus®)	1.5	24	None
Combinations			
70/30 (70% NPH, 30% regular)	0.5–1.0	13–18	Dual
70/30 (NovoLog® mix, 70% NPA, 30% aspart)	0.05–0.15	13–18	Dual
50/50 (50% NPH, 50% regular)	0.5–1.0	13–18	Dual
75/25 (Humalog® mix, 75% NPL, 25% lispro)	0.05–0.15	13–18	Dual

insulin pulses each constitute approximately 50% of the average total daily dose (0.6–0.7 U/kg) in intensive-therapy regimens. As mentioned above, intermediate or long-acting insulin in one or two daily injections is used as basal insulin, and short or rapid-acting insulins are used to cover the meals.

An insulin algorithm can be used by the patient to adjust the rapid-acting insulin dose based on the blood glucose level and the estimated amount of carbohydrate to be eaten. A typical regimen would call for 1–2 extra units of insulin for each 50-mg/dl increment in blood glucose above the dose called for by the preprandial target of 80–120 mg/dl, or 1 U more for each 15 g of extra carbohydrate to be ingested above the usual amount of carbohydrate prescribed by the nutrition plan.

The insulin glargine has virtually no peak, which may make it the ideal basal insulin for intensive insulin therapy; it apparently is associated with less nocturnal hypoglycemia [56]. Similar improvement in fasting blood glucose with insulin glargine compared with NPH insulin was reported [57].

Treatment of Type 2 diabetes

Patients with Type 2 diabetes have insulin resistance and deficiency. The goals for glycemic control are the same as in Type 1 and are summarized in Table 13.6. Treatment should include: (i) patient education (glucose monitoring, diet, and exercise), (ii) evaluation for vascular and neurological complications, (iii) measures aimed at minimizing cardiovascular risk factors, and (iv) avoidance of drugs that can aggravate the abnormalities in insulin or lipid metabolism.

Blood glucose monitoring

A standard number of daily glucose checks by patients is not set. One needs to individualize the advice so that the number of measurements requested is appropriate to each patient's therapy and physician's need for information necessary to adjust the treatment. Typically, at least fasting blood glucose and 2-h postprandial blood glucose (2 h after the heaviest meal of the day) should be monitored.

Nutrition

Nutritional therapy is an essential component of successful diabetes management and can improve many aspects of Type 2 diabetes, including obesity, hypertension, dyslipidemia, and insulin release and responsiveness. Consensus guidelines recommend that the calories should consist of < 30% total fat, < 10% saturated fat, < 10% polyunsaturated fat, 10–15% monounsaturated fat, 10–20% protein, and 50–55% carbohydrate [54].

Weight loss of as little as 5–10% produces significant decreases in plasma glucose and HbA_{1c} over 1–3 months [58]. Despite the clear benefit of weight loss, only a few patients with Type 2 diabetes are able to attain and maintain substantial weight loss [59]. This difficulty has probably a physiological basis since weight loss lowers the metabolic rate, thereby retarding further weight loss.

Exercise

Regular exercise, such as walking 45–60 min at a brisk pace three to five times a week, improves insulin sensitivity and facilitates insulin action; increases energy expenditure; reduces the risk of future cardiovascular disease; facilitates control of hypertension; enhances the patient's sense of well-being and physical fitness; and improves dyslipidemia. Clinicians may consider an exercise–stress electrocardiogram in all individuals > 35 years old to detect silent ischemic heart disease.

Pharmacological therapy

Treatment options for management of Type 2 diabetes have increased significantly over the past several years. However, nonpharmacological treatments (diet and exercise) need to be emphasized indefinitely because none of the drug therapies will have their maximum impact otherwise.

Table 13.9 summarizes the antidiabetic oral drugs mostly used in the USA and Table 13.10 summarizes some of the characteristics of antidiabetic

Table 13.9 Antidiabetic oral drugs used in the USA

Drugs	Duration of effect (h)	Lowest effective single dose (mg)	Maximum daily dose (mg)
Sulfonylureas			
Glyburide (DiaBeta®, Micronase®)	16–24	1.25	20
Micronized glyburide (Glynase®)	12–24	1.5	12
Glipizide (Glucotrol®)	12–24	5	40
Glipizide-GITS (Glucotrol-XL®)	24	5	20
Glimepiride (Amaryl®)	24	0.5	8
Biguanides			
Metformin (Glucophage®)	5–6	500	2500
Thiazolidinediones			
Pioglitazone (Actos®)	+ 24	15	45
Rosiglitazone (Avandia®)	+ 24	2	8
α-Glucosidase inhibitors			
Acarbose (Precose®)	6	25	300
Miglitol (Glyset®)	6	25	300
Meglitidinides			
Repaglinide (Prandin®)	0.5–2	0.5	16
D-phenylalanine derivative			
Nateglinide (Starlix®)	0.5–2	60	360

Table 13.10 Characteristics of antidiabetic oral drugs

	Sulfonylureas	Meglitidinides/ D-phenylalanine	Thiazolidinediones	α-Glucosidase inhibitors	Biguanides
Mechanism	Increase pancreatic insulin release	Increase pancreatic insulin release (coincidentally with meals)	Improve insulin sensitivity	Slow digestion of complex carbohydrates, oligosaccharides, and disaccharides	Decrease hepatic glucose output (major). Improves insulinx insulin
Hypoglycemia potential	Yes	Yes	No	No	No
Weight gain	Yes	Yes	Yes	No	No (may be associated with weight loss)
Side-effects	Hypoglycemia Hypersensitivity +	Hypoglycemia +	Edema +	Flatulence Diarrhea +++	Nausea Diarrhea ++
Monotherapy effect	+++	+++ (especially in postprandial hyperglycemia)	++	+	+++
Impact of renal status	++	−	−	+	+++ Risk of lactic acidosis
Impact of hepatic status	++	+	+	++	++
Effect on lipids					
Triglyceride	Lower	Lower	Lower	Lower	Lower
HDL-cholesterol	Minimum	Minimum	Raise	Minimum	Raise
Total cholesterol	Minimum	Minimum	Minimum	Minimum	Lower
Lower HbA$_{1c}$ (%)	1.5–2.0	0.5–0.7	0.5–2.0	0.5–1.0	1.5–2.0

oral drugs. Despite the multitude of pharmacological agents available, as shown in Table 13.9, for treatment of Type 2 diabetes mellitus, none of it can alone be expected adequately to control hyperglycemia indefinitely. Despite all of the medications, there appear to be secondary failures after initial response. These are recognized by deterioration of glycemic control. These failures may occur because of disease progression (mostly), lack of dietary adherence, and intercurrent illness. It is very important to address this issue with the patient from the first visit to the clinic so the patient expects to be put on combination of oral antidiabetic drugs or insulin at some point, as the disease tends to progress over time.

The use of antidiabetic drugs as monotherapy

Sulfonylureas
Most patients who are of normal weight or only moderately obese are begun on a sulfonylurea, which usually lowers FPG by 50–70 mg/day.

Meglitidinides, phenylalanine derivatives, and α-glucosidase inhibitors
Patients who have mainly postprandial hyperglycemia (as shown with their blood glucose monitoring 2 h after meals) are candidates for these agents. They lower postprandial glucose by 50–70 mg/dl.

Biguanides
Patients with marked obesity may benefit from metformin because it is not associated with weight gain on improvement in glycemic control, and a modest weight loss may be seen. Among responders, metformin lowers FPG by 50–70 mg/dl.

Thiazolidinediones
These agents are mostly used in the combination treatment. When used as monotherapy, they can lower FPG by 50–70 mg/dl.

The use of antidiabetic drugs as combination therapy
The combination treatment is becoming more popular as a result of the improved understanding of the pathogenesis of hyperglycemia in Type 2 diabetes mellitus. The availability of combination therapies supports the logic of attacking two or more different causes of hyperglycemia simultaneously—for example, reducing insulin resistance in the liver with metformin while increasing insulin secretion with a sulfonylurea.

Various combinations of oral drugs may be considered in patients who have not responded to a single drug alone:
Sulfonylurea + metformin
Sulfonylurea + thiazolidinedione
Metformin + thiazolidinedione

Metformin + meglitinide
Meglitinide + thiazolidinedione
Sulfonylurea + metformin + thiazolidinedione
Repaglinide or nateglinide + metformin + thiazolidinedione
Acarbose + any other drug
Miglitol + sulfonylurea
Insulin + any other drug

Examples of therapeutic strategies in Type 2 diabetes

1 If fasting plasma glucose > 250 mg/dl and patient is symptomatic, always start insulin at least for a few weeks until symptoms of hyperglycemia are relieved.

2 If fasting plasma glucose < 250 mg/dl and the patient is asymptomatic, initiate education and try 4 weeks of diet and exercise. Evaluate every 1–2 weeks. If treatment targets are not met, advance to next step.

3 Add one of the antidiabetic drugs. See 'The use of antidiabetic drugs as monotherapy'. If hyperglycemia persists or worsens, advance to next step within 1 month.

4 Combination of oral antidiabetic drugs. If not adequate, advance to next step within 1 month.

5 Oral drug(s) and bedtime insulin (NPH, Lente, or glargine). If not adequate, advance to next step.

6 Multiple-dose insulin therapy.

Aspirin and diabetes treatment

We have addressed the increased atherosclerotic risk of diabetes above. There is evidence that aspirin is beneficial as primary and secondary strategy to prevent cardiovascular events in nondiabetic and diabetic individuals.

The evidence for secondary prevention

In the Hypertension Optimal Treatment (HOT) Trial, aspirin significantly reduced cardiovascular events by 15% and myocardial infarction by 36%. The relative effects of aspirin were similar in nondiabetic and diabetic subjects [60].

The Early Treatment Diabetic Retinopathy Study (ETDRS) consisted of patients with Type 1 and Type 2 diabetes. The relative risk for myocardial infarction in the first 5 years in patients randomized to aspirin therapy was lowered significantly to 0.72 [61].

The Anti-Platelet Trialists (APT) have reported a meta-analysis of 145 prospective controlled trials of antiplatelet therapy in men and women after myocardial infarction, stroke or transient ischemic attack, or positive cardiovascular history (vascular surgery, angioplasty, angina, etc.).

Reductions in vascular events were about one-quarter in each of these categories, and diabetic subjects had risk reductions that were comparable to nondiabetic individuals [62].

The evidence for primary prevention

The US Physicians' Health Study was a primary prevention trial in which a low-dose aspirin regimen was compared with placebo in male physicians. There was a 44% reduction in the risk of myocardial infarction in the treated group, and subgroup analyses in the diabetic physicians revealed a reduction in myocardial infarction from 10.1% (placebo) to 4.0% (aspirin), yielding a relative risk of 0.39 for the diabetic men on aspirin therapy [63].

If no contraindications exist, low-dose aspirin therapy should be used as a primary and secondary prevention strategy in men and women with diabetes. Unfortunately, in a survey of 1503 adults with diabetes conducted between 1988 and 1994, only 20% took aspirin regularly [64]. Aspirin therapy should not be recommended for patients under the age of 21 years because of the increased risk of Reye's syndrome associated with aspirin use in this population.

Guidelines for diabetes care

HbA$_{1c}$

HbA$_{1c}$ provides a single number that reflects average glycemic control over the preceding 2–3 months.

1 Check every 6 months in patients with Type 2 diabetes whose glycated hemoglobin is in the desirable range.

2 Check every 3 months in patients with Type 1 diabetes and in patients with Type 2 diabetes whose control is not satisfactory.

3 Target level = 7% per ADA. However, the American College of Endocrinology (ACE) recommends the primary target for HbA$_{1c}$ to be < 6.5% [13].

4 Action required for ≥ 8% per ADA guidelines (Table 13.6).

Microalbuminuria

The normal rate of albumin excretion is < 20 mg/day (15 µg/min); values between 30 and 300 mg/day (20–200 µg/min) in a patient with diabetes indicate microalbuminuria. Values > 300 mg/day (200 µg/min) represent overt proteinuria.

1 Type 2 diabetes: yearly 24-h urine albumin; the first examination is at the diagnosis of the disease.

2 Type 1 diabetes: yearly 24-h urine albumin; the first examination is 5 years after diagnosis. Note that screening can be more simply achieved by a timed urine collection or an early morning specimen to minimize changes in urine volume that occur during the day. Microalbuminuria is unlikely if the albumin excretion rate is < 20 μg/min in a timed collection or the urine albumin concentration is < 20–30 mg/l in a random specimen. Higher values may represent false-positive results, and should be confirmed by a 24-h collection or by repeated early morning measurements. This can be avoided by calculation of the albumin-to-creatinine ratio in an untimed urine specimen. A value above 30 μg of albumin/mg of creatinine suggests that albumin excretion is > 30 mg/day and therefore that microalbuminuria is probably present.

3 Action if albumin > 30 mg/g creatinine; consider ACE inhibitors (or angiotensin II receptor antagonists) and aggressively control blood pressure to ≤ 125/75.

LDL-cholesterol

1 Check yearly or more often as necessary.
2 Goal < 100 mg/dl.
3 Action required for level > 130 mg/dl. Consider statins as first-line therapy.

HDL-cholesterol

1 Check yearly or more often as necessary.
2 Goal > 45 mg/dl. If low, consider niacin or fibrates.

Triglycerides

1 Check yearly or more often as necessary.
2 Goal < 150 mg/dl.
3 Action required for level > 400 mg/dl. Consider niacin or fibrates, or fish oil.

Blood pressure

1 Every visit, minimum every 6 months.
2 Goal < 130/80; if renal impairment is present, the goal is ≤ 125/75.

Foot examination

1 Every visit for diabetes care.
2 At least once a year by a podiatrist.

Dilatated eye examination

1 Type 2 diabetes: yearly; the first examination is at the diagnosis of the disease.
2 Type 1 diabetes: yearly; the first examination is 5 years after diagnosis.

Smoking assessment

Yearly, if current smoker, counseling for cessation at each visit.

Note that a survey in the USA found the prevalence of cigarette smoking was higher among diabetic patients than nondiabetic subjects, even after adjusting for age, sex, race, and educational level (27.3% among people with diabetes vs. 25.9% among people without diabetes) [65]. In a cohort of over 3055 patients from the UKPDS, the estimated hazard ratio for CAD for smokers was 1.4 [66].

Evidence for tight glucose control in the hospital

An estimated 6 million hospitalizations per year in the USA are accompanied by hyperglycemia (with and without diabetes) [67,68]. In an acute illness, a generalized stress response is initiated. The levels of counterregulatory hormones (including epinephrine, norepinephrine, glucagon, cortisol, and growth hormone) increase. This, in turn, can increase levels of circulating serum glucose, free fatty acids, and ketone bodies by accelerating catabolism, hepatic gluconeogenesis, and lipolysis. In addition, acute illness may result in acidosis from lactate or ketone body accumulation. Acidosis leads to progressive insulin resistance causing additional impairment in carbohydrate metabolism. Dramatic changes in dietary intake, activity levels, and pharmacological interventions can even worsen the hyperglycemia.

Studies in the areas of stroke, myocardial infarction, bypass surgery, and nosocomial infections all show a tremendous potential to reduce morbidity, mortality, lengths of stay, and added costs among hospitalized patients with hyperglycemia. Unfortunately, hyperglycemia is often overlooked when a hospitalized patient is acutely ill and facing a life-threatening illness such as a stroke or myocardial infarction.

Acute hyperglycemia, regardless of the presence of diabetes, predicts increased risk of in-hospital mortality after ischemic stroke in nondiabetic patients and increased risk of poor functional recovery in nondiabetic stroke survivors; nondiabetic stroke survivors whose admission glucose level was > 121–144 mg/dl (6.7–8 mmol/l) had a greater risk of poor functional recovery [69].

In one study, only 43% of the patients with an admission glucose value of > 120 mg/dl were able to return to work, whereas 76% of patients with lower glucose values regained employment [70]. In another one, a plasma glucose level > 144 mg/dl within the first 24 h of admission was a risk factor independent of age, stroke type, and stroke severity that doubled the mortality risk [71].

Even transient hyperglycemia in the setting of acute stroke is a significant predictor of worse outcome. Patients with transient hyperglycemia had larger ischemic lesions on computed tomography than diabetics and had higher 30-day mortality than normoglycemics. One-year mortality was similar in transient hyperglycemics and diabetics, and both were significantly higher than in normoglycemics [72].

When determining the goals for glycemic control in a hospitalized patient, there are two main considerations: (i) avoiding hypoglycemia, and (ii) avoiding hyperglycemia.

Initial considerations in selecting the optimal regimen for glycemic control in the inpatient with diabetes are:

1 the type of diabetes (patients with Type 1 diabetes must always receive treatment with insulin even if they are nothing by mouth (NPO));
2 nutritional status (is the patient eating or is he/she NPO?);
3 the type of outpatient treatment.

The patient is NPO

Stop all oral antidiabetic drugs (if the patient is on these prior to admission) and start the patient on D_5W IV and regular insulin by intravenous infusion. Adjust the insulin drip to keep the blood glucose as close to normal as possible.

The patient is eating

If the patient is on insulin, continue the same regimen as outside the hospital and adjust the treatment on a daily basis. Avoid 'sliding scale' insulin coverage as it often results in erratic rather than improved glycemic control [73]. If the patient is on oral antidiabetic drugs, these can be continued and tighter blood glucose, if needed, can be established by adding insulin. When the patient is taken for a procedure that involves the administration of i.v. dye, the patient must be well hydrated and the oral antidiabetic drugs must be discontinued the day of the procedure and not resumed until the patient starts eating and the renal function is not compromised.

Targeted glycemic control (80–110 mg/dl) should be attempted in the setting of acute stroke, unless contraindicated. In patients with diabetes, relative contraindications to tight control in the setting of stroke include a history of coma or seizures in the presence of hypoglycemia or a concurrent unstable cardiac status. In a study of 1548 patients admitted to the intensive care unit, the morbidity and mortality in the intensive insulin therapy group (maintenance of blood glucose at a level between 80 and 110 mg/dl) vs. the conventional therapy group (maintenance of blood glucose at a level between 180 and 200 mg/dl) was reduced by 45% and 34%, respectively, over 12 months [74].

Insulin resistance

Insulin resistance can occur in nondiabetic individuals as well as diabetics and the frequency of this physiological phenomenon is likely to increase with the increasing obesity in North American populations. Improving insulin sensitivity may be associated with a decreased stroke risk. A secondary analysis of data from the UKPDS group found that treatment with metformin was associated with a decreased number of strokes (3.3 events/1000 patient-years) compared with treatment with insulin or sulfonylureas (6.2 events/1000 patient-years) ($P = 0.032$) [75].

Summary

Diabetes mellitus has a tremendous impact on our society. Diabetic complications are common and have devastating consequences. Future development of blindness, kidney failure, and amputation can be markedly lessened by attention to therapies and preventive approaches demonstrated to be effective. The increased use of medications such as ACE inhibitors also holds the promise of decreasing stroke in this population.

References

1 Kiers L, Davis SM, Larkins R *et al.* Stroke topography and outcome in relation to hyperglycemia and diabetes. *J Neurol Neurosurg Psychiatry* 1992; 55: 263–70.
2 O'Neill PA, Davies I, Fullerton KJ *et al.* Stress hormone and blood glucose response following acute stroke in the elderly. *Stroke* 1991; 22: 842–7.
3 Jorgensen HS, Nakayama H, Raaschou HO *et al.* Stroke in patients with diabetes. The Copenhagen Stroke Study. *Stroke* 1994; 25: 1977–84.
4 Center for Disease Control and Prevention. National estimates and general information on diabetes in the United States. *Diabetes Facts Sheet.* Atlanta: US Department Health and Human Services, Center for Disease Control and Prevention, 1997.
5 American Diabetes Association. Economic consequences of diabetes mellitus in the US 1997. *Diabetes Care* 1998; 21: 296–309.
6 Harris MI, Flegal KM, Cowie CC *et al.* Prevalence of diabetes, impaired fasting glucose, and impaired glucose tolerance in US adults. The Third National Health and Nutrition Examination Survey, 1988–1994. *Diabetes Care* 1998; 21: 518–26.
7 American Diabetes Association. Self monitoring of blood glucose. *Diabetes Care* 1994; 7: 81–6.
8 King H, Aubert RE, Herman WH. Global burden of diabetes 1995–2025: prevalence, numerical estimates, and projections. *Diabetes Care* 1998; 21: 1414–21.

9   Report of the Expert Committee on the Diagnosis and Classification of Diabetes Mellitus. *Diabetes Care* 1997; 20: 1183–97.

10 Alberti KG, Zimmet PZ. Definition, diagnosis and classification of diabetes mellitus and its complications. Part 1: diagnosis and classification of diabetes mellitus provisional report of a WHO consultation. *Diabet Med* 1998; 15: 539–53.

11 American Diabetes Association. Clinical Practice Recommendations 1998: Screening for type 2 diabetes. *Diabetes Care* 1998; 21 (Suppl. 1): S1–S22.

12 American Diabetes Association. Position statement: screening for diabetes. *Diabetes Care* 2001; 24 (Suppl. 1): S21–S27.

13 *ACE Consensus Conference on Guidelines for Glycemic Control.* Washington, DC: The American College of Endocrinology, 2001.

14 Levetan CS, Passaro MD, Jablonski KA *et al*. Effect of physician specialty on outcomes in diabetic ketoacidosis. *Diabetes Care* 1999; 22: 1790–5.

15 Quinn M, Angelico MC, Warram JH *et al*. Familial factors determine the development of diabetic nephropathy in patients with IDDM. *Diabetologia* 1996; 39: 940–5.

16 Klein R, Klein BE. Vision disorders in diabetes. *Diabetes in America*. DHHS Publication Number 85-1468. Washington, DC: United States Government Printing Office, 1985.

17 Klein R, Klein BE, Moss SE *et al*. Association of ocular disease and mortality in a diabetic population. *Arch Ophthalmol* 1999; 117: 1487–95.

18 The Diabetic Retinopathy Study Research Group. Preliminary report on effects of photocoagulation therapy. *Am J Ophthalmol* 1976; 81: 383–96.

19 Photocoagulation for diabetic macular edema. Early Treatment Diabetic Retinopathy Study report number 1. *Arch Ophthalmol* 1985; 103: 1796–806.

20 US renal data system. USRDS 1998 Annual Data Report. Bethesda, MD: National Institutes of Health, National Institute of Diabetes and Digestive and Kidney Diseases, 1998.

21 Ritz E, Stefanski A. Diabetic nephropathy in type 2 diabetes. *Am J Kidney Dis* 1996; 27: 167–94.

22 Mogensen CE. Prediction of clinical diabetic nephropathy in IDDM patients. Alternatives to microalbuminuria? *Diabetes* 1990; 39: 761–7.

23 Ismail N, Becker B, Strzelczyk P *et al*. Renal disease and hypertension in noninsulin-dependent diabetes mellitus. *Kidney Int* 1999; 55: 1–28.

24 Ravid M, Savin H, Jutrin I *et al*. Long-term stabilizing effect of angiotensin-converting enzyme inhibition on plasma creatinine and on proteinuria in normotensive type II diabetic patients. *Ann Intern Med* 1993; 118: 577–81.

25 Tuominen JA, Ebeling P, Koivisto VA. Long-term lisinopril therapy reduces exercise-induced albuminuria in nonalbuminuric normotensive IDDM patients. *Diabetes Care* 1998; 21: 1345–8.

26 Joint National Committee. The sixth report of the Joint National Committee on Detection, Evaluation, and Treatment of High Blood Pressure. *Arch Intern Med* 1997; 157: 2413–46.

27 Greene DA, Feldman EL, Stevens MJ *et al*. Diabetic neuropathy. In: Porte D, Sherwin R, Rifkin H, eds. *Diabetes Mellitus.* East Norwalk, CT: Appleton Lange, 1995.

28 Dyck PJ, Kratz KM, Karnes JL *et al*. The prevalence by staged severity of various types of diabetic neuropathy, retinopathy, and nephropathy in a population-based cohort: The Rochester Diabetic Neuropathy Study. *Neurology* 1993; 43: 817–24.

29 The Diabetes Control and Complications Trial Research Group. The effect of intensive treatment of diabetes on the development and progression of long-term complications in insulin-dependent diabetes mellitus. *N Engl J Med* 1993; 329: 977–8.

30 Reichard P, Pihl M, Rosenqvist U *et al*. Complications in IDDM are caused by elevated blood glucose level: Stockholm Diabetes Intervention Study (SDIS) at 10-year follow-up. *Diabetologia* 1996; 39: 1483–8.

31 Intensive blood-glucose control with sulfonylureas or insulin compared with conventional treatment and risk of complications in patients with type 2 diabetes (UKPDS 33). UK Prospective Diabetes Study (UKPDS) Group. *Lancet* 1998; 352: 837–53.

32 Ohkubo Y, Kishikawa H, Araki E *et al*. Intensive insulin therapy prevents the progression of diabetic microvascular complications in Japanese patients with noninsulin-dependent diabetes mellitus: a randomized prospective 6-year study. *Diabetes Res Clin Pract* 1995; 28: 103–17.

33 Wake N, Hisashige A, Katayama T *et al*. Cost-effectiveness of intensive insulin therapy for type 2 diabetes: a 10-year follow-up of the Kumamoto study. *Diabetes Res Clin Pract* 2000; 48: 201–10.

34 Grundy SM, Benjamin IJ, Burke GL *et al*. Diabetes and cardiovascular disease: a statement for healthcare professionals from the American Heart Association. *Circulation* 1999; 100: 1134–46.

35 Haffner SM, Lehto S, Ronnemaa T *et al*. Mortality from coronary heart disease in subjects with type 2 diabetes and in nondiabetic subjects with and without prior myocardial infarction. *N Engl J Med* 1998; 339: 229–34.

36 Kannel W, McGee D. Diabetes and cardiovascular risk factors: The Framingham Study. *Circulation* 1979; 59: 8–13.

37 Gu K, Cowie CC, Harris MI. Diabetes and decline in heart disease mortality in US adults. *JAMA* 1999; 281: 1291–7.

38 Granger CB, Califf RM, Young S *et al*. Outcome of patients with diabetes mellitus and acute myocardial infarction treated with thrombolytic agents. *J Am Coll Cardiol* 1993; 21: 920–5.

39 Niakan E, Harati Y, Rolak L *et al*. Silent myocardial infarction and diabetic cardiovascular autonomic neuropathy. *Arch Intern Med* 1986; 146: 2229–30.

40 Murabito JM, D'Agostino RB, Silbershatz H *et al*. Intermittent claudication: a risk profile from the Framingham Heart Study. *Circulation* 1997; 96: 44–9.

41 Jude EB, Oyibo SO, Chalmers N *et al*. Peripheral arterial disease in diabetic and nondiabetic patients: a comparison of severity and outcome. *Diabetes Care* 2001; 24: 1433–7.

42 Criqui MH, Langer RD, Fronek A *et al*. Mortality over a period of 10 years in patients with peripheral arterial disease. *N Engl J Med* 1992; 326: 381–6.

43 Barrett-Connor E, Khaw K. Diabetes mellitus: an independent risk factor for stroke. *Am J Epidemiol* 1988; 128: 116–24.

44 Elkind MS, Sacco RL. Stroke risk factors and stroke prevention. *Semi Neurol* 1998; 18: 429–39.

45 Lindegard B, Hillbom M. Associations between brain infarction, diabetes, and alcoholism: observations from the Gothenberg Population Cohort Study. *Acta Neurol Scand* 1987; 75: 195–200.

46 Weinberger J, Biscarra V, Weisberg MK *et al*. Factors contributing to stroke in patients with atherosclerotic disease of the great vessels: the role of diabetes. *Stroke* 1983; 16: 709–12.

47 Saito I, Folsom AR, Brancati FL *et al*. Nontraditional risk factors for coronary heart disease incidence among persons with diabetes: The Atherosclerosis Risk in Communities (ARIC) Study. *Ann Intern Med* 2000; 133: 81–91.

48 Despres JP, Lamarche B, Mauriege P *et al*. Hyperinsulinemia as an independent risk factor for ischemic heart disease. *N Engl J Med* 1996; 334: 952–7.

49 Jokl R, Laimins M, Klein RL *et al*. Arterial thrombosis and atherosclerosis in diabetes. Platelet plasminogen activator inhibitor 1 in patients with type II diabetes. *Diabetes Care* 1994; 17: 818–23.

50 Parulkar AA, Pendergrass ML, Granda-Ayala R *et al*. Nonhypoglycemic effects of thiazolidinediones. *Ann Intern Med* 2001; 134: 61–71.

51 Van Haelst PL, van Doormaal JJ, May JF *et al*. Secondary prevention with fluvastatin decreases levels of adhesion molecules, neopterin and C-reactive protein. *Eur J Intern Med* 2001; 12: 503–9.

52 United Kingdom Prospective Diabetes Study Group. Tight blood pressure control and risk of macrovascular and microvascular complications in type 2 diabetes: UKPDS 38. *Br Med J* 1998; 317: 703–13.

53 American Diabetes Association. Standards of medical care for patients with diabetes mellitus. *Diabetes Care* 2001; 24 (Suppl. 1): S33–S43.

54 American Diabetes Association. Nutrition recommendations and principles for people with diabetes mellitus. *Diabetes Care* 2001; 24 (Suppl. 1): S44–S47.

55 The Diabetes Control and Complications Trial Research Group. Weight gain associated with intensive therapy in the Diabetes Control and Complications Trial. *Diabetes Care* 1988; 11: 567–73.

56 Ratner RE, Hirsch IB, Neifing JL *et al*. Less hypoglycemia with insulin glargine in intensive therapy for type 1 diabetes. *Diabetes Care* 2000; 23: 639–43.

57 Rosenstock J, Park G, Zimmerman J. Basal insulin glargine (HOE 901) versus NPH insulin in patients with type 1 diabetes on multiple daily insulin regimens. U. S. Insulin Glargine Type 1 Diabetes Investigator Group. *Diabetes Care* 2000; 23: 1137–42.

58 Wing RR, Koeske R, Epstein LH *et al*. Long-term effects of modest weight loss in type II diabetic patients. *Arch Intern Med* 1987; 147: 1749–53.

59 Henry RR, Schaeffer L, Olefsky JM. Glycemic effects of intensive caloric restriction and isocaloric refeeding in noninsulin-dependent diabetes mellitus. *J Clin Endocrinol Metab* 1985; 61: 917–25.

60 Hansson L, Zanchetti A, Carruthers SG *et al*. Effects of intensive blood-pressure lowering and low dose aspirin on patients with hypertension: principal results of the Hypertension Optimal Treatment (HOT) randomized trial. *Lancet* 1998; 351: 1755–62.

61 ETDRS Investigators. Aspirin effects on mortality and morbidity in patients with diabetes mellitus. Early Treatment Diabetic retinopathy Study Report 14. *JAMA* 1992; 268: 1292–300.

62 Antiplatelet Trialists' Collaboration. Collaborative overview of randomized trials of antiplatelet therapy I. Prevention of death, myocardial infarction, and stroke by prolonged antiplatelet therapy in various categories of patient. *Br Med J* 1994; 308: 81–106.

63 Steering Committee of the Physicians' Health Study Research Group. Final report on the aspirin component of the ongoing Physicians' Health Study. *N Engl J Med* 1989; 321: 129–35.

64 Aspirin use among adults with diabetes: estimates from the Third National Health and Nutrition Examination Survey. *Diabetes Care* 2001; 24: 197–201.

65 Ford ES, Malarcher AM, Herman WH *et al*. Diabetes mellitus and cigarette smoking: findings from the 1989 National Health Interview Survey. *Diabetes Care* 1994; 17: 688–92.

66 Turner RC, Millns H, Neil HA *et al*. Risk factors for coronary artery disease in noninsulin dependent diabetes mellitus: United Kingdom prospective diabetes study (UKPDS. 23). *Br Med J* 1998; 316: 823–8.

67 Levetan CS, Passaro M, Jablonski K *et al*. Unrecognized diabetes among hospitalized patients. *Diabetes Care* 1998; 21: 246–9.

68 *US Center for Health Statistics: 1997 National Hospital Discharge Survey (Public Use Data Tape)*. Washington, DC: US Department of Health and Human Services, 1999.

69 Capes SE, Hunt D, Malmberg K *et al*. Stress hyperglycemia and prognosis of stroke in nondiabetic and diabetic patients: a systematic overview. *Stroke* 2001; 32: 2426–32.

70 Pulsinelli WA, Levy DE, Sigsbee B *et al*. Increased damage after ischemic stroke in patients with hyperglycemia with or without established diabetes mellitus. *Am J Med* 1983; 74: 540–3.

71 Weir CJ, Murray GD, Dyker AG *et al*. Is hyperglycemia an independent predictor of poor outcome after acute stroke? Results of a long-term follow up study. *Br Med J* 1997; 314: 1303–6.

72 Szczudlik A, Slowik A, Turaj W *et al*. Transient hyperglycemia in ischemic stroke patients. *J Neurol Sci* 2001; 189: 105–11.

73 Queale WS, Alexander JS, Brancati FL. Glycemic control and sliding scale insulin use in medical inpatients with diabetes mellitus. *Arch Intern Med* 1997; 157: 545–52.

74 Van den Berghe G, Wouters P, Weekers F *et al*. Intensive insulin therapy in critically ill patients. *N Engl J Med* 2001; 345: 1359–67.

75 Kernan WN, Inzucchi SE, Viscoli CM, Brass LM, Bravata DM, Horwitz RI. Insulin resistance and risk for stroke. *Neurology* 2002; 59: 809–15.

CHAPTER 14

Hypertension Treatment

John M. Flack, Neel Patel, Vishal Mehra, Samar Nasser

Hypertension is a risk factor for stroke

The cerebral circulation is highly pressure-sensitive. Accordingly, hypertension is a major risk factor for stroke [1] as well as for recurrent stroke in stroke survivors [2]. In fact, hypertension is the most important modifiable risk factor for stroke. Blood pressure (BP) levels, particularly systolic blood pressure (SBP), rise with advancing age while diastolic blood pressure (DBP) plateaus in the mid sixth decade of life and is incrementally lower at older ages. Despite lower DBP with advancing age, stroke risk escalates rapidly at older ages in parallel with the rise in SBP and the widening of the pulse pressure (SBP–DBP). The age-related escalation of stroke risk, however, is not surprising since lower DBP at older ages is attributable to a loss in arterial elasticity in the major arterial conduit vessels [3] and has also been linked to a high burden of carotid atherosclerosis [4]. Obviously, these age-related pathological vascular changes facilitate the expression of ischemic cerebral injury.

Blood pressure as a prognostic factor in acute stroke

Higher blood pressure levels after acute ischemic stroke have been linked to poor clinical outcomes [5,6]. An observational study using the Intravenous Nimodipine West European Stroke Trial (INWEST) found that high initial BP poststroke predicted poor functional outcome at 21 days [6]. In patients with intracranial hemorrhage (ICH) mean BP on admission (and volume of the hematoma) in patients with putaminal and thalamic hemorrhage were linked to higher mortality [7]. Similar findings were reported in another study in patients with supratentorial intracerebral hemorrhage as hypertension, along with the inverse of age, blood glucose and hematoma volume, were the strongest predictors of first-day mean arterial pressure (MAP), and MAP (particularly if > 145 mmHg) was related to worse 28-day survival [8]. Another study by Dandapani and coworkers

[9] found that markedly elevated BP (MAP > 145 mmHg) on admission and MAP < 125 mmHg within 2–6 h of admission were associated with improved mortality and less severe morbidity. Nevertheless, the data regarding the prognostic significance of BP on stroke outcomes have been conflicting. For example, other poststroke studies have shown either no [10,11] or favorable [12] prognostic significance of BP level on stroke outcomes. The aforementioned differences in the relation of BP with stroke outcome may relate to differences in stroke type, severity, or possibly other methodological factors.

Circadian BP variation and BP variability also are abnormal poststroke. Cardiac baroreceptor activity is impaired after acute stroke leading to increased BP variability [13]. Also, the normal nocturnal declines in BP, both systolic and diastolic, are markedly attenuated to absent [14] or may even reverse [15]. Circadian BP variation appears to predict functional recovery after stroke. One study examined the influence of circadian BP patterns on early (1 week) neurological recovery poststroke and found the difference between the daytime and night-time BP levels related positively to functional recovery (Rankin scale) and neurological improvement (Scandinavian stroke scale) [16].

Autoregulation of cerebral blood flow

The physiological rationale both for and against treatment of hypertension in the various settings of acute cerebral ischemia depends upon understanding the relationship of systemic BP with cerebral blood flow (CBF) across a broad range of systemic pressures (Fig. 14.1). Under normal circumstances, CBF is ~ 50 ml/100 g per min [17]. The maintenance of CBF relatively constant across a broad range of systemic perfusion pressures, cerebral autoregulation of blood flow, is an important protective mechanism for maintaining normal cerebral oxidative metabolism. In normal, nonhypertensive persons, cerebral autoregulation keeps CBF constant between MAP of 60 and 150 mmHg [18]. This is accomplished, relatively rapidly, by dilatation (when BP falls) and constriction (when BP rises) of cerebral resistance vessels [19,20]. These rapidly occurring changes in CBF are mediated by directionally appropriate changes in cerebrovascular resistance (CVR) [18]. Within the BP limits of normal autoregulation of CBF, CBF is proportional to cerebral oxidative metabolism and is highly sensitive to ambient pCO_2; higher levels of carbon dioxide increase CBF. In chronic hypertension the entire autoregulatory curve may be shifted to the right [21,22]. The lower limit of the autoregulatory curve is shifted rightward (toward higher pressures), in part, because the pressure-related hypertrophy diminishes the maximum dilatatory capacity of cerebral resistance vessels. On the other hand, the upper limit of the autoregulatory curve shifts rightward because pressure-related hypertrophy/

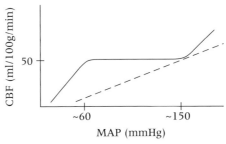

Fig. 14.1 Relation of systemic perfusion pressure to cerebral blood flow. In nonhypertensives between mean arterial pressure (MAP) 60–150 mmHg, there is little variation in cerebral blood flow (CBF) in response to changes in MAP. Chronic hypertension shifts the entire CBF autoregulatory curve to the right. In both normotensives and hypertensives the overall shape of the CBF autoregulatory curve is sigmoidal. The dotted line depicts the distortion of the normal CBF autoregulatory curve into essentially a linear relation within the 'ischemic penumbra' during acute brain ischemia. The ischemic penumbra is the non-infarcted and injured but potentially viable brain tissue that is adjacent to the infarcted area.

remodelling allows these same arterial resistance vessels to withstand much higher systemic pressures before their structural and functional integrity is compromised and CBF rises. Successful long-term antihypertensive treatment over many weeks to months can shift the CBF autoregulatory curve leftward back to a near normal range of MAP [23].

Reductions in MAP below the lower limit of CBF autoregulation

As systemic perfusion pressure falls below the lower limits of CBF autoregulation, cerebral resistance vessels have dilatated maximally but are unable to prevent the fall in CBF. As CBF falls, cerebral oxidative metabolism can be maintained via increased oxygen extraction resulting in a wider arteriovenous oxygen difference. Nevertheless, neurological symptoms—lethargy, confusion, somnolence, seizures, obtundation—only develop after the reductions in CBF exceed the maximum compensatory capacity of augmented oxygen extraction [19].

Increases in MAP above the upper limit of CBF autoregulation

As systemic perfusion pressure rises within the normal range of cerebral autoregulation, cerebral resistance vessels constrict. When systemic perfusion pressure exceeds the upper limits of CBF autoregulation, then CBF increases dramatically. Abnormally high CBF can cause vasogenic brain edema potentially leading to increased intracranial pressure (ICP) [24,25]. Raised ICP has two important physiological effects. First, systemic BP rises in response to raised ICP to maintain effective cranial perfusion pressure (CPP). Second, CBF may fall as a consequence of raised ICP that reduces CPP, although this tendency is counterbalanced, at least partially, by the reflex rise in systemic perfusion pressure. Symptoms of central nervous system (CNS) dysfunction—seizures, lethargy, stupor, coma, etc.,—may occur as BP rises above the upper limits of the CBF autoregulatory curve.

Blood pressure and cerebral blood flow regulation during acute brain ischemia

Blood pressure reflexively rises during acute brain ischemia and brain trauma. However, the early rise in BP clearly preceeds the peak increase in intracranial pressure that typically occurs 3–5 days postinfarct [26,27]. Large cerebellar strokes can obstruct the flow of cerebrospinal fluid and result in ICP shortly after the infarct [28]. During acute brain ischemia, even during transient ischemic attacks (TIAs), autoregulation of CBF disrupts ischemic areas of the brain that surround the already infarcted area [29]. The non-infarcted viable area around the infarct has been labeled the 'ischemic penumbra' [30,31]. Thus, this injured yet potentially viable area of brain tissue is highly dependent upon systemic perfusion pressure to maintain blood flow and oxygen delivery to maintain cerebral oxidative metabolism. Simply put, the disruption of CBF in ischemic brain areas is reflected in a more linear, as opposed to the normal sigmoidal, relationship between systemic perfusion pressure and CBF. The disruption of CBF autoregulation appears to vary according to the area of the brain that develops ischemia. Accordingly, disordered CBF autoregulation appears to be greater for brainstem ischemic lesions than for hemispheric lesions; severe hemispheric lesions cause greater disruption of autoregulation than minor hemispheric lesions, and subcortical lesions cause more disruption than cortical ischemic insults [29]. Stroke type can also impact whether CBF autoregulation is impaired or not. Autoregulation of CBF may not be impaired in small ICH (< 45 ml) [32]. However, larger volume ICH may lead to disrupted autoregulation of CBF because of raised intracranial pressure (and decreased CPP) and as a consequence of neuronal injury [32]. Also, persons with subarachnoid haemorrhage (SAH) often manifest abnormal cerebral autoregulation [33]; impairment of cerebral autoregulation appears to precede arterial vasospasm in ICH and, in turn, this impairment further disrupts cerebral autoregulation and reduces CPP [33]. Table 14.1 defines important cerebral hemodynamic parameters and their interrelationships.

This disruption of CBF autoregulation occurring with acute brain ischemia may last for weeks, or perhaps even longer. Even TIA has been

Table 14.1 Definitions of cerebral hemodynamic parameters

CPP = MAP – ICP

CBF = CPP/CVR

MAP ≅ CPP (when ICP is normal)

MAP » CPP (when ICP is elevated)

CPP, Cranial perfusion pressure; MAP, mean arterial pressure; ICP, intracranial pressure; CBF, cerebral blood flow; CVR, cerebrovascular resistance.

associated with alterations in CBF autoregulation [34]. The disruption of CBF autoregulation in areas of brain ischemia coupled with excessively high systemic perfusion pressures can significantly increase blood flow, facilitate brain edema formation, and potentially raise ICP. A significant proportion of persons with acute stroke may ultimately develop elevated ICP; therefore, the rise in systemic perfusion pressure might also help maintain CPP and therefore CBF in ischemic areas of the brain when ICP is elevated. The greatest poststroke systemic BP elevations appear to be associated with intracranial hematomas [15,35].

Therapeutic considerations and implications

The clinical imperative to emergently lower elevated BP by pharmacological means depends on these four assumptions: (i) that elevated BP triggered the acute ischemic event; (ii) that persistently elevated BP may cause infarct extension, hemorrhagic transformation of ischemic strokes, or further bleeding in ICH; (iii) that BP elevations have caused new or worsening target-organ injury (e.g. heart failure); and/or (iv) that BP elevations are severe enough to cause imminent injury to pressure-sensitive target organs in persons without such injury. However, the potential risks of persistently elevated BP in the setting of acute brain ischemia must be counterbalanced against the very real risks of iatrogenic harm when BP is emergently lowered [36,37]. A clear understanding of altered autoregulation of CBF as well as an understanding of the natural history of BP poststroke can prevent therapeutic misadventures that may result in disastrous clinical consequences for the patients with acute brain ischemia complicated by elevated BP.

If BP lowering by pharmacological means is to be undertaken emergently, several important issues with significant therapeutic implications must be addressed: (i) via what route should therapy be administered; (ii) what drugs should be used as well as avoided; (iii) what are appropriate BP targets; and (iv) over what time frame should BP goals be obtained?

The relative paucity of adequately powered randomized, controlled clinical trials of hypertension treatment with assessment of relevant neurological, functional status, and cardiovascular clinical endpoints undermines optimal therapeutic decision-making during brain ischemia, at least with regard to the decision to acutely lower BP.

Natural history of blood pressure levels poststroke

Clearly, hypertension is the major risk factor for stroke. Furthermore, approximately 80% of patients with acute stroke have elevated BP at the time of hospital admission [38] even in patients without antecedent hypertension, though admission BP levels are higher among those with chronic hypertension [38,39]. Blood pressure falls significantly during the first 4 days after acute stroke and continues to fall spontaneously through 7–10 days poststroke [35,39,40]. In one large series of acute stroke patients, the fall in BP averaged 20/10 mmHg by day 10 [38].

Major considerations regarding therapy in acute brain ischemia

A multiplicity of factors should be considered when deciding on whether to treat hypertension in patients with acute brain ischemia. These factors relate to the type of stroke, patient clinical characteristics, the decision to intervene pharmacologically or not, the route of drug administration, the physical location of drug administration within the hospital, the drug class of the chosen agent(s), and the status of other pressure-sensitive target organs. The overarching aim of therapeutic interventions to lower BP, albeit modestly, during acute brain ischemia is to prevent further brain injury as well as to avoid, or at least minimize, pressure-related complications in other target organs such as the heart, kidneys, and peripheral vasculature. These aims can best be accomplished by lowering BP by means that do not disrupt CBF autoregulation and therefore preserve CBF. Also, when excessive BP reductions occur, the ability rapidly to reverse brain hypoperfusion and systemic hypotension is desirable.

During the initial assessment of the patient with acute brain ischemia, BP will be elevated more often than not. Though the precise mechanism(s) underlying this elevation of BP remains poorly elucidated and incompletely understood, there is some suggestion that increased sympathetic nervous system (SNS) activity and/or an imbalance of sympathetic and parasympathetic nervous system tone may be important [41,42]. Despite the fact that elevated BP, over the long term, is a risk factor for stroke, elevations in BP at the time of admission appear to represent a response to acute brain ischemia more often than actually being the precipitating factor of the acute ischemic event. Thus, antihypertensive therapy is not automatically required in the setting of acute brain ischemia and elevated BP.

In these situations, the clinician should carefully search for some indication of previous BP control such as chart documentation of previous BP levels, evidence of target-organ damage such as retinopathy, left ventricular enlargement, proteinuria, reduced kidney function, or evidence of worsening target-organ function (e.g. new onset or worsening heart failure). The presence of any or all of these conditions suggests chronically elevated BP and a likely shift of the lower and upper limits of normal CBF autoregulation to higher levels of BP. The decision to initiate BP-lowering therapy should be undertaken with careful consideration of prior BP control levels as well as the status of other pressure-sensitive target organs such as the heart, kidney, and the peripheral as well as the microvasculature. Another key consideration is stroke type. Cerebral autoregulation appears to be impaired in most types of brain ischemia with the exception of small to moderate volume ICH.

Blood pressure treatment thresholds and other considerations in acute brain ischemia

There is no clear consensus on how to manage BP during and immediately after acute brain ischemia. Nevertheless, there is some guidance for the practitioner in this situation. American Heart Association guidelines for management of the patient with acute ischemic stroke do not recommend acute pharmacological interventions to emergently lower BP during stroke unless the mean arterial BP is > 130 mmHg or the SBP is > 220 mmHg [26]; even when BP exceeds these levels the guideline recommends cautious treatment and therapeutic intervention to lower BP, *per se*, will not always be necessary. In fact, the majority of stroke patients will not need new or intensified antihypertensive drug therapy [26]. These recommendations seem both reasonable and prudent in the absence of definitive clinical trials. Table 14.2 displays potential indications for acute pharmacological intervention to lower BP during acute brain ischemia.

How should BP be lowered and by how much?

If therapeutic intervention is deemed necessary, then how should BP be lowered and by how much? There are several general caveats regarding antihypertensive treatment in acute brain ischemia. A major physiological reason to consider treatment is that persistently elevated BP may cause excessive CBF leading to brain edema formation, raised ICP, infarct extension into the ischemic penumbra, and/or hemorrhagic transformation of ischemic or embolic stroke. In the setting of ICH, there is legitimate concern that persistent BP elevations might cause persistent intracerebral bleeding and hematoma expansion [43–45]; however, it appears that the bleeding typically stops within 6–12 h of the initial bleed [46]. Even in

Table 14.2 Potential indications for acute pharmacological intervention during acute brain ischemia

Severe BP elevation   MAP > 130 or SBP > 220 mmHg
Use of thrombolytic therapy   Target BP < 185/110 mmHg

New/worsening target-organ injury
  Heart failure
  New/worsening azotemia
  Aortic dissection

Cerebral edema Papilledema [1] ?Embolic stroke

MAP, Mean arterial pressure; SBP, systolic blood pressure.

the setting of acute embolic stroke there is evidence in an experimental rabbit model that BP treatment with intravenous labetalol minimizes hemorrhagic transformation [47]. On the other hand, these possibilities must be balanced against the risk of iatrogenic cerebral hypoperfusion leading to worsened neurological symptoms [37,48–50] or increased mortality [51] occurring in response to reductions in BP.

When acute pharmacological intervention to lower BP is undertaken the first guiding principle is that BP reductions should be gradual and reasonably predictable. Therefore, reductions in MAP by ~ 10–15% followed by reassessment of overall clinical and neurological status seem reasonable and prudent. Acute intervention with oral antihypertensives is generally avoided, although in persons without impaired sensorium and/or swallowing difficulties, oral outpatient antihypertensive medications should be continued. When it is not feasible to continue ambulatory medications via the oral route, then either the same (or similar) medications should be administered via either the intravenous route or via a feeding tube. Continuation of oral sedating orally sympatholytics such as clonidine is probably not advisable—yet neither is abrupt discontinuation, since this can result in severe rebound hypertension. Perhaps in this situation, and in the absence of contraindications to their use, intravenous β-blockers can be prescribed instead.

Attempting to lower BP acutely with oral agents such as clonidine or short-acting nifedipine should certainly be avoided. Clonidine can cause sedation and drowsiness and therefore may confuse the clinical assessment of the patient experiencing acute stroke. Short-acting nifedipine can abruptly and precipitously lower BP; and, the BP response to this agent is highly unpredictable. This increases the likelihood of overzealous BP lead-ing to a potentially deleterious fall in CBF into the ischemic penumbra that may depress cerebral oxidative metabolism and result in further neuronal injury. Also, calcium antagonists may impair autoregulation of CBF lead-ing to reductions in CBF as BP falls [36,51] and raise ICP [52]. Thus, calcium antagonists are not indicated for emergent BP lowering in persons with acute brain ischemia. However, a clear exception to this recommen-dation is in the setting of SAH when nimodipine is indicated to combat arterial spasm. In general, rapidly acting oral antihypertenisve agents lead to highly variable reductions in BP and, in most cases of acute brain ischemia, should be avoided. Another potential complication of precipit-ous BP lowering is the development of ischemia of other target organs such as the myocardium. Finally, the rapid and sizeable reduction in BP may activate the SNS, leading to constriction of the larger preresistance cerebral vessels thereby reducing CBF despite compensatory dilatation of the smaller intracerebral resistance vessels.

The ideal antihypertensive agent for emergent BP lowering during acute brain ischemia would gradually lower BP and, if BP fell excessively, the hypotensive effect could be reversed rather quickly (e.g. seconds to minutes) or CBF would be maintained despite the reductions in systemic pressure. Furthermore, the ideal hypotensive agent for acute therapeutic intervention would be administered via the intravenous route, would not raise ICP, and would avoid significant dilatation of cerebral resistance vessels that might lead to a 'steal' syndrome by shunting blood flow away from injured, acutely ischemic, though still potentially viable, areas of the brain (ischemic penumbra). The hypotensive effect of both intravenous nitroglycerin and nitroprusside can be reversed rather quickly by titration of the infusion rate; however, both drugs can raise ICP [53,54]. In addi-tion, nitroprusside can theoretically cause an intracranial [55,56] and/or a coronary 'steal' syndrome, i.e. shunting of blood flow away from ischemic areas as a consequence of arteriolar vasodilatation. Sodium nitroprusside can also impair autoregulation of CBF leading to reductions in CBF [57,58]. Nevertheless, nitroprusside has been used successfully in indi-viduals experiencing acute ICH [59,60]. The clinician should remain cognizant of the fact that even if CBF autoregulation remains intact, the BP range within which CBF autoregulation is normal has probably been shifted to the right (toward higher systemic pressures).

A body of clinical and experimental data exists for at least two other intravenous antihypertensive agents, labetalol (alpha beta blocker) and enalapril [angiotensin converting enzyme (ACE) inhibitor], regarding their ability to lower BP during acute cerebral ischemia without impairing CBF. Intravenous labetalol has been used without complications to lower severely elevated BP in persons with TIA, hypertensive encephalopathy, and ICH [61–63]. Another study in patients with essential hypertension shed light on why labetalol safely lowers BP in situations of acute brain ischemia. Pearson and coworkers [63] compared the effect of intravenous injections of diazoxide 300 mg and labetalol 150 mg on BP and CBF; despite rapid reductions in BP in both groups (labetalol slightly greater than diazoxide), a reduction in CBF was observed with diazoxide but not labetalol. Furthermore, labetalol does not appear to either raise ICP [64] or negatively affect autoregulation of CBF [65].

ACE inhibitors appear to have no deleterious impact on autoregulation of CBF [52]; in fact, at least in animal studies, these agents appear to shift both the lower and upper limits of the CBF autoregulatory curve downward (toward lower BP levels). It has been speculated that the mechanism underlying the downward shift of the entire CBF autoregulatory curve relates to diminution of angiotensin II-mediated constriction of the larger cerebral vessels that control the influx of blood into the smaller cerebral resistance vessels that mediate CBF autoregulation [66]. One small human clinical study of regional CBF in 12 patients within 5 days of acute stroke found no change in mean hemispheric CBF 1 h after administration of 25 mg of captopril. However, there was no reduction in BP either in this study, making the therapeutic implications of this study less clear. In a study of 14 patients with normal pressure hydrocephalus 1 h after 50 mg of oral captopril, MAP was reduced from 109 to 93 mmHg without change in the arteriovenous oxygen difference (an estimate of CBF change) or ICP. Figure 14.2 shows a suggested algorithm outlining the approach to emergent BP lowering during acute brain ischemia.

Drugs to avoid

Antihypertensive drugs that dilatate cerebral resistance vessels and/or raise ICP are best avoided in the setting of acute brain ischemia. Drugs with these characteristics tend to impair CBF into the ischemic penumbra. Accordingly, hydralazine is a powerful cerebral vasodilatator, raises ICP, and appears to impair autoregulation of CBF [52,67–69]. The raised ICP uncouples the close relationship of systemic perfusion pressure with CPP, and the activation of the SNS in response to the intense peripheral arterial vasodilatation can constrict the larger cerebral preresistance vessels. Both of these physiological effects probably underlie the observed reductions in CBF after administration of hydralazine. For similar reasons, short-acting calcium antagonists such as nifedipine should not be used to emergently lower BP during acute brain ischemia. Though not commonly used in contemporary medical practice, diazoxide is another drug to avoid, as it can significantly decrease CBF as it lowers BP. Nitroglycerin effectively lowers BP and importantly reduces coronary ischemia—however, because it raises ICP this agent should be avoided, if at all possible, in the setting of acute brain ischemia.

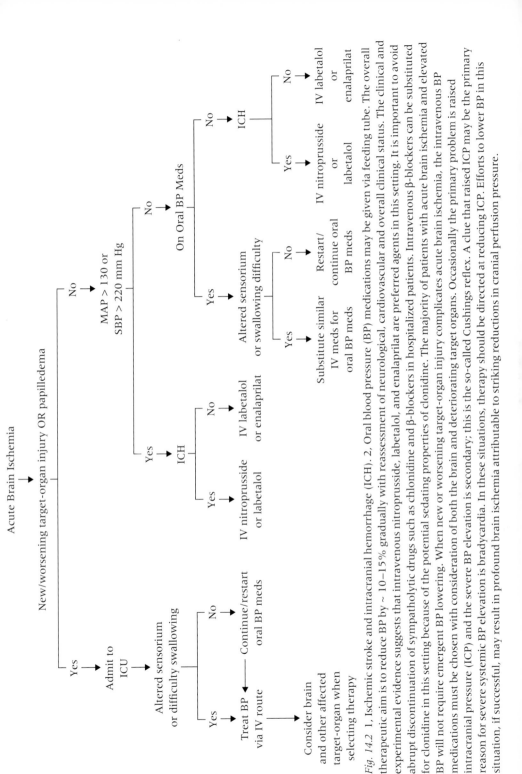

Fig. 14.2 1, Ischemic stroke and intracranial hemorrhage (ICH). 2, Oral blood pressure (BP) medications may be given via feeding tube. The overall therapeutic aim is to reduce BP by ~ 10–15% gradually with reassessment of neurological, cardiovascular and overall clinical status. The clinical and experimental evidence suggests that intravenous nitroprusside, labetalol, and enalaprilat are preferred agents in this setting. It is important to avoid abrupt discontinuation of sympatholytic drugs such as clonidine and β-blockers in hospitalized patients. Intravenous β-blockers can be substituted for clonidine in this setting because of the potential sedating properties of clonidine. The majority of patients with acute brain ischemia and elevated BP will not require emergent BP lowering. When new or worsening target-organ injury complicates acute brain ischemia, the intravenous BP medications must be chosen with consideration of both the brain and deteriorating target organs. Occasionally the primary problem is raised intracranial pressure (ICP) and the severe BP elevation is secondary; this is the so-called Cushings reflex. A clue that raised ICP may be the primary reason for severe systemic BP elevation is bradycardia. In these situations, therapy should be directed at reducing ICP. Efforts to lower BP in this situation, if successful, may result in profound brain ischemia attributable to striking reductions in cranial perfusion pressure.

Antihypertensive drug therapy and stroke prevention

Primary stroke prevention

In placebo-controlled clinical trials, antihypertensive drug therapy with a variety of antihypertensive drug classes including diuretics [70,71], β-blockers [72], calcium antagonists [73,74], and ACE inhibitors [75,76] have all been shown to lower stroke risk in hypertensive patients initially free of stroke [77,78]. The Heart Outcomes Prevention Evaluation (HOPE) study, in which blood pressure was relatively well controlled prior to study entry, evaluated ramipril in patients at increased risk of vascular events and has been discussed in a previous chapter.

There are long-term clinical trial data suggesting that stroke risk reduction may not occur equally when BP is lowered with the various antihypertensive drug classes. For example, meta-analyses of hypertension stroke endpoint trials strongly suggest that diuretics and calcium antagonists are highly effective antistroke agents, and that calcium antagonists, dihydropridine and rate-lowering considered together, might be slightly better than diuretics [70,79,80]. A similar, though statistically insignificant, trend (7%) in favor of amlodipine preventing stroke more effectively than chlorthalidone was seen in the recently completed Antihypertensive and Lipid-Lowering Treatment to Prevent Heart Attack Trial (ALLHAT) study [70]. Also, in the ALLHAT study the diuretic chlorthalidone had a 15% lower stroke risk than lisinopril, an ACE inhibitor. The stroke risk differential in favor of chlorthalidone over lisinopril was 40% in African-Americans. However, there is one interpretational caveat. That is, the ACE inhibitor lowered SBP less effectively than chlorthalidone by the end of the study. In the overall cohort, the difference was 2 mmHg, among persons > 65 years 3 mmHg, and in African-Americans it was 4 mmHg—these BP lowering differences were even larger during earlier study years. In ALLHAT the calcium antagonist, amlodipine, was not compared directly with the ACE inhibitor, lisinopril. These data may be interpreted by some as further evidence that ACE inhibitors should be avoided in African-Americans. However, our interpretation is different. We believe these data are consistent with the thesis that ACE inhibitors will not protect against stroke unless SBP is adequately controlled. Furthermore, we have previously argued vigorously against the use of race or ethnicity as a surrogate for BP response or target-organ protection with ACE inhibitors, or for that matter, any hypertensive drug class in individual patients [81].

A meta-analysis in older hypertensives by Messerli and coworkers [82] showed that β-blockers were less effective than thiazide diuretics for lowering stroke risk—however, it should be pointed out that this same analysis found that β-blockers less effectively lowered BP than diuretic-based regimens. The recently reported Losartan Intervention for Endpoint (LIFE) Reduction study enrolled 9193 men and women with a mean of age of 66.9 years with SBP 160–200 mmHg and DBP < 90 mmHg (average 174/98 mmHg). Follow-up averaged 4.7 years. Participants were randomized to either once daily atenolol or losartan; hydrochlorothiazide was the add-on drug in both treatment arms. The angiotensin receptor blocker losartan more effectively prevented stroke than did the β-blocker atenolol [83]. Total stroke was 25% lower (10.8 strokes/1000 patient-years vs. 14.5) despite comparable reductions in BP of 30/17 and 29/17 mmHg from baseline in the losartan and atenolol groups, respectively. This intriguing finding merits further study. A large body of clinical trial evidence suggests, however, that effective BP lowering, not drug selection, is responsible for most of the stroke risk reduction during antihypertensive treatment.

Secondary stroke prevention

Data regarding prevention of recurrent stroke via pharmacological BP lowering are sparse. A pooled analysis across nine randomized clinical trials that included some stroke survivors reported a significant 29% reduction in risk of recurrent stroke [84]. The Perindopril Protection Against Recurrent Stroke (PROGRESS) [2] study enrolled 6105 persons with a history of either ischemic stroke, ICH, stroke of unknown type, TIA or amaurosis fugax, and has been discussed previously in this volume. This study highlighted the importance of lowering BP in reducing recurrent ischemic brain events and major vascular complications in stroke survivors. Over 4 years of follow-up, combination therapy with perindopril and indapamide lowered blood pressure 12/5 mmHg and reduced recurrent stroke risk by 43%. Also, the risk of cognitive decline and the composite of cognitive decline and dementia were reduced 19% and 19%, respectively [85].

There are several notes of caution for the practitioner when prescribing antihypertensive drug therapy in persons with chronic brain ischemia or poststroke patients. There are some data suggesting that CBF, though not cerebral oxidative metabolism, is depressed in persons with chronic atherothrombotic brain infarction [86]; this suggests that increased arterial oxygen extraction has occurred to compensate for reduced CBF to maintain cerebral oxidative metabolism. There are also data in persons with chronic cerebral ischemia linking pharmacological reductions in BP to potential adverse clinical outcomes [87]. In persons with severe carotid artery stenosis, particularly older individuals, antihypertensive drug therapy may reduce CBF (enalapril < isradipine) [88,89]. Finally, some poststroke patients manifest excessive nocturnal dipping of BP that has been linked to silent and clinical cerebral ischemia [90]. However, by no means has it been proven that the excessive nocturnal dipping in BP is attributable to antihypertensive drug therapy; in fact, there does not appear to be a direct causal link. Nevertheless, all of these cautionary factors can complicate BP treatment in the poststroke or chronic brain ischemia patient.

Isolated systolic hypertension

Isolated systolic hypertension (ISH) is the major form of hypertension in elderly individuals and represents a significant portion of the burden of inadequately treated hypertension in North America. Previous studies estimate that 65% of hypertension in the elderly is due to ISH.

A recent study from the First National Health and Nutrition Examination Survey Follow-up Study (NHANES) evaluated the long-term (20 years) stroke risk for both ISH, defined as a systolic BP > 160 mmHg and DBP < 90 mmHg, as well as borderline ISH, defined as SBP between 140 and 159 mmHg and DBP < 90 mmHg [91]. Among 12 344 participants between the ages of 25 and 74 years, 493 were classified as having ISH and 1241 were categorized as borderline ISH. Following adjustment for conventional vascular risk factors, there was an increased risk of stroke in both patients with ISH (relative risk 2.7) and borderline ISH (relative risk 1.4). The risk was increased for both ischemic stroke and ICH. The stroke risk was independently associated with older age, diabetes mellitus, and SBP > 180 mmHg.

In terms of treatment, more than one study in the past has demonstrated the value of treating ISH in terms of stroke reduction. The Systolic Hypertension in the Elderly (SHEP) trial showed that a diuretic-based regimen was associated with a decreased rate of stroke (36% reduction), myocardial infarction (MI), and congestive heart failure [92]. In terms of stroke subtypes, both ischemic and hemorrhagic strokes were reduced, and for ischemic stroke subtypes there was a greater reduction in lacunar strokes (relative risk 0.53) and cryptogenic events (relative risk 0.64) compared with atherosclerotic stroke (relative risk 0.99) [93].

The Syst-Eur Trial enrolled 4695 patients with ISH and baseline SBP between 160 and 219 mmHg and DBP < 95 mmHg [94]. The patients were assigned to treatment with the calcium channel blocker nitrendipine or placebo, with the possible addition of enalapril and HCTZ. The active treatment group had a decrease in BP of 23 mmHg systolic and 7 mmHg diastolic, with the between-group difference being 10.1 mmHg systolic and 4.5 mmHg diastolic. This was associated with a 42% risk reduction for stroke (13.7 strokes per 1000 patient-years vs. 7.9, $P = 0.003$) and a 44% risk reduction for nonfatal stroke. Cardiac events were also reduced to a significant degree, with fatal and nonfatal cardiovascular events declining by 31%.

A recent subgroup analysis from the LIFE trial mentioned above also showed the value of losartan treatment in patients with ISH and left ventricular hypertrophy [95]. In this trial, 1326 patients were classified as having ISH and despite comparable BP reduction, the group assigned to treatment with losartan had a 25% risk reduction compared with atenolol-based treatment for stroke, MI, or vascular death (25.1 events per 1000 patient-years vs. 35.4 events, $P = 0.02$). The reduction in stroke alone was 40% ($P = 0.02$).

Therefore, the data are quite compelling that treatment of ISH is warranted and many HTN authorities would recommend a target SBP of at least < 140 mmHg for these patients. Additional studies to evaluate treatment of patients with borderline ISH are needed.

Blood pressure targets

The optimal blood pressure for different stroke subtypes is not completely established. Some clinicians have recommended 'liberalizing' BP treatment up to approximately 140/80 for patients with large-vessel occlusions (e.g. carotid occlusion) or intracranial atherosclerosis.

For patients with lacunar infarctions, a multicentre trial has been launched to compare aggressive BP lowering to < 130 mmHg with 'conventional' lowering to < 150 mmHg. This study will provide important information regarding therapeutic BP targets in secondary stroke prevention.

Summary

Pharmacological BP lowering prevents initial and recurrent stroke. Though some differences in stroke risk reduction have been observed between various antihypertensive drug classes, the totality of evidence suggests that the magnitude of BP lowering is much more important than the drugs used to lower BP. Most hypertensives will require more than a single drug to achieve target BP levels. Antihypertensive agents with the strongest evidence supporting primary stroke prevention are the calcium antagonists and thiazide diuretics. These agents will frequently be used in multidrug antihypertensive drug regimens, especially thiazide diuretics. In complex (> 2) drug regimens it will be virtually impossible to control BP without inclusion of a diuretic. Angiotensin receptor blockers will probably play an increasingly important role in stroke prevention.

In the setting of acute brain ischemia, the majority of individuals will have elevated BP, though only a minority of them will need emergent pharmacological BP lowering. Intravenous labetalol and enalaprilat have the most substantial evidence in acute brain ischemia; in ICH sodium nitroprusside and labetalol have the most evidence in support of their use. In acute brain ischemia, modest BP reductions of 10–15% should be the goal of therapy.

References

1 Collins R, Peto R, MacMahon S *et al.* Blood pressure, stroke, and coronary heart disease. Part 2, Short-term reductions in blood pressure: overview of randomised drug trials in their epidemiological context. *Lancet* 1990; 335: 827–38.

2 PROGRESS Collaborative Group. Randomised trial of a perindopril-based blood-pressure-lowering regimen among 6105 individuals with previous stroke or transient ischaemic attack. *Lancet* 2001; 358: 1033–41.

3 Benetos A, Waeber B, Izzo J *et al.* Influence of age, risk factors, and cardiovascular and renal disease on arterial stiffness: clinical applications. *Am J Hypertens* 2002; 15: 1101–8.

4 Sutton-Tyrrell K, Alcorn HG, Wolfson SK Jr, Kelsey SF, Kuller LH. Predictors of carotid stenosis in older adults with and without isolated systolic hypertension. *Stroke* 1993; 24: 355–61.

5 Dawson SL, Manktelow BN, Robinson TG *et al.* Which parameters of beat-to-beat blood pressure and variability best predict early outcome after acute ischemic stroke? *Stroke* 2000; 31: 463–8.

6 Ahmed N, Wahlgren G. High initial blood pressure after acute stroke is associated with poor functional outcome. *J Int Med* 2001; 249: 467–73.

7 Terayama Y, Tanahashi N, Fukuuchi Y *et al.* Prognostic value of admission blood pressure in patients with intracerebral hemorrhage. Keio Cooperative Stroke Study. *Stroke* 1997; 28: 1185–8.

8 Fogelholm R, Avikainen S, Murros K. Prognostic value and determinants of first-day mean arterial pressure in spontaneous supratentorial intracerebral hemorrhage. *Stroke* 1997; 28: 1396–400.

9 Dandapani BK, Suzuki S, Kelley RE, Reyes-Iglesias Y, Duncan RC. Relation between blood pressure and outcome in intracerebral hemorrhage. *Stroke* 1995; 26: 21–4.

10 Carlberg B. The prognostic value of admission blood pressure in patients with acute stroke. *Stroke* 1993; 24: 1372–5.

11 Fiorelli M, Alperovitch A, Argentino C *et al.* Prediction of long-term outcome in the early hours following acute ischemic stroke. Italian Acute Stroke Study Group. *Arch Neurol* 1995; 52: 250–5.

12 Allen CMC. Predicting the outcome of acute stroke: a prognostic score. *J Neurol Neurosurg Psychiatry* 1984; 47: 475–80.

13 Robinson TG, James M, Youde J *et al.* Cardiac baroreceptor sensitivity is impaired after acute stroke. *Stroke* 1997; 28: 1671–6.

14 Dawson SL, Evans SN, Manktelow BN *et al.* Diurnal blood pressure change varies with stroke subtype in the acute phase. *Stroke* 1998; 29: 1519–24.

15 Lip GY, Zarifis J, Farooqi IS *et al.* Ambulatory blood pressure monitoring in acute stroke. The West Birmingham Stroke Project. *Stroke* 1997; 28: 31–5.

16 Bhalla A, Wolfe CD, Rudd AG. The effect of 24-hour blood pressure levels on early neurological recovery after stroke. *J Int Med* 2001; 250: 121–30.

17 Kety SS, Hafkenschiel JH, Jeffers WA, Leopold IH, Shenkin HA. The blood flow, vascular resistance, and oxygen consumption of the brain in essential hypertension. *J Clin Invest* 1948; 27: 511–4.

18 Powers WJ. Acute hypertension after stroke: the scientific basis for treatment decisions. *Neurology* 1993; 43: 461–7.

19 Strandgaard S, Haunso S. Can differences in cerebral and coronary autoregulation and O_2 extraction explain why antihypertensive treatment prevents stroke but not myocardial infarction? *Ann Clin Res* 1988; 20 (Suppl. 48): 10–3.

20 Strandgaard S, Paulson OB. Regulation of cerebral blood flow in health and disease. *J Cardiovasc Pharmacol* 1992; 19 (Suppl. 6): S89–S93.

21 Strandgaard S, Olesen J, Skinhoj E, Lassen NA. Autoregulation of brain circulation in severe arterial hypertension. *Br Med J* 1973; 1: 507–10.

22 Strandgaard S, Paulson OB. Cerebral blood flow and its pathophysiology in hypertension. *Am J Hypertens* 1989; 2: 486–92.

23 Strandgaard S. Autoregulation of cerebral blood flow in hypertensive patients. The modifying influence of prolonged antihypertensive treatment on the tolerance to acute, drug induced hypotension. *Circulation* 1976; 53: 720–7.

24 Spence JD, Del Maestro RF. Hypertension in acute ischemic strokes. *Treat Arch Neurol* 1985; 42: 1000–2.

25 Johansson BB, Nilsson B. Cerebral vasomotor reactivity in normotensive and spontaneous hypertensive rats. *Stroke* 1979; 10: 572–6.

26 Adams HP Jr. Guidelines for the management of patients with acute ischemic stroke: a synopsis. A Special Writing Group of the Stroke Council, American Heart Association. *Heart Dis Stroke* 1994; 3: 407–11.

27 Plum F. Brain swelling and edema in cerebral vascular disease. *Res Publ Assoc Res Nerv Ment Dis* 1961; 41: 318–48.

28 Busse O, Laun A, Agnoli AL. Obstructive hydrocephalus in cerebellar infarcts. *Fortschr Neurol Psychiatr* 1984; 52: 164–71.

29 Meyer JS, Shimazu K, Fukuuchi Y. Impaired neurogenetic cerebrovascular control and dysautoregulation after stroke. *Stroke* 1973; 4: 461–7.

30 Pulsinelli W. Pathophysiology of acute ischaemic stroke. *Lancet* 1992; 339: 533–6.

31 Fisher M. Characterizing the target of acute stroke therapy. *Stroke* 1997; 28: 866–72.

32 Powers WJ, Zazulia AR, Videen TO *et al.* Autoregulation of cerebral blood flow surrounding acute (6–22 hours) intracerebral hemorrhage. *Neurology* 2001; 57: 18–24.

33 Lang EW, Diehl RR, Mehdorn HM. Cerebral autoregulation testing after aneurysmal subarachnoid hemorrhage: the phase relationship between arterial blood pressure and cerebral blood flow velocity. *Crit Care Med* 2001; 29: 158–63.

34 Hartmann A. Prolonged disturbances of regional cerebral blood flow in transient ischemic attacks. *Stroke* 1985; 16: 932–9.

35 Harper G, Castleden CM, Potter JF. Factors affecting changes in blood pressure after acute stroke. *Stroke* 1994; 25: 1726–9.

36 Lisk DR, Grotta JC, Lamk LM *et al*. Should hypertension be treated after acute stroke? A randomized controlled trial using single photon emission computed tomography. *Arch Neurol* 1993; 50: 855–62.

37 Fischberg GM, Lazano E, Rajamani K, Ameriso S, Fisher MJ. Stroke precipitated by moderate blood pressure reduction. *J Emerg Med* 2000; 19: 339–46.

38 Wallace JD, Levy LL. Blood pressure after stroke. *J Am Med Assoc* 1981; 246: 2177–80.

39 Britton M, Carlsson A, de Faire U. Blood pressure course in patients with acute stroke and matched controls. *Stroke* 1986; 17: 861–4.

40 Morfis L, Schwartz RS, Poulos R *et al*. Blood pressure changes in acute cerebral infarction and hemorrhage. *Stroke* 1997; 28: 1401–5.

41 Sander D, Winbeck K, Klingelhofer J, Etgen T, Conrad B. Prognostic relevance of pathological sympathetic activation after acute thromboemobolic stroke. *Neurology* 2001; 57: 833–8.

42 Eames PJ, Blake MJ, Dawson SL, Panerai RB, Potter JF. Dynamic cerebral autoregulation and beat to beat blood pressure control are impaired in acute ischaemic stroke. *J Neurol Neurosurg Psychiatry* 2002; 72: 467–72.

43 Broderick J, Brott T, Tomsick T *et al*. Ultra-early evaluation of intracerebral homorrhage. *J Neurosurg* 1990; 72: 195–9.

44 Bae HG, Lee KS, Yun IG *et al*. Rapid expansion of hypertensive interacerebral hemorrhage. *Neurosurgery* 1992; 31: 35–41.

45 Venkatesh A, Deibert E, Diringer MN. Hemodynamic monitoring in the neurological intensive care unit. *Neurol India* 2001; 49 (Suppl. 1): S9–18.

46 Mayer SA. Ultra-early hemostatic therapy for intracerebral hemorrhage. *Stroke* 2003; 34: 224–9.

47 Fagan SC, Bowes MP, Lyden PD, Zivin JA. Acute hypertension promotes hemorrhagic transformation in a rabbit embolic stroke model: effect of labetalol. *Exp Neurol* 1998; 150: 153–8.

48 Britton M, de Faire U, Helmers C. Hazards of therapy for excessive hypertension in acute stroke. *Acta Med Scand* 1980; 207: 253–87.

49 Lavin P. Management of hypertension in patients with acute stroke. *Arch Intern Med* 1986; 146: 66–8.

50 Ahmed N, Nasman P, Wahlgren NG. Effect of intravenous nimodipine on blood pressure and outcome after acute stroke. *Stroke* 2000; 31: 1250–5.

51 Kaste M, Fogelhoim R, Erila T *et al*. A randomized, double-blind, placebo-controlled trial of nimodipine in acute ischemic hemispheric stroke. *Stroke* 1994; 25: 1348–53.

52 Strandgaard S, Paulson OB. Antihypertensive drugs and cerebral circulation. *Eur J Clin Invest* 1996; 26: 625–30.

53 Ghani GA, Sung YF, Weinstein MS, Tindall GT, Fleischer AS. Effects of intravenous nitroglycerin on the intracranial pressure and volume pressure response. *J Neurosurg* 1983; 58: 562–5.

54 Anile C, Zanghi F, Bracali A, Maira G, Rossi GF. Sodium nitroprusside and intracranial pressure. *Acta Neurochir* 1981; 58: 203–11.

55 Phillips SJ, Whisnant JP. Hypertension and the brain. The National High Blood Pressure Education Program. *Arch Intern Med* 1992; 152: 938–45.

56 Strandgaard S, Paulson OB. Hypertensive disease and the cerebral circulation. In: Laragh JH, Brenner BM., eds. *Hypertension: Pathophysiology, Diagnosis, and Management.* New York: Raven Press, Publishers, 1990: 399–416.

57 Candia GJ, Heros RC, Lavyne MH, Zervas NT, Nelson CN. Effect of intravenous sodium nitroprusside on cerebral blood flow and intracranial pressure. *Neurosurgery* 1978; 3: 50–3.

58 Brown FD, Hanlon K, Crockard HA, Mullan S. Effect of sodium nitroprusside on cerebral blood flow in conscious human beings. *Surg Neurol* 1977; 7: 67–70.

59 Marshman LA, Morice AH, Thompson JS. Increased efficacy of sodium nitroprusside in middle cerebral arteries following acute subarachnoid hemorrhage: indications for its use after rupture. *J Neurosurg Anesthesiol* 1998; 10: 171–7.

60 Cressman MD, Gifford RW Jr. Hypertension and stroke. *J Am Coll Cardiol* 1983; 1: 521–7.

61 Wilson DJ, Wallin JD, Vlachakis ND *et al.* Intravenous labetalol in the treatment of severe hypertension and hypertensive emergencies. *Am J Med* 1983; 75: 95–102.

62 Patel RV, Kertland HR, Jahns BE, Zarowitz BJ, Mlynarek ME, Fagan SC. Labetalol: response and safety in critically ill hemorrhagic stroke patients. *Ann Pharmacother* 1993; 27: 180–1.

63 Pearson RM, Griffith DN, Woollard M, James IM, Havard CW. Comparison of effects on cerebral blood flow of rapid reduction in systemic arterial pressure by diazoxide and labetalol in hypertensive patients: preliminary findings. *Br J Clin Pharmacol* 1979; 8: 195S–198S.

64 Van Aken H, Puchstein C, Schweppe M, Heinecke A. Effect of labetalol on intracranial pressure in dogs with and without intracranial hypertension. *Acta Anesth Scand* 1982; 26: 615–9.

65 Olsen KS, Svendsen LB, Larsen FS, Paulson OB. Effect of labetalol on cerebral blood flow, oxygen metabolism and autoregulation in healthy humans. *Br J Anesth* 1995; 75: 51–4.

66 Postiglione A, Bobkiewicz T, Vinholdt-Pedersen E, Lassen NA, Paulson OB, Barry DI. Cerebrovascular effects of angiotensin converting enzyme inhibition involve large artery dilatation in rats. *Stroke* 1991; 22: 1362–8.

67 Overgaard J, Skinhoj E. A paradoxical cerebral hemodynamic effect of hydralazine. *Stroke* 1975; 6: 402–4.

68 Schroeder T, Sillesen H. Dihydralazine induces marked cerebral vasodilatation in man. *Eur J Clin Invest* 1987; 17: 214–7.

69 Barry DI, Strandgaard S. Acute effects of antihypertensive drugs on autoregulation of cerebral blood flow in spontaneously hypertensive rats. *Progr Appl Microcirc* 1985; 8: 206–12.

70 ALLHAT officers and coordinators for the ALLHAT Collaborative Research Group. Major outcomes in high-risk hypertensive patients randomized to

angiotensin-converting enzyme inhibitor or calcium channel blocker vs. diuretic: The Antihypertensive and Lipid-Lowering Treatment to Prevent Heart Attack Trial (ALLHAT). *JAMA* 2002; 18: 2981–7.

71 Hall WD. Risk reduction associated with lowering systolic blood pressure. Review of clinical trial data. *Am Heart J* 1999; 138: 225–30.

72 Psaty BM, Smith NL, Siscovick DS *et al*. Health outcomes associated with antihypertensive therapies used as first-line agents. A systematic review and meta-analysis. *JAMA* 1997; 277: 739–45.

73 Staessen JA, Wang JG, Thijs L. Calcium-channel blockade and cardiovascular prognosis: recent evidence from clinical outcome trials. *Am J Hypers* 2002; 15: 85S–93S.

74 Opie LH, Schall R. Evidence-based evaluation of calcium channel blockers for hypertension. Equality of mortality and cardiovascular risk relative to conventional therapy. *J Am Coll Cardiol* 2002; 39: 315–22.

75 Bosch J, Yusuf S, Pogue J *et al.*, on behalf of the HOPE Investigators. Use of ramipril in preventing stroke: double blind randomized trial. *Br Med J* 2002; 324: 1–5.

76 Yusuf S, Sleight P, Pogue J, Bosch J, Davies R, Dagenais G. Effects of an angiotensin-converting-enzyme inhibitor, ramipril, on cardiovascular events in high-rish patients. The Heart Ouctcomes Prevention Evaluation Study Investigators. *N Engl J Med* 2000; 342: 145–53.

77 Staessen JA, Wang JG, Thijs L. Cardiovascular protection and blood pressure reduction: a meta-analysis. *Lancet* 2001; 358: 1305–15.

78 Staessen JA, Wang JG, Thijs L, Fagard R. Overview of the outcome trials in older patients with isolated systolic hypertension. *J Hum Hypertens* 1999; 13: 859–63.

79 Neal B, MacMahon S, Chapman N. Effects of ACE inhibitors, calcium antagonists, and other blood pressure-lowering drugs: results of prospectively designed overviews of randomised trials: Blood Pressure Lowering Treatment Trialists' Collaboration. *Lancet* 2000; 356: 1955–64.

80 Pahor M, Psaty BM, Alderman MH *et al*. Health outcomes associated with calcium antagonists compared with other first-line antihypertensive therapies. a meta-analysis of randomised controlled trials. *Lancet* 2000; 356: 1949–54.

81 Flack JM, Mensah GA, Ferrario CM. Using angiotensin converting enzyme inhibitors in African-American hypertensives. a new approach to treating hypertension and preventing target-organ damage. *Curr Med Res Opin* 2000; 16: 66–79.

82 Messerli FH, Grossman E, Goldbourt U. Are beta-blockers efficacious as first-line therapy for hypertension in the elderly? A systematic review. *JAMA* 1998; 279: 1903–7.

83 Dahlof B, Devereux RB, Kjeldsen SE *et al*. Cardiovascular morbidity and mortality in the Losartan Intervention For Endpoint reduction in hypertension study (LIFE): a randomized trial against atenolol. *Lancet* 2002; 359: 995–1003.

84 Gueyffier F, Boissel J-P, Boutitie F *et al*. Effect of antihypertensive treatment in patients having already suffered from stroke. *Stroke* 1997; 28: 2557–62.

85 Tzourio C, Anderson C, Chapman N *et al.* Effects of blood pressure lowering with perindopril and inadpamide therapy on dementia and cognitive decline in patients with cerebrovascular disease. *Arch Intern Med* 2003; 163: 1069–75.

86 Nakane H, Ibayashi S, Fujii K, Irie K, Sadoshima S, Fujishima M. Cerebral blood flow and metabolism in hypertensive patients with cerebral infarction. *Angiology* 1995; 46: 801–10.

87 Mori S, Sadoshima S, Fujii K *et al.* Decrease in cerebral blood flow with blood pressure reductions in patients with chronic stroke. *Stroke* 1993; 24: 1376–81.

88 Fagan SC, Robert S, Ewing JR, Levine SR, Ramadan NM, Welch KM. Cerebral blood flow changes with enalapril. *Pharmacotherapy* 1992; 12: 319–23.

89 Akopov SE, Simonian NA. Comparison of isradipine and enalapril effects on regional carotid circulation in patients with hypertension with unilateral internal carotid artery stenosis. *J Cardiovasc Pharmacol* 1997; 30: 562–70.

90 Kario K, Pickering TG, Matsuo T *et al.* Stroke prognosis and abnormal nocturnal blood pressure falls in older hypertensives. *Hypertension* 2001; 38: 852–7.

91 Qureshi AI, Suri FK, Mohammad Y, Guterman LR, Hopkins LN. Isolated and borderline isolated systolic hypertension relative to long-term risk and type of stroke. *Stroke* 2002; 33: 2781–8.

92 SHEP Cooperative Research Group. Prevention of stroke by antihypertensive drug treatment in older persons with isolated systolic hypertension. *JAMA* 1991; 265: 3255–64.

93 Perry HM, Davis BR, Price TR *et al.* Effect of treating isolated systolic hypertension on the risk of developing various types and subtypes of stroke. *JAMA* 2000; 284: 465–71.

94 Staessen JA, Fagard R, Thijs L *et al.* Randomised double-blind comparison of placebo and active treatment for older patients with isolated systolic hypertension. *Lancet* 1997; 350: 757–64.

95 Kjeldsen S, Dahlof B, Devereux RB *et al.* Effects of losartan on cardiovascular morbidity and mortality in patients with isolated systolic hypertension and left ventricular hypertrophy. *JAMA* 2002; 288: 1491–8.

CHAPTER 15

Other Medical Therapies

Bradley S. Jacobs, Mar Castellanos, Ramesh Madhavan

Medical therapies for prevention of transient ischemic attack (TIA) and ischemic stroke have mostly focused on treatment of some of the well-proven, modifiable risk factors, such as diabetes and hypertension, and various antithrombotic regimens. However, over the past several years the roles of other risk factors and medical therapies for TIA and stroke prevention have been elucidated. In this chapter, we will discuss some of the pathophysiological and epidemiological bases of some of these more recently suggested risk factors and medical therapies that may offer further potential for TIA and ischemic stroke prevention. Most studies have looked at stroke and TIA together or stroke alone, thus the application of the results to prevention of TIA alone may be presumed, but not proven.

Hyperhomocysteinemia

Elevated levels of total plasma homocysteine have been associated with an increased risk of vascular disease [1]. Initially, an enzyme deficiency of cystathionine β-synthase (an enzyme responsible for homocysteine metabolism) was discovered to be responsible for severe hyperhomocysteinemia (> 100 μM) and homocysteinuria that was associated with vascular disease. McCully first noted that different enzyme deficiency states associated with homocysteinuria were associated with vascular disease and then postulated that elevated homocysteine levels were responsible for the vascular disease [2]. Experimental animal studies have shown that these very high levels of serum homocysteine were probably responsible for the resultant vascular disease [3].

High levels of homocysteine that result in vascular disease are associated with rare severe enzyme deficiencies or dysfunction, whereas mild to moderate elevations of homocysteine are more common in the general population. The role that these smaller elevations of homocysteine (> 10–15 μM) play in the development of vascular disease is less clear. Over the past 20 years, attempts have been made to assess whether these mild to moderate

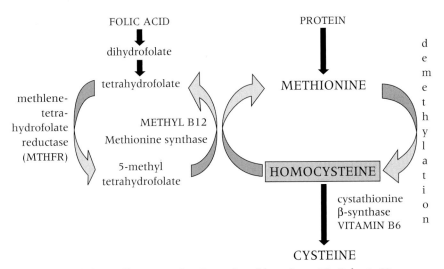

Fig. 15.1 Metabolism of homocysteine. Reproduced from Sacco RL, Roberts JK, Jacobs BS. Homocysteine as a risk factor for ischemic stroke: an epidemiological story in evoltution. *Neuroepidemiology* 1998; 17: 167–73 with permission from S. Karger AG, Basel.

elevations are related to vascular disease. Several case–control and prospective studies found an increased risk of vascular disease with mildly elevated levels of homocysteine [1]. An assumption has been that even this mild hyperhomocysteinemia, whatever the etiology, was probably causally responsible for the increased risk of vascular disease (just as with the higher levels).

Homocysteine is an amino acid metabolite of methionine. Two important pathways for disposal of homocysteine are through remethylation to methionine or conversion to cysteine (Fig. 15.1). The important enzymes in these pathways are methylenetetrahydrofolate reductase and cystathionine β-synthase, respectively. Important vitamin cofactors include folic acid, vitamin B6, and vitamin B12. Deficiencies or dysfunction of these enzymes or deficiencies of these vitamins may cause elevated homocysteine levels. In addition, impaired renal function has been shown to be related to decreased clearance of homocysteine from the blood and resultant hyperhomocysteinemia.

Several less intuitive factors have been shown to be associated with elevated homocysteine levels. Perhaps the most important study investigating these relationships is the Hordaland Homocysteine Study [4]. In this Norwegian study, 7591 men and 8585 women without a known history of hypertension, diabetes, coronary heart disease, or cerebrovascular disease were selected from the National Population Registry. Elevated homocysteine was associated with male sex, older age, increasing amounts of cigarettes smoked, higher total cholesterol levels, higher blood pressure, higher heart rate, low levels of physical activity, lower intakes of vitamin supplements, and lower dietary intakes of fruits and vegetables. The reasons for some of these associations are not clear. These are all potential confounders of the relationship between homocysteine and vascular disease.

Laboratory assays for plasma homocysteine generally measure the total concentration of free thiol, disulfide, and mixed disulfide forms of homocysteine, which are collectively termed 'homocysteine' or 'total plasma homocysteine'. Fasting total plasma homocysteine is the most common and convenient test to perform. Total plasma homocysteine increases after protein meals or methionine loading, which provides the basis for the 'post-methionine loading' test for hyperhomocysteinemia. In this test, total plasma homocysteine is measured 2 h after oral administration of methionine. This test may have greater sensitivity than measurement of fasting total plasma homocysteine for detecting moderate hyperhomocysteinemia caused by abnormalities of homocysteine trans-sulfuration [5]. Specialized tests for detection of specific DNA mutations in cystathionine β-synthase or 5,10-methylenetetrahydrofolate reductase are available.

If the homocysteine is elevated, testing levels of folate, vitamin B12, and vitamin B6 may be helpful in determining whether specific supplementation with one of these vitamins may be most efficacious. Additionally, further work-up for an etiology of these deficiencies may be warranted—especially vitamin B12 deficiency.

Management of patients with severe hyperhomocysteinemia (> 100 μM) and homocysteinuria (most often diagnosed in children) is directed toward lowering the total plasma homocysteine concentration with vitamin supplementation. Initial therapy for severe hyperhomocysteinemia consists of oral administration of large doses of pyridoxine (250–1200 mg daily). Because only about 50% of patients with homozygous deficiency of cystathionine β-synthase respond to pyridoxine, additional therapeutic measures are often employed. These include dietary methionine restriction, supplementation with folic acid or vitamin B12, and administration of the methyl donor, betaine.

For moderate hyperhomocystinemia (15–100 μM) or 'high normal' homocysteinemia (10–15 μM), lowering of homocysteine has not yet been proven to reduce the risk of stroke in randomized controlled trials. There are several trials addressing homocysteine reduction for stroke prevention, including the Bergen Vitamin Study, Vitamin Intervention for Stroke Prevention Trial (VISP) [5a], and Vitamins To Prevent Stroke Study (VITATOPS) [5b]. Because the treatment with vitamin supplementation is relatively benign, based on clinical observational studies it is reasonable to treat pending completion of these trials. Current recommendations [6] advocate checking serum homocysteine levels in patients at 'high risk' of vascular disease with a goal level of < 10 μM. If the level is elevated then further blood testing for specific vitamin deficiencies (folate, B12, and B6) may be considered and vitamin supplementation specifically directed toward these deficiencies. If no clear deficiencies are found, a diet rich in these vitamins may be considered—fortified cereals, leafy green vegetables, fruits, legumes, poultry, beef, fish, artichoke, asparagus, beans, and cabbage. A daily multivitamin may be considered at this time as well (or after re-testing levels following dietary change). If still elevated, daily folic acid 1–2 mg, vitamin B6 25–100 mg, and vitamin B12 0.5–1 mg may be tried. If still elevated, higher doses of these vitamins, in particular folic acid, up to 15 mg daily may be employed. If still elevated, then betaine 3 g twice a day can be attempted.

Cholesterol and statins

Cholesterol and stroke

Dyslipidemia is a well-established risk factor for coronary artery disease and peripheral vascular disease, presumably by contributing to atherosclerosis. Its relationship to stroke has been more controversial [7–9].

Several prospective studies have not shown a relationship between total cholesterol and cerebral infarction [10–12], while others have [13,14]. Several studies have shown an inverse association with cerebral hemorrhage [10,13,15], while one showed a positive association [16]. A review of prospective cohort studies found no clear relationship between plasma total cholesterol levels and stroke (both infarction and hemorrhage) [17]. However, there was a weak positive association between cholesterol and the risk of ischemic stroke and a weak negative association with hemorrhagic stroke [17,18].

Several suggestions for the inconsistent results and lack of association seen in prior studies have been proposed [9,14]. All stroke subtypes were studied together, not only those that would be more strongly related to atherosclerosis. Many studies of stroke risk were performed in patients who developed coronary heart disease, and this limits the interpretation of these studies for several reasons. Studies of coronary heart disease were mainly conducted with middle-aged men, while the population most at risk of stroke is older. Persons in these studies most probably succumbed to coronary heart disease rather than going on to develop stroke. Finally, persons diagnosed with coronary heart disease may be treated with risk factor intervention and are less likely to have stroke later in life.

Recent studies, focusing on ischemic stroke and TIA and specific lipoprotein classes, have been more valuable. A population-based case–control study in northern Manhattan showed increased HDL levels associated with a reduced risk of ischemic stroke [19]. A prospective case–control study in

Israel demonstrated higher total cholesterol, higher LDL, and lower HDL to be associated with an increased risk of ischemic stroke or TIA [20]. Furthermore, extracranial carotid stenosis has been associated with dyslipidemia. Carotid atherosclerosis has been positively associated with total cholesterol [21,22] and LDL [23–25] and inversely associated with HDL [23,26,27].

Statins and stroke

Statins competitively inhibit the liver enzyme HMG-CoA reductase which is the last regulated step in cholesterol synthesis. Statins lower LDL levels by upregulating LDL receptor activity and reducing entry of LDL into the circulation [28]. Other possible beneficial effects of statins include improved endothelial function, decreasing cholesterol accumulation in macrophages, increased antioxidant capacity of plasma, improved stabilization of atherosclerotic plaque, and prevention of thrombus formation [29]. Statins may also have an effect on inflammation. Some studies have shown statin therapy to lower C-reactive protein (CRP) [30,31] and attenuate the risk of recurrent coronary events in persons with high CRP [32].

There are currently six statins on the market: atorvastatin, fluvastatin, lovastatin, pravastatin, simvastatin and rosouvastatin. The most common adverse effects include gastrointestinal upset, muscle aches, and hepatitis. Rare effects include myopathy, rhabdomyolysis, rash, peripheral neuropathy, insomnia, bad or vivid dreams, and difficulty sleeping or concentrating. Hepatotoxicity occurs in < 1% of patients when given high doses. Hepatitis induced by statins is accompanied by fatigue, sluggishness, anorexia, and weight loss with moderate elevation of serum aminotransferases. These symptoms subside quickly after the drug is discontinued [28].

Severe myopathy occurs in approximately 0.08% of persons taking the currently available statins [33]. Cerivastatin was withdrawn from the market after the Food and Drug Administration received reports of death of 31 people taking the drug who developed rhabdomyolysis (12 who concomitantly used gemfibrozil) and subsequently there were indications that as many as 100 deaths were linked [33]. The rate of fatal rhabdomyolysis was about 16–80 times more frequent with cerivastatin compared with other statins [34].

Several trials of statins in patients with coronary heart disease have shown that statins reduce the risk of stroke in these patients. In a meta-analysis [35] of 13 trials, 442 strokes occurred in 20 438 study participants. An overall stroke risk reduction of 31% (odds ratio 0.69; 95% confidence interval 0.57, 0.83) was determined. The authors calculated that approximately 40 strokes could be prevented when using statins in 10 000 patients with coronary artery disease over 'a considerable length of time'. The major randomized controlled trials are presented in Table 15.1. The Prospective Pravastatin Pooling (PPP) project [36] was a prospectively

Table 15.1 Major randomized, placebo-controlled trials of statins

Study	n	Age (years)	Inclusion criteria	Follow-up period (years)	Drug	All-cause mortality—number needed to treat	Major coronary events—number needed to treat	Stroke or TIA—number needed to treat
Scandinavian Simvastatin Survival Study (SSSS) [81]	4444 (82% men)	35–70	Post myocardial infarction	5.4	Simvastatin 20–40 mg/day	29 for 5 years to prevent 1 death	12 for 5 years to prevent 1 event	65 for 5 years to prevent 1 event
Cholesterol and Recurrent Events (CARE) study [38]	4159 (86% men)	21–75	Post myocardial infarction	5	Pravastatin 40 mg/day or placebo	125 for 5 years to prevent 1 death	33 for 5 years to prevent 1 event	86 for 5 years to prevent 1 stroke
Long-term Intervention with Pravastatin in Ischemic Disease (LIPID) study [39]	9014 (83% men)	31–75	Post myocardial infarction or unstable angina	6	Pravastatin 40 mg/day or placebo	33 for 6 years to prevent 1 death	28 for 6 years to prevent 1 event	127 for 6 years to prevent 1 stroke
West of Scotland Coronary Prevention Study (WOSCOP) [37]	6595 men	45–64	High risk with no myocardial infarction	5	Pravastatin 40 mg/day or placebo	Not significant	44 for 5 years to prevent 1 event	Not significant

defined analysis of three of these large randomized, placebo-controlled trials of pravastatin for coronary heart disease prevention that included 19 768 patients, with 598 patients having stroke during 5 years of follow-up. The primary prevention trial in hypercholesterolemic men [WOSCOPS (West of Scotland Coronary Prevention Study) [37]] did not show a significant reduction in stroke risk. However, the two secondary prevention trials, CARE (Cholesterol And Recurrent Events) [38] and LIPID (Long-term Intervention with Pravastatin in Ischemic Disease) [39] individually demonstrated reductions in nonfatal and total stroke rates. The combined data of the latter two trials showed a 22% reduction in total strokes ($P = 0.01$). When all three trials were combined, a 20% reduction ($P = 0.01$) in total stroke was noted. From the WOSCOPS trial, 3333 patients per year would need to be treated to prevent one stroke. From the combined CARE and LIPID trials, 588 patients with coronary heart disease per year would need to be treated to prevent one stroke.

While these trials have shown stroke risk reduction with statins, it is important to remember that the primary aim of these trials was to assess coronary heart disease prevention. All but the WOSCOPS trial were secondary prevention trials in patients with coronary heart disease. This limits the applicability of the results of these trials to patients with coronary heart disease and not necessarily patients with stroke and without coronary heart disease. The stroke risk reduction in patients with coronary heart disease may be related to risk reduction of recurrent coronary heart disease and subsequent reduction of stroke.

Trials of statins for recurrent stroke prevention in patients without a history of coronary heart disease are underway. One of these is the Stroke Prevention by Aggressive Reduction in Cholesterol Levels (SPARCL) [40] with atorvastatin. The British Heart Foundation/Medical Research Council Heart Protection Study (BHF/MRC-HPS) utilized simvastatin in a broad range of patients with either established vascular disease or vascular risk factors [41]. In this study, 20 536 patients were enrolled and treated with either simvastatin 40 mg or placebo. During a 5-year treatment period, there was an observed 18% reduction in death for coronary reasons (5.7% vs. 6.9%, $P = 0.0005$), and reductions of approximately one-quarter in fatal or nonfatal stroke (4.3% vs. 5.7%, $P < 0.0001$).

Approximately one-sixth of the patients in the HPS study were enrolled with a history of stroke. These patients, along with other important subgroups, showed benefit with simvastatin treatment. For patients with previous stroke, the event rate for major vascular events was reduced from 29.8% to 24.7%. Interestingly, even those patients with a LDL level of < 116 mg/dl showed benefit, suggesting that the non-LDL-lowering properties of statins were useful in this population.

While further studies are being completed, the use of the guidelines set forth by the Third Report of the National Cholesterol Education Program

Table 15.2 ATP III classification of optimal lipoprotein profile

Total cholesterol	
< 200	Desirable
200–239	Borderline high
≥ 240	High
LDL-cholesterol	
< 100	Optimal
100–129	Near or above optimal
130–159	Borderline high
160–189	High
≥ 190	Very high
HDL-cholesterol	
< 40	Low
≥ 60	High

(NCEP) Expert Panel on Detection, Evaluation, and Treatment of High Blood Cholesterol in Adults [42] is recommended. New definitions of desirable lipid values are defined (Table 15.2). These guidelines propose various degrees of intervention and treatment based on the risk profile of the patient. Tightest control of hypercholesterolemia is recommended for patients with coronary heart disease or coronary heart disease risk equivalents. Risk equivalents include diabetes, other clinical forms of atherosclerotic disease (peripheral artery disease, abdominal aortic aneurysm, and symptomatic carotid artery disease), or the presence of multiple risk factors that confer a 10-year risk for coronary heart disease of > 20%. For these persons, a target LDL goal of < 100 mg/dl is recommended. Complete information about these guidelines and a program for handheld computers may be found at the website www.nhlbi.nih.gov

ACE inhibitors

A complete discussion of the role of hypertension and its treatment may be found in another chapter, while this section will pertain more specifically to the role of angiotensin converting enzyme inhibitors (ACE-I) in stroke prevention. In brief, hypertension is a powerful, prevalent and treatable independent risk factor for TIA and stroke [43]. It is well established that the reduction of systolic, diastolic, or both in hypertensive subjects substantially reduces stroke risk [44–46].

Although it is clear that lowering blood pressure reduces the risk of stroke, it is less clear whether the class of agent used is of importance. A meta-analysis of randomized controlled trials found β-blockers and high-dose diuretics to be effective in stroke prevention [47]. Overviews of trials comparing calcium antagonist-based regimens with those based on other antihypertensive drugs suggested that a calcium antagonist-based regimen may be slightly more effective in reducing stroke risk [48]. A recent population-based case–control study suggested that thiazide diuretics were better than other medications for stroke prevention [49].

Angiotensin II is a potent peripheral vasoconstrictor, inhibits renin secretion, and stimulates aldosterone release, thus increasing blood pressure. ACE is the same as kinase II that breaks down bradykinin, a potent vasodepressor. ACE-I block the conversion of angiotensin I to angiotensin II and prevent the breakdown of bradykinin, thus lowering blood pressure. Other beneficial effects of ACE-I that have been proposed include antagonizing proliferation of smooth muscle cells, antagonizing the rupture of plaque, improving vascular endothelial function, reducing left ventricular hypertrophy, and enhancing fibrinolysis [50].

Two recent randomized controlled trials of ACE-I have fueled interest in the use of this class of medication for stroke prevention. The trials are the Heart Outcomes Prevention Evaluation (HOPE) Study [50] and the Perindopril Protection Against Recurrent Stroke Study (PROGRESS) [51].

The HOPE study was a randomized, placebo-controlled trial of ramipril 10 mg each day in 9297 'high-risk' patients with a composite primary outcome of myocardial infarction, stroke, or death from cardiovascular causes. High-risk patients were 55 years or older and had a history of coronary artery disease, stroke, peripheral vascular disease, or diabetes plus at least one other risk factor (hypertension, elevated total cholesterol, low HDL-cholesterol, cigarette smoking, or microalbuminuria). Patients were excluded if they had a low ejection fraction, were taking an ACE-I or vitamin E (another part of the study examined the efficacy of vitamin E supplementation), had uncontrolled hypertension or overt nephropathy, or suffered a myocardial infarction or stroke within 4 weeks of enrollment. A primary endpoint was reached by 14.0% of the ramipril group compared with 17.8% of the placebo group (relative risk 0.78, $P < 0.001$).

In a more detailed analysis of stroke outcome in the study [52], the relative risk of any stroke was reduced by 32% and the relative risk of fatal stroke was reduced by 61% in the ramipril group compared with the placebo group. Fewer patients in the ramipril group than in the placebo group (2.2% vs. 3.4%) had an ischemic stroke (relative risk 0.64, 0.50–0.82). A total of 190 (4.1%) patients in the ramipril group had a TIA compared with 227 (4.9%) in the placebo group (relative risk 0.83, 0.68–1.00). The effect was observed early and the benefit continued to increase throughout the 4.5-year study period. The reduction was consistent across different subtypes of stroke and in various subgroups examined and it was independent of the modest reduction in blood pressure seen with ramipril.

The HOPE study demonstrated the value of ramipril for the primary prevention of stroke. The study was not powered to determine the effectiveness of ramipril for secondary prevention. Approximately 11% of patients had a history of stroke at study entry and these patients showed benefit from ramipril treatment, along with other important subgroups.

The results of PROGRESS confirmed the efficacy of the ACE inhibitors (in combination with a diuretic) in the secondary prevention of stroke [51]. In this study, 6105 patients were randomized and 3051 received 'active treatment' with a perindopril-based regimen. Active treatment included perindopril 4 mg for all treated patients. The responsible physician chose whether indapamide 2.5 mg (or placebo) should be used in addition to perindopril (or placebo) prior to the start of the study. In other words, patients received perindopril, perindopril plus indapamide, single placebo, or double placebo. Patients in the active treatment group received perindopril or perindopril plus indapamide, while patients in the placebo group received either single placebo or double placebo. Of persons in the active treatment group, 58% receive indapamide in addition to perindopril.

Active treatment was associated with a significant 28% relative risk reduction in the primary outcome of total stroke (fatal and nonfatal). A significant stroke risk reduction of 43% was noted in the group of patients who received the combination of perindopril and indapamide, but there was not a significant reduction in patients receiving perindopril alone. The benefits of the active treatment were consistently observed in both hypertensive (defined as systolic > 160 or diastolic > 90) and nonhypertensive patients. Active treatment reduced total stroke by 32% in hypertensive subjects and by 27% in nonhypertensive subjects. Perindopril plus indapamide reduced total stroke risk by 44% in hypertensive and by 42% in nonhypertensive participants.

Single therapy with perindopril was not shown to be efficacious for stroke prevention, but this study may have lacked the ability to prove so, as this was not the primary aim of the study. The single therapy group was significantly less hypertensive and probably had a lower risk of stroke. As pointed out by the authors and in the accompanying commentary [53], the group characteristics of patients who received combination therapy differed from patients receiving single therapy. Patients in the combination therapy group possibly represented a group with a greater risk for vascular events, thus making risk reduction with antihypertensive therapy easier to demonstrate.

While the HOPE study raises the possible role of ramipril in stroke prevention, it is important to consider that these results were found in a specific population of high-risk patients. While HOPE points out that ramipril may have effects beyond that expected for its antihypertensive properties, PROGRESS does not clearly show perindopril to have a similar effect. However, this may at least partially be related to differences in study design. PROGRESS does demonstrate the importance of hypertension treatment in the prevention of recurrent stroke. The 43% risk reduction with combination therapy occurred with a blood pressure reduction of 12/5, suggesting that blood pressure reduction to a moderate degree can result in significant event reduction. With combination perindopril and indapamide therapy, for every 14 patients treated for 5 years, approximately one stroke could be prevented [54].

Another category of medication which may be especially appealing for stroke reduction is the angiotensin receptor blockers (ARBs). The Losartan Intervention For Endpoint reduction in hypertension study (LIFE) evaluated a losartan-based treatment regimen vs. an atenolol-based strategy [55]. Overall, 9193 patients with hypertension (160–200/95–115 mmHg) and left ventricular hypertrophy on ECG were enrolled. Despite similar reductions in blood pressure (30/17 in the losartan group and 29/17 in the atenolol group), there was a 25% risk reduction for the endpoint of fatal or nonfatal stroke (232 and 309 in the losartan and atenolol groups, respectively). This suggests that losartan has pharmacological properties which provide additional protection from stroke compared with a β-blocker-based regimen.

Undiagnosed and poorly controlled hypertension is very common [56]. In one study of survivors of stroke and myocardial infarction, 53% of patients with hypertension were poorly controlled and 11% without a prior diagnosis of hypertension were hypertensive (> 140/90) [57]. Diagnosis and treatment of hypertension is an underutilized instrument for stroke prevention. Several classes of antihypertensives hold large potential for preventing stroke and TIA. While ACE-I may have some beneficial effects beyond lowering blood pressure, further research is required to discern whether expensive drugs such as some ACE-Is are clearly better than some less expensive drugs, such as diuretics [53].

Cigarette smoking

In the USA, 20.7% was the median prevalence of cigarette smoking among the states in the year 2000. Compared with 1991, 14 of 47 states noted an increase in smoking, whereas only one state noted a decrease [58]. Smoking accelerates the process of atherosclerosis and is an independent risk factor for peripheral vascular disease, coronary heart disease and stroke [59,60]. The Framingham prospective study demonstrated a relative risk of cerebral infarction of 1.6 in men and 1.9 in women [59]. A significant dose–response relationship was noted, with persons smoking more than 40 cigarettes per day having twice the risk compared with persons smoking less than 10 cigarettes per day. A meta-analysis of 32 studies demonstrated a relative risk of infarct of 1.9 and a dose–response as well [61]. Several mechanisms of how smoking may predispose to vascular disease have been proposed. Included are increased fibrinogen, increased thrombin generation, increased platelet activation, and endothelial dysfunction [62].

One of the most striking aspects of cigarette smoking as a vascular disease risk factor is that some studies have shown it to be a completely reversible and curable condition. In the Framingham study 51% of persons quit smoking over 26 years. The risk of stroke declined significantly within 2 years of quitting and reverted to the same as nonsmokers within 5 years [59]. Another study in middle-aged British men showed similar results [63].

While the condition is reversible, smoking cessation is not quite as 'simple' as treatment for other vascular disease risk factors. Most persons (70%) wish to quit completely and about 46% attempt to quit each year [64]. However, the success rates are poor: 7% have long-term success by quitting on their own and 15–30% have success with guideline-recommended counselling and treatment [64]. Recognition and advice to quit from physicians may be an important motivator for smokers. A good resource for strategies of counselling and pharmacotherapy may be found in the *Clinical Practice Guideline for Treating Tobacco Use and Dependence* from the US Public Health Service [64].

Physical inactivity

Regular exercise reduces the risk of premature death and cardiovascular disease [65,66], but its effectiveness in stroke prevention has only more recently become more accepted. Earlier studies suggested physical inactivity is a weak, non-independent risk factor for stroke, present in only certain populations [67,68]. The British Regional Heart Study demonstrated that physical activity was inversely associated with stroke independent of other vascular risk factors [69]. The Northern Manhattan Stroke Study also demonstrated that physical activity was significantly protective for stroke after adjustment for other vascular risk factors and regardless of age, sex and race-ethnicity [70]. The Physicians Health Study demonstrated that exercise vigorous enough to work up a sweat was associated with decreased stroke risk in men, but not independent of other stroke risk factors [71].

The intensity of physical activity necessary to bring about a reduction in stroke risk is not clear. Some studies have not shown a significantly increased effect with increased intensity of activity [68,69]. However, the Nurses' Health Study [72] and the Northern Manhattan Stroke Study [73] both showed a dose–response relationship. This difficulty in finding a dose–response relationship could be related to variations in the methods used to assess physical activity.

Physical activity generally appears to have an effect independent of other stroke risk factors. Some of its effect is mediated through control of risk factors such as hypertension [74], diabetes [75], cardiovascular disease [65,66], and lower body weight. Other possible mechanisms of how physical activity lowers the risk of stroke include reducing plasma fibrinogen [76], reducing platelet adhesiveness and aggregability [77], and increasing HDL [78].

Studies have not uniformly delineated the optimal length and intensity of physical activity for stroke prevention. However, the benefits of even modest physical activity, such as walking, are apparent for both cardiovascular disease and stroke prevention. The Centers for Disease Control and Prevention and the National Institutes of Health recommend exercise for at least 30 min of moderate intensity on most, and preferably all, days of the week [79,80].

References

1 Beresford SAA, Boushey CJ. Homocysteine, folic acid, and cardiovascular disease risk. In: Bendich A, Deckelbaum RJ, eds. *Preventive Nutrition: the Comprehensive Guide for Health Professionals*. Totowa, NJ: Humana Press Inc., 1997: 193–224.

2 McCully KS. Vascular pathology of homocystinemia: implications for the pathogenesis of atherosclerosis. *Am J Pathol* 1969; 56: 111–28.

3 Boushey CJ, Beresford SA, Omenn GS, Motulsky AG. A quantitative assessment of plasma homocysteine as a risk factor for vascular disease. Probable benefits of increasing folic acid intakes. *JAMA* 1995; 274: 1049–57.

4 Nygard O, Vollset SE, Refsum H *et al*. Total plasma homocysteine and cardiovascular risk profile. The Hordaland Homocysteine Study. *JAMA* 1995; 274: 1526–33.

5 D'Angelo A, Selhub J. Homocysteine and thrombotic disease. *Blood* 1997; 90: 1–11.

5a Toole JF, Malinow MR, Chambless LE *et al*. Lowering homocysteine in patients with ischemic stroke to prevent recurrent stroke, myocardial infarction, and death: the Vitamin Intervention for Stroke Prevention (VISP) randomized controlled trial. *JAMA* 2004; 291: 565–75.

5b VITATOPS Trial Study Group. The VITATOPS (Vitamins to Prevent Stroke) Trial: rationale and design of an international, large, simple, randomised trial of homocysteine-lowering multivitamin therapy in patients with recent transient ischaemic attack or stroke. *Cerebrovasc Dis* 2002; 13: 120–6.

6 Malinow MR, Bostom AG, Krauss RM. Homocysteine, diet, and cardiovascular diseases: a statement for healthcare professionals from the Nutrition Committee, American Heart Association. *Circulation* 1999; 99: 178–82.

7 Demchuk AM, Hess DC, Brass LM, Yatsu FM. Is cholesterol a risk factor for stroke?: Yes. *Arch Neurol* 1999; 56: 1518–20.

8 Landau WM. Is cholesterol a risk factor for stroke?: No. *Arch Neurol* 1999; 56: 1521–4.

9 Gorelick PB, Schneck M, Berglund LF, Feinberg W, Goldstone J. Status of lipids as a risk factor for stroke. *Neuroepidemiology* 1997; 16: 107–15.

10 Ueshima H, Iida M, Shimamoto T *et al*. Multivariate analysis of risk factors for stroke. Eight-year follow-up study of farming villages in Akita, Japan. *Prev Med* 1980; 9: 722–40.

11 Tanaka H, Hayashi M, Date C *et al*. Epidemiologic studies of stroke in Shibata, a Japanese provincial city: preliminary report on risk factors for cerebral infarction. *Stroke* 1985; 16: 773–80.

12 Salonen JT, Puska P, Tuomilehto J, Homan K. Relation of blood pressure, serum lipids, and smoking to the risk of cerebral stroke. A longitudinal study in Eastern Finland. *Stroke* 1982; 13: 327–33.

13 Iso H, Jacobs DR Jr, Wentworth D, Neaton JD, Cohen JD. Serum cholesterol levels and six-year mortality from stroke in 350,977 men screened for the multiple risk factor intervention trial. *N Engl J Med* 1989; 320: 904–10.

14 Benfante R, Yano K, Hwang LJ, Curb JD, Kagan A, Ross W. Elevated serum cholesterol is a risk factor for both coronary heart disease and thromboembolic stroke in Hawaiian Japanese men. Implications of shared risk. *Stroke* 1994; 25: 814–20.

15 Kagan A, Popper JS, Rhoads GG. Factors related to stroke incidence in Hawaii Japanese men. The Honolulu Heart Study. *Stroke* 1980; 11: 14–21.

16 Lindenstrom E, Boysen G, Nyboe J. Influence of total cholesterol, high density lipoprotein cholesterol, and triglycerides on risk of cerebrovascular disease: the Copenhagen City Heart Study. *Br Med J* 1994; 309: 11–5.

17 Cholesterol, diastolic blood pressure, and stroke: 13,000 strokes in 450,000 people in 45 prospective cohorts. Prospective studies collaboration. *Lancet* 1995; 346: 1647–53.

18 Law MR, Thompson SG, Wald NJ. Assessing possible hazards of reducing serum cholesterol. *Br Med J* 1994; 308: 373–9.

19 Sacco RL, Benson RT, Kargman DE *et al*. High-density lipoprotein cholesterol and ischemic stroke in the elderly: the Northern Manhattan Stroke Study. *JAMA* 2001; 285: 2729–35.

20 Koren-Morag N, Tanne D, Graff E, Goldbourt U. Low- and high-density lipoprotein cholesterol and ischemic cerebrovascular disease: the bezafibrate infarction prevention registry. *Arch Intern Med* 2002; 162: 993–9.

21 Fine-Edelstein JS, Wolf PA, O'Leary DH *et al*. Precursors of extracranial carotid atherosclerosis in the Framingham Study. *Neurology* 1994; 44: 1046–50.

22 Reed DM, Resch JA, Hayashi T, MacLean C, Yano K. A prospective study of cerebral artery atherosclerosis. *Stroke* 1988; 19: 820–5.

23 Salonen R, Seppanen K, Rauramaa R, Salonen JT. Prevalence of carotid atherosclerosis and serum cholesterol levels in eastern Finland. *Arteriosclerosis* 1988; 8: 788–92.

24 Grotta JC, Yatsu FM, Pettigrew LC *et al*. Prediction of carotid stenosis progression by lipid and hematologic measurements. *Neurology* 1989; 39: 1325–31.

25 Heiss G, Sharrett AR, Barnes R, Chambless LE, Szklo M, Alzola C. Carotid atherosclerosis measured by B-mode ultrasound in populations: associations

with cardiovascular risk factors in the ARIC study. *Am J Epidemiol* 1991; 134: 250–6.

26 Crouse JR, Toole JF, McKinney WM *et al.* Risk factors for extracranial carotid artery atherosclerosis. *Stroke* 1987; 18: 990–6.

27 Prati P, Vanuzzo D, Casaroli M *et al.* Prevalence and determinants of carotid atherosclerosis in a general population. *Stroke* 1992; 23: 1705–11.

28 Knopp RH. Drug treatment of lipid disorders. *N Engl J Med* 1999; 341: 498–511.

29 Gorelick PB. Stroke prevention therapy beyond antithrombotics. unifying mechanisms in ischemic stroke pathogenesis and implications for therapy: an invited review. *Stroke* 2002; 33: 862–75.

30 Ridker PM, Rifai N, Pfeffer MA, Sacks F, Braunwald E. Long-term effects of pravastatin on plasma concentration of C-reactive protein. The Cholesterol and Recurrent Events (CARE) Investigators. *Circulation* 1999; 100: 230–5.

31 Albert MA, Danielson E, Rifai N, Ridker PM. Effect of statin therapy on C-reactive protein levels: the pravastatin inflammation/CRP evaluation (PRINCE): a randomized trial and cohort study. *JAMA* 2001; 286: 64–70.

32 Ridker PM, Rifai N, Clearfield M *et al.* Measurement of C-reactive protein for the targeting of statin therapy in the primary prevention of acute coronary events. *N Engl J Med* 2001; 344: 1959–65.

33 Pasternak RC, Smith SC Jr, Bairey-Merz CN, Grundy SM, Cleeman JI, Lenfant C. ACC/AHA/NHLBI clinical advisory on the use and safety of statins. *J Am Coll Cardiol* 2002; 40: 567–72.

34 Staffa JA, Chang J, Green L. Cerivastatin and reports of fatal rhabdomyolysis. *N Engl J Med* 2002; 346: 539–40.

35 Blauw GJ, Lagaay AM, Smelt AH, Westendorp RG. Stroke, statins, and cholesterol. A meta-analysis of randomized, placebo-controlled, double-blind trials with HMG-CoA reductase inhibitors. *Stroke* 1997; 28: 946–50.

36 Byington RP, Davis BR, Plehn JF *et al.* Reduction of stroke events with pravastatin: the Prospective Pravastatin Pooling (PPP) Project. *Circulation* 2001; 103: 387–92.

37 Shepherd J, Cobbe SM, Ford I, Isles CG *et al.* Prevention of coronary heart disease with pravastatin in men with hypercholesterolemia. West of Scotland Coronary Prevention Study Group. *N Engl J Med* 1995; 333: 1301–7.

38 Sacks FM, Pfeffer MA, Moye LA *et al.* The effect of pravastatin on coronary events after myocardial infarction in patients with average cholesterol levels. Cholesterol and Recurrent Events Trial investigators. *N Engl J Med* 1996; 335: 1001–9.

39 The Long-Term Intervention with Pravastatin in Ischaemic Disease (LIPID) Study Group. Prevention of cardiovascular events and death with pravastatin in patients with coronary heart disease and a broad range of initial cholesterol levels. *N Engl J Med* 1998; 339: 1349–57.

40 Amarenco P, Bogousslavsky J, Callahan AS *et al.* Design and baseline characteristics of the stroke prevention by aggressive reduction in cholesterol levels (SPARCL) study. *Cerebrovasc Dis* 2003; 16: 389–95.

41 MRC/BHF Heart Protection Study of cholesterol-lowering with simvastatin in 20,536 high-risk individuals: a randomised placebo-controlled trial. *Lancet* 2002; 360: 7–22.

42 Executive Summary of The Third Report of The National Cholesterol Education Program (NCEP) Expert Panel on Detection, Evaluation, and Treatment of High Blood Cholesterol In Adults (Adult Treatment Panel III). *JAMA* 2001; 285: 2486–97.

43 Goldstein LB, Adams R, Becker K *et al.* Primary prevention of ischemic stroke: a statement for healthcare professionals from the Stroke Council of the American Heart Association. *Stroke* 2001; 32: 280–99.

44 Collins R, Peto R, MacMahon S *et al.* Blood pressure, stroke, and coronary heart disease. Part 2, Short-term reductions in blood pressure: overview of randomised drug trials in their epidemiological context. *Lancet* 1990; 335: 827–38.

45 Prevention of stroke by antihypertensive drug treatment in older persons with isolated systolic hypertension. Final results of the Systolic Hypertension in the Elderly Program (SHEP). SHEP Cooperative Research Group. *JAMA* 1991; 265: 3255–64.

46 Staessen JA, Fagard R, Thijs L *et al.* Randomised double-blind comparison of placebo and active treatment for older patients with isolated systolic hypertension. The Systolic Hypertension in Europe (Syst-Eur) Trial Investigators. *Lancet* 1997; 350: 757–64.

47 Psaty BM, Smith NL, Siscovick DS *et al.* Health outcomes associated with antihypertensive therapies used as first-line agents. A systematic review and meta-analysis. *JAMA* 1997; 277: 739–45.

48 Neal B, MacMahon S, Chapman N. Effects of ACE inhibitors, calcium antagonists, and other blood-pressure-lowering drugs: results of prospectively designed overviews of randomised trials. Blood Pressure Lowering Treatment Trialists' Collaboration. *Lancet* 2000; 356: 1955–64.

49 Klungel OH, Heckbert SR, Longstreth WT Jr *et al.* Antihypertensive drug therapies and the risk of ischemic stroke. *Arch Intern Med* 2001; 161: 37–43.

50 The Heart Outcomes Prevention Evaluation Study Investigators. Effects of an angiotensin-converting-enzyme inhibitor, ramipril, on cardiovascular events in high-risk patients. *N Engl J Med* 2000; 342: 145–53.

51 PROGRESS Collaborative Group. Randomised trial of a perindopril-based blood-pressure-lowering regimen among 6,105 individuals with previous stroke or transient ischaemic attack. *Lancet* 2001; 358: 1033–41.

52 Bosch J, Yusuf S, Pogue J *et al.* Use of ramipril in preventing stroke: double blind randomised trial. *Br Med J* 2002; 324: 699.

53 Staessen JA, Wang J. Blood-pressure lowering for the secondary prevention of stroke. *Lancet* 2001; 358: 1026–7.

54 Messerli FH, Hanley DF Jr, Gorelick PB. Blood pressure control in stroke patients: what should the consulting neurologist advise? *Neurology* 2002; 59: 23–25.

55 Dahlof B, Devereux RB, Kjeldsen SE *et al.* Cardiovascular morbidity and mortality in the Losartan Intervention for Endpoint reduction in hypertension study (LIFE): a randomised trial against atenolol. *Lancet* 2002; 359: 995–1003.

56 Burt VL, Cutler JA, Higgins M *et al.* Trends in the prevalence, awareness, treatment, and control of hypertension in the adult US population. Data from the Health Examination Surveys, 1960 to 1991. *Hypertension* 1995; 26: 60–9.

57 Qureshi AI, Suri MF, Guterman LR, Hopkins LN. Ineffective secondary prevention in survivors of cardiovascular events in the US population: report from the Third National Health and Nutrition Examination Survey. *Arch Intern Med* 2001; 161: 1621–8.

58 Nelson DE, Bland S, Powell-Griner E *et al.* State trends in health risk factors and receipt of clinical preventive services among US adults during the 1990s. *JAMA* 2002; 287: 2659–67.

59 Wolf PA, D'Agostino RB, Kannel WB, Bonita R, Belanger AJ. Cigarette smoking as a risk factor for stroke. The Framingham Study. *JAMA* 1988; 259: 1025–9.

60 Robbins AS, Manson JE, Lee IM, Satterfield S, Hennekens CH. Cigarette smoking and stroke in a cohort of U.S. male physicians. *Ann Intern Med* 1994; 120: 458–62.

61 Shinton R, Beevers G. Meta-analysis of relation between cigarette smoking and stroke. *Br Med J* 1989; 298: 789–94.

62 Bottcher M, Falk E. Pathology of the coronary arteries in smokers and non-smokers. *J Cardiovasc Risk* 1999; 6: 299–302.

63 Wannamethee SG, Shaper AG, Whincup PH, Walker M. Smoking cessation and the risk of stroke in middle-aged men. *JAMA* 1995; 274: 155–60.

64 A clinical practice guideline for treating tobacco use and dependence: a US Public Health Service report. The Tobacco Use and Dependence Clinical Practice Guideline Panel, Staff, and Consortium Representatives. *JAMA* 2000; 283: 3244–54.

65 Powell KE, Thompson PD, Caspersen CJ, Kendrick JS. Physical activity and the incidence of coronary heart disease. *Annu Rev Public Health* 1987; 8: 253–87.

66 Berlin JA, Colditz GA. A meta-analysis of physical activity in the prevention of coronary heart disease. *Am J Epidemiol* 1990; 132: 612–28.

67 Abbott RD, Rodriguez BL, Burchfiel CM, Curb JD. Physical activity in older middle-aged men and reduced risk of stroke: the Honolulu Heart Program. *Am J Epidemiol* 1994; 139: 881–93.

68 Kiely DK, Wolf PA, Cupples LA, Beiser AS, Kannel WB. Physical activity and stroke risk: the Framingham Study. *Am J Epidemiol* 1994; 140: 608–20.

69 Wannamethee G, Shaper AG. Physical activity and stroke in British middle aged men. *Br Med J* 1992; 304: 597–601.

70 Sacco RL, Gan R, Boden-Albala B *et al.* Leisure-time physical activity and ischemic stroke risk: the Northern Manhattan Stroke Study. *Stroke* 1998; 29: 380–7.

71 Lee IM, Hennekens CH, Berger K, Buring JE, Manson JE. Exercise and risk of stroke in male physicians. *Stroke* 1999; 30: 1–6.

72 Hu FB, Stampfer MJ, Colditz GA *et al.* Physical activity and risk of stroke in women. *JAMA* 2000; 283: 2961–7.

73 Sacco RL, Gan R, Boden-Albala B *et al.* Leisure-time physical activity and ischemic stroke risk: the Northern Manhattan Stroke Study. *Stroke* 1998; 29: 380–7.

74 Kokkinos PF, Narayan P, Colleran JA *et al.* Effects of regular exercise on blood pressure and left ventricular hypertrophy in African-American men with severe hypertension. *N Engl J Med* 1995; 333: 1462–7.

75 Hu FB, Sigal RJ, Rich-Edwards JW *et al.* Walking compared with vigorous physical activity and risk of type 2 diabetes in women: a prospective study. *JAMA* 1999; 282: 1433–9.

76 Lakka TA, Salonen JT. Moderate to high intensity conditioning leisure time physical activity and high cardiorespiratory fitness are associated with reduced plasma fibrinogen in eastern Finnish men. *J Clin Epidemiol* 1993; 46: 1119–27.

77 Wang JS, Jen CJ, Chen HI. Effects of exercise training and deconditioning on platelet function in men. *Arterioscler Thromb Vasc Biol* 1995; 15: 1668–74.

78 Williams PT. High-density lipoprotein cholesterol and other risk factors for coronary heart disease in female runners. *N Engl J Med* 1996; 334: 1298–303.

79 Pate RR, Pratt M, Blair SN *et al.* Physical activity and public health. A recommendation from the Centers for Disease Control and Prevention and the American College of Sports Medicine. *JAMA* 1995; 273: 402–7.

80 NIH Consensus Development Panel on Physical Activity and Cardiovascular Health. Physical activity and cardiovascular health. *JAMA* 1996; 276: 241–6.

81 Randomised trial of cholesterol lowering in 4444 patients with coronary heart disease: the Scandinavian Simvastatin Survival Study (4S). *Lancet* 1994; 344: 1383–9.

CHAPTER 16

Thrombolysis for Acute Transient Ischemic Attack and Mild Stroke

Michael R. Frankel, James Bichsel

The management of patients with transient ischemic attack (TIA) or mild ischemic stroke symptoms is focused on stroke prevention and treatment of associated risk factors. However, decisions to use thrombolytic therapy may arise in these patients in the Emergency Department (ED). This chapter will explore the relationship between TIA or mild stroke and administration of thrombolytic therapy.

Thrombolytic therapy and TIA

In 1996, the Food and Drug Administration (FDA) approved recombinant tissue plasminogen activator (rt-PA) for patients with acute ischemic stroke. The benefit of intravenous (i.v.) rt-PA was demonstrated in two randomized, double-blind, placebo-controlled trials that were consecutively performed and funded by the National Institutes of Neurological Disorders and Stroke (NINDS) [1]. Entitled Part 1 and Part 2 of the NINDS rt-PA Stroke Study, both trials used identical entry criteria (see Table 16.1) and enrolled patients with acute stroke symptoms to receive i.v. rt-PA or placebo over 1 h. The initiation of the infusion was within 3 h of symptom onset and patients were managed according to a standardized set of guidelines (see Table 16.2). The longterm benefit of rt-PA was demonstrated in each of the two trials. Overall, there were 624 patients enrolled and those treated with rt-PA were 37–62% more likely than placebo-treated patients to achieve a favorable outcome at 3 months [1]. The absolute differences between groups were robust and statistically significant in favor of rt-PA in each of the two studies and for each of the four outcome scales used. For example, based on the Modified Rankin scale, 43% of rt-PA-treated patients vs. 27% of placebo-treated patients had no disability at 3 months. Overall, absolute differences in favor of rt-PA-treated patients ranged between 13% and 16% depending on the outcome scale used. This means

Table 16.1 Criteria for the use of intravenous tissue plasminogen activator (t-PA) in acute ischemic stroke

---

Inclusions

Ischemic stroke with a clearly defined symptom onset

No evidence of intracranial blood on brain computed tomography scan

180 min or less from the time of symptom onset to initiation of i.v. t-PA

Measurable neurological deficit

Exclusions

Rapidly improving or minor stroke symptoms

Stroke or serious head trauma within 3 months

Major surgery within 14 days

History of intracranial hemorrhage

Systolic blood pressure > 185 mmHg or diastolic blood pressure > 110 mmHg at the time of treatment initiation

Aggressive BP treatment, i.e. continuous i.v. infusion of an antihypertensive to achieve above goal

Suspected subarachnoid hemorrhage despite a normal computed tomography scan

Gastrointestinal or GU tract hemorrhage within 21 days

Arterial puncture at a noncompressible site within 7 days

Seizure at the onset of stroke

Use of heparin within 48 h and an elevated partial thromboplastin time

PT > 15 s, platelet count < 100 000, glucose < 50 or > 400

Dosing and infusion of rt-PA

0.9 mg/kg i.v., not to exceed 90 mg

10% given as bolus over 1 min; remainder infused over 1 h

Data from [1]. BP, blood pressure; GU, genitourinary; PT, prothrombin time.

Table 16.2 Management guidelines after initiation of recombinant tissue plasminogen activator (rt-PA) therapy

---

No anticoagulants or antiplatelet agents for 24 h

No volume expanders

Blood pressure monitoring for the first 24 h: every 15 min for 2 h after starting infusion, every 30 min for 6 h, then every hour from the eighth hour until 24 h after t-PA started

Aggressive blood pressure management to maintain BP < 185/110 mmHg

Neurological checks for signs of deterioration at each blood pressure measurement

---

Data from [7].

that for every 100 patients treated with rt-PA, at least 13 more will have no disability or be functionally independent as a result of treatment. Similar findings were also found at 1 year [2]. Although patients with rapidly resolving symptoms or minor stroke symptoms were excluded from entering the study, it is likely that some patients who were having a TIA were enrolled.

There are several questions that arise in the acute setting that are pertinent to thrombolytic therapy in patients who may be having a TIA. What is the likelihood of administering rt-PA to a TIA patient within a population of patients being considered for thrombolysis? What is the risk of using rt-PA in a patient who is having a TIA? Is it possible to determine which patients are going to recover spontaneously, thereby avoiding the risk and expense of using rt-PA?

What is the likelihood of administering rt-PA to a TIA patient when using the NINDS criteria for determining eligibility?

The long-standing definition of TIA requires symptoms to resolve by 24 h [3]. In the NINDS studies, 3% of placebo patients were neurologically normal at 24 h, thereby defining the percentage of TIA patients who meet criteria for administering rt-PA [4]. Because the randomization process for the trials created two closely matched groups of patients, it is likely that 3% of the patients treated with rt-PA were destined to have a spontaneous recovery in the absence of thrombolytic therapy. However, because rt-PA favorably alters the natural history of cerebral ischemia, there were more patients in the rt-PA group (12%) at 24 h who were neurologically normal [4].

Prior studies have shown that the majority of TIAs will resolve within 1 h [3,5,6]. This phenomenon explains why only a small percentage of patients with TIA were enrolled in the NINDS study. In the Cooperative Study of Transient Ischemic Attacks, the median duration of carotid distribution TIAs was 14 min and that of vertebrobasilar TIAs was 8 min [3]. Only 14% of events which lasted more than 1 h eventually qualified as a TIA by resolving completely within 24 h. Hence the vast majority of vascular events lasting more than 1 h will result in deficits which are likely to be permanent. This fact has great importance for decision making with i.v. rt-PA.

The time it takes for stroke symptom recognition, transportation to the ED, rapid assessment of stroke signs in the ED, obtaining a noncontrast computed tomography (CT) scan of the head and applying the criteria for treatment with i.v. rt-PA means that the vast majority of patients will be treated after 60 min from symptom onset. Thus, most patients with TIA are unlikely to be eligible for treatment with i.v. rt-PA. Equally important is the relationship between neurological dysfunction lasting more than 1 h and the high likelihood of a permanent deficit. In order to maximize benefit from i.v. rt-PA, it is critical that patients be rapidly assessed and treated according to accepted guidelines in order to minimize longterm disability from stroke [7–10]. Waiting for symptoms to resolve spontaneously will diminish benefit since time from symptom onset to initiation of rt-PA infusion correlates with benefit from rt-PA [11]. Furthermore, data from the NINDS study and pooled data from the six large clinical trials of i.v. rt-PA show that patients with more severe neurological deficits present earlier in the 6-h time window [12]. These analyses show that the benefit of rt-PA was greater the earlier it was initiated, even though patients who were treated earlier had a greater severity of neurological dysfunction. Thus, the risk of waiting for symptoms to resolve spontaneously will adversely affect a group of patients who have the greatest chance for benefit and the most to gain from treatment with rt-PA.

What is the risk of using rt-PA in a patient who is having a TIA?

Overall, the risk of symptomatic intracerebral hemorrhage (SICH), defined as neurological deterioration within 36 h from symptom onset and a CT showing intracranial blood, was 6.4% in the rt-PA group in the NINDS study [1]. After the FDA approval for stroke, additional studies have shown similar and often lower rates of SICH (see Table 16.3) [13–21].

Table 16.3 Risk of symptomatic intracerebral hemorrhage (ICH) with i.v. recombinant tissue plasminogen activator (rt-PA)

Study	Setting	No. of patients	Symptomatic ICH, %
NINDS (rt-PA arm) [1]	Phase III randomized clinical trial	312	6
Phase IV studies			
Houston [13]	Three hospitals	30	7
Multicenter survey [14]	13 US centres	189	6
OSF network [15]	14 hospitals in Illinois	75	5
Cleveland [16]	29 Cleveland area hospitals	70	16
STIC study [17]	31 hospitals in Minnesota	252	7
Greater Cincinnati [18]	16 hospitals	109	2
Cologne [19]	Single academic referral center	150	4
STARS Study [20]	57 medical centres in the USA	389	3
CASES [21]	68 centres in Canada	450	4
All series		1714	5

Modified with permission, from Warach S. Thrombolysis in stroke beyond three hours: Targeting patients with diffusion and perfusion MRI. *Ann Neurol* 2002; 51: 11–13.

Table 16.4 Relationship between stroke severity and risk of symptomatic intracerebral hemorrhage (SICH) in patients treated with recombinant tissue plasminogen activator (rt-PA) in Part A and Part B of the NINDS rt-PA Stroke Study

Baseline NIHSS Score	*SICH, %*
1–5	2
6–10	3
11–15	5
16–20	4
> 20	17
All patients	6

Data from [22].

Within the NINDS studies, the best predictor of SICH was severity of stroke symptoms as measured by the NIH Stroke Scale (NIHSS) score [22]. Table 16.4 shows the risk of SICH in relation to stroke severity. For patients with the mildest stroke symptoms, the risk of rt-PA is about 2% [22]. Since patients with TIA are unlikely to have significant parenchymal damage, their risk is probably no more than the risk for patients with the mildest deficits enrolled in the NINDS studies. Thus, it is likely that the risk of treating a patient with a TIA is probably no more than 2% and may be as low as the risk of using rt-PA in patients with acute myocardial infarction (1%) [23].

As previously mentioned, about 3% of patients who are eligible for rt-PA are patients with a TIA. Applying this percentage to a population of patients who meet the criteria for treatment with i.v. rt-PA provides an estimate of the adverse impact of SICH related to treating the occasional patient who is having a TIA. For every 1000 patients treated with rt-PA for acute ischemic stroke, there will be 30 who were destined to have spontaneous resolution by 24 h. Causing an SICH in this group of patients is of great concern to the treating physician. Physicians want to minimize the chance of treating a patient with rt-PA who is destined to have a normal recovery without treatment. Combining the likelihood of treating a TIA patient with the risk of SICH, we see that for every 1000 patients treated with rt-PA, about two patients (6% risk of SICH when treating 30 patients with TIA) will have an SICH who would have had a normal recovery without treatment. This represents a liberal estimate, since it is quite likely that the risk of SICH after rt-PA in patients with TIA is closer to the risk of treating patients with the mildest neurological deficits—approximately 2%. Thus, a more likely estimate of risk is that for every 1000 patients treated with rt-PA, one patient who was destined to have a TIA will suffer the consequences of an SICH.

Table 16.5 Comparison of risks and benefits of different stroke therapies

	rt-PA for acute ischemic stroke [1]	CEA for symptomatic ICA stenosis (70–99%) [24]	CEA for asymptomatic ICA stenosis (60–99%) [26]
Risk per 1000 patients treated	60 patients with SICH	60 patients with stroke	20 patients with stroke
Benefit per 1000 patients treated	160 more people with no disability*	170 ipsilateral strokes prevented	60 strokes prevented
Number needed to treat to create one excellent outcome	Six patients	Six patients	17 patients
Frequency and risk of treating patients with TIA Number of TIA patients per 1000 treated with procedure	30	500	NA
Risk of treating patient with TIA	2% (SICH)	6% (stroke or death)	NA
Number of TIA patients who have a serious complication per 1000 treated with the procedure	One (SICH) (2% of 30)	30 (stroke or death) (6% of 500)	NA

*Based on Modified Rankin Scale at 3 months. At 1 year, the number is 130 [2].
rt-PA, Recombinant tissue plasminogen activator; CEA, carotid endarterectomy; SICH, symptomatic intracerebral hemorrhage; TIA, transient ischemic attack.

Is this risk acceptable? Most physicians who treat patients with acute ischemic stroke are nonsurgeons and therefore unaccustomed to performing therapeutic interventions that have immediate but acceptable risk. Reviewing complication rates from other accepted procedures offered to patients with stroke (see Table 16.5) helps put this risk in perspective and will now be discussed.

The North American Symptomatic Carotid Endarterectomy Trial (NASCET) compared carotid endarterectomy (CEA) with aspirin in 659 patients with symptomatic stenosis and established the benefit of CEA in patients with high-grade (70–99%) symptomatic stenosis [24]. At 2 years, the rate of ipsilateral stroke was 9% and 26% in the surgical and medical treatment groups, respectively, yielding a relative benefit of 65% and an absolute benefit of 17% in favor of surgery. This benefit occurred even though there was a surgical complication rate of about 6% (stroke). Thus, 60 strokes per 1000 CEAs performed on symptomatic internal carotid artery stenosis are attributable to the procedure. Of these 60 patients, some were destined to have a stroke even without surgery. To determine this, one can extrapolate the natural history of high-grade symptomatic carotid stenosis from the medical arm of the study. Over 2 years, patients on aspirin alone had an ipsilateral stroke rate of 26%. Thus, about 15 of the 60 patients with perioperative stroke were destined to have a stroke even if they had not had surgery. For every 1000 CEAs performed on symptomatic patients with high-grade stenosis, about 45 people—who would have been alive and without a recurrent stroke if they had not undergone the procedure—will have a stroke related to the CEA. This represents a small group of patients who do not need surgery and are harmed by the treatment. Yet, despite the risk of surgery, it is clear that more patients with symptomatic, high-grade carotid stenosis will benefit from CEA than if treated with aspirin alone. This is because the benefit of reducing the risk of recurrent stroke is much greater than the immediate but acceptable risk of surgery. At the present time, the complication rate from CEA is the best that can be achieved given our current state of technology and understanding about the ability of surgeons to perform this procedure. While we may speculate about how to improve patient selection through advances in imaging or through better surgical or endovascular techniques, the critieria used in NASCET to select patients for CEA remain the method with the most evidence for reducing the impact of recurrent stroke in patients with carotid stenosis despite the risk of the procedure.

In a similar risk analysis, t-PA for acute ischemic stroke is a favorable treatment modality despite an increased risk. As mentioned above, the rate of SICH was 6% in the NINDS rt-PA Stroke Study (see Table 16.3). Thus, for every 1000 patients treated with rt-PA, 60 will have a SICH. However, some of these 60 patients were destined to have a poor outcome if they had not been treated with rt-PA. To determine this, we look at the placebo groups from the NINDS studies and find that about 50% of patients had a poor outcome, defined as severe disability or death [25]. Thus, 30 patients (per 1000 treated with rt-PA) who would have had a functional outcome of moderate disability or better if they had not been treated with rt-PA will have a SICH. If one looks at the subgroup of patients with favorable outcome, there will be 15 patients with SICH (per 1000 treated with rt-PA) who would have had no disability (Modified Rankin score of 0 or 1) if they had not been treated with rt-PA. Yet, despite this risk, a substantial proportion of patients will benefit from rt-PA if they meet the criteria for treatment (see Table 16.1). Obviously, the risk/benefit assessment is similar to the situation noted above with CEA. Although we can speculate about improving the criteria for patient selection through more sophisticated neuroimaging, the criteria used in the NINDS study remain the method of patient selection with the best evidence for reducing the disability caused by acute ischemic stroke.

Another aspect of comparing the risk of CEA with the risk of rt-PA relates to the baseline level of function prior to therapeutic intervention. By definition, patients who are candidates for thrombolytic therapy have a significant neurological deficit in order to meet criteria for enrollment and are at high risk for longterm disablity. On the other hand, patients who are candidates for CEA may be neurologically normal or have a nondisabling deficit but are at high risk of recurrent stroke. Of the patients entered into NASCET, over half had a recent TIA as their reason for enrollment. Thus, many of the perioperative complications from CEA done for symptomatic stenosis are on patients who have no neurological deficit related to their carotid stenosis at baseline.

If we look at CEA for asymptomatic carotid stenosis, the risks appear more acceptable but the absolute benefit is much less [26]. The risk of perioperative stroke in patients with asymptomatic stenosis is about 2%; however, the absolute benefit is only 6%. For every 1000 patients who have CEA for asymptomatic stenosis 60 strokes will be prevented. This compares with 170 strokes prevented per 1000 procedures for patients with high-grade, symptomatic stenosis and 160 patients whose strokes are essentially cured per 1000 treated with rt-PA for acute ischemic stroke (see Table 16.5).

There are limitations to the comparison of rt-PA therapy with CEA. Thrombolysis for acute stroke is a therapeutic procedure for neurologically impaired patients who are at risk of longterm disability. The treatment decreases this burden by increasing the number of patients who are functionally independent without increasing the number who are dependent. CEA is a preventive surgery for patients who are neurologically normal (asymptomatic or recent TIA) or only mildly impaired (nondisabling stroke) and the treatment reduces the risk of recurrent stroke in these patients. Although thrombolysis and CEA are different treatment modalities with different indications and outcome measures, the assessment of risk and benefit is similar.

Is it possible to identify patients with acute stroke symptoms who are going to recover spontaneously, thereby avoiding the risk and expense of using rt-PA?

Advances in neuroimaging (see p. 359) have shown tremendous promise in depicting ischemic brain tissue that is at risk of infarction. However, the ability of these techniques to identify accurately patients who are going to recover spontaneously is not yet established. A simpler technique involves application of two of the exclusion criteria from the NINDS studies—the presence of minor stroke symptoms and rapid improvement in stroke symptoms (see Table 16.1). Although these criteria help diminish the chance of treating a patient who is going to recover spontaneously, several caveats are worth noting. In the NINDS studies, patients had to have a measureable deficit on the NIHSS and meet the criteria in Table 16.1 in order to be enrolled into the study; however, there were no absolute

NIHSS score criteria for entry. This is important to note, since a significant shortcoming of the NIHSS is that patients with identical scores may have varying degrees of stroke severity. For example, on the NIHSS scale, severe aphasia is counted as 2 points, which is the same score given to a patient with drift and mild ataxia in one limb [27]. Yet most clinicians and patients would consider severe aphasia to be more disabling. By weighting these symptoms equally, the NIHSS score gives a skewed impression of the severity of stroke for patients with low NIHSS scores. Rather than an absolute cut-off for the use of the NIHSS to determine eligibility for rt-PA, guidelines for the definition of minor stroke symptoms include the following examples: pure sensory symptoms, isolated dysarthria, isolated facial weakness or isolated ataxia [4]. Although excluding patients with minor stroke symptoms or rapid improvement will minimize the chance of treating a patient who does not need rt-PA, overuse of these two exclusions can deprive patients of the chance of avoiding longterm disability.

In a recent study, data were collected on a series of patients with acute ischemic stroke who presented within 3 h and were excluded from rt-PA therapy [28]. For 31% of the cohort, rt-PA was withheld because the stroke symptoms were considered too mild or were rapidly improving. According to the authors, 'a recurring reason was the improvement of motor symptoms, but resolution was not as complete as the treating physician had hoped, leaving the patient either profoundly dysphasic or with disabling neglect and/or inattention'. [28] A third of the patients excluded due to mild stroke symptoms or rapid improvement were dependent or dead by the time of discharge (defined as Modified Rankin score > 2). If they had been treated with i.v. rt-PA it is quite possible that many would be alive and independent. While indiscriminate use of rt-PA is certainly not recommended, fear of SICH may create an over-application of these two exclusion criteria. The risk of SICH from i.v. rt-PA in patients who are improving or have mild stroke symptoms is probably between 1 and 2%. Based on the data from Barber *et al.* [28], the risk of not treating may be much greater. Obviously, there needs to be careful consideration of the significance of the neurological deficit and the temporal pattern of spontaneous improvement in order to avoid excluding patients who will benefit from thrombolysis.

Thrombolysis in mild stroke

Does rt-PA improve the outcome of patients with mild neurological deficits?

The NINDS rt-PA Stroke Study Group published an analysis of factors that might affect the response to rt-PA and found no variable or combination of variables that identified patients who were unlikely to respond

[29]. Although the NINDS rt-PA trials were not designed to have enough statistical power to answer questions about subgroups, the data show that all patient subgroups appear to benefit.

An analysis of the effect of rt-PA in patients with mild neurological deficits enrolled in the NINDS studies was recently completed (NINDS rt-PA Stroke Study Group, unpublished data). Since there is no established definition of mild stroke in the literature, several definitions were determined prior to performing the exploratory analysis (see Table 16.6) and were based on factors readily available to the clinician making a decision about t-PA, namely clinical presentation, CT results, and presumed stroke subtype. Each of these definitions of mild stroke showed benefit for rt-PA over placebo (odds ratio = 2.0, $P < 0.001$).

Overall, baseline NIHSS scores ranged from 1 to 37, with a median of 14 [1]. A score of ≤ 9 marked the least severe quartile of patients (definition 1). The 3-month outcome for patients in this subgroup showed that 73% of rt-PA-treated patients vs. 56% of placebo-treated patients had no disability at 3 months. A second analysis (definition 2) also showed benefit for rt-PA in patients with NIHSS scores of ≤ 9 after omitting patients who had symptoms of more severe stroke such as impaired consciousness, aphasia or neglect. The third definition of mild stroke took into consideration the prognosis for patients with clinical characteristics of subcortical ischemia by excluding patients with evidence of cortical deficits which may be a marker of more severe stroke. This definition identified about two-thirds of the patients enrolled into the two trials and showed benefit of rt-PA.

Table 16.6 also shows the percentage of patients with mild stroke symptoms at the time of study entry who had an undesirable outcome at 90 days defined as moderate disability or worse. In all three of the definitions of mild stroke, patients were less likely to have an undesirable outcome. This is a relevant observation since physicians are reluctant to use rt-PA in patients with mild symptoms for fear of inducing a bad outcome in a patient who has a good natural history without treatment. These data show that patients with mild stroke symptoms not only are more likely to have a favorable outcome with rt-PA but are also less likely to have an undesirable outcome. This beneficial effect is despite an increased risk of SICH.

What is the risk of using rt-PA in patients with mild stroke symptoms?

The risks of SICH in mild stroke are listed in Table 16.6. The risk of rt-PA ranges from 2 to 3% and is at least half the risk of rt-PA for all patients enrolled. Thus, despite the small risk of rt-PA, more patients with mild stroke symptoms will benefit when treated with rt-PA according to accepted selection criteria and management guidelines. Deviating from these guidelines may increase the risk of SICH [14,16].

Table 16.6 Mild stroke in the NINDS rt-PA Stroke Trials (Parts 1 and 2 combined)*

| | | Outcome at 90 days (%) | | | |
| | | Favorable outcome: no disability | Moderate disability or worse | | |
Mild stroke† Definition	Treatment group (n)	MRS‡ ≤ 1	MRS‡ ≥ 3	Mortality at 90 days (%)	SICH§ (%)
1	Placebo (78)	56	26	5	0
	t-PA (99)	73	18	1	3
2	Placebo (70)	57	26	6	0
	t-PA (91)	73	18	0	2
3	Placebo (201)	34	53	15	0
	t-PA (206)	53	39	8	2

*Unpublished data. Obtained with permission from the National Institutes of Neurological Disorders and Stroke (NINDS) rt-PA Stroke Study Group.

†Mild stroke definitions:

Definition 1: All patients with the lowest National Institutes of Health Stroke Scale (NIHSS) score severity quartile (NIHSS score ≤ 9). This definition analyzes the group of patients with the lowest quartiles of NIHSS scores independent of the spheres of neurological deficit involved.

Definition 2: All patients with NIHSS score = 9 (least severe quartile of stroke severity), deleting all those with aphasia, extinction/neglect, or impaired consciousness. This definition takes the least severe quartile of patients and further eliminates those with selected items that are generally not involved with mild infarcts.

Definition 3: All patients with only motor deficits (can include dysarthria and/or ataxia) with or without sensory deficits. These patients can only have a combination of motor, coordination, and sensory deficits without any deficits in the spheres of language, level of consciousness, extinction/neglect, horizontal eye movements, or visual fields. The approach was an attempt to capture those patients with primarily subcortical ischemic events.

‡MRS, Modified Rankin Scale.
MRS = 0: No symptoms at all.
MRS = 1: No significant disability despite symptoms.
MRS = 2: Slight disability. Unable to carry out all previous activities but able to look after own affairs without assistance.
MRS = 3: Moderate disability. Requiring some help but able to walk without assistance.
MRS = 4: Moderately severe disability. Unable to walk without assistance.
MRS = 5: Severe disability. Bedridden, constant care.
MRS = 6: Death.
§SICH, Symptomatic intracerebral hemorrhage. Defined as neurological deterioration within 36 h of treatment with a computed tomography showing intracranial blood [1].

It is important to note that the overall benefit found in the NINDS studies was not due soley to the effect on patients with mild deficits. It has been suggested that the benefit of rt-PA is primarily for patients with syndromes of middle cerebral artery branch occlusion [30]. Although no data from the NINDS rt-PA Stroke Study Group have been published to support this conclusion, there are data showing that no particular subgroup is more or less likely to benefit from rt-PA [29]. For example, if the data are analyzed after excluding patients with mild deficit (NIHSS score ≤ 9, definition 1), the benefit of rt-PA in patients with more severe stroke remains. For those with an NIHSS score of > 9, 29% of the rt-PA-treated patients vs. 17% of the placebo-treated patients had no disability at 3 months [29]. Thus, there is a 70% greater likelihood of a having no disability at 3 months when rt-PA is given to patients with moderate to severe stroke symptoms (NIHSS > 9). This benefit is despite an increased risk of SICH in patients with more severe symptoms (see Table 16.4).

Although the longterm prognosis in patients with small-vessel stroke is better than in those with large-vessel strokes, the outcome of patients with lacunar stroke in the NINDS studies showed that about half of patients in the placebo group had some degree of disability at 3 months [1]. Thus, although the definition of mild stroke will include some patients with lacunar syndromes, many patients with lacunar stroke do not have a favorable outcome. Patients with small-vessel stroke who were treated with rt-PA were more likely to achieve a favorable outcome compared with placebo-treated patients with the same stroke subtype. As published in the original paper, 63% of patients with the small-vessel subtype treated with rt-PA vs. 40% of those treated with placebo had no disability at 90 days. However, it should be noted that only 81 patients were classified as small-vessel occlusive stroke. Although the numbers are small, the relative and absolute benefit is similar to that seen with the definitions of mild stroke in Table 16.6.

Advances in non-invasive neurovascular imaging in acute stroke

Can neuroimaging reliably identify patients who will recover spontaneously?

Non-invasive neurovascular imaging can provide information about regional perfusion, arterial patency and evidence of ischemic injury (see Table 16.7). In theory, certain patterns may identify patients who are likely to recover spontaneously [31–34]. For example, the presence of patent arteries in the absence of a perfusion deficit might obviate the need for thrombolytic therapy. However, this is a pattern that could be seen

Table 16.7 Non-invasive neurovascular imaging for acute ischemic stroke

---

Computed tomography (CT)
Noncontrast CT [35]
CT angiography [36]
CT perfusion [37]
Xenon CT [38]

Magnetic resonance imaging (MRI) [31–34]
T1, T2, FLAIR sequences
Diffusion weighted imaging
Perfusion weighted imaging
MR spectroscopy
MR angiography

Ultrasound
Carotid Doppler
Transcranial Doppler [39]

Single-photon emission computed tomography (SPECT) [40]

---

with small-vessel ischemia and i.v. rt-PA appears beneficial for these patients (see discussion above).

The ideal imaging modality to identify patients with acute stroke symptoms who are destined to have a full recovery does not yet exist. However, in the near future, advances in neurovascular imaging may give clinicians a higher level of confidence about predicting outcome and provide appropriate refinement of clinical decision making regarding reperfusion therapy [34]. At the present time, noncontrast CT remains the imaging modality of choice. It provides a rapid and sensitive assessment of the presence of hemorrhage and may show signs of early ischemia. Although subtle early ischemic changes do not appear to alter the potential benefit or risk of using rt-PA in the first 3 h, the presence of obvious subacute low attenuation on CT representing early ischemic changes should prompt the clinician to re-assess the time of symptom onset, as it usually takes more than 1 or 2 h to detect obvious hypodensity [35].

Multimodal magnetic resonance imaging (MRI), which includes diffusion weighted imaging (DWI), perfusion imaging, and high speed MRA, provides additional information in the setting of acute stroke [31–34]. Because imaging patients by MRI can prolong the door to needle time for thrombolysis and potentially limit benefit, special considerations must be made to assure rapid imaging. Also, the sensitivity of MRI for detecting intracranial hemorrhage remains a matter of controversy [33]. In select cases, particularly those with diagnostic uncertainty, MRI can help affirm the clinical impression of acute ischemic stroke. DWI is able to depict early ischemic changes, even before detection on T2-weighted MRI sequences. Likewise, for patients who have large-vessel occlusive disease, perfusion MRI can show tissue at risk of infarction. Although initial reports suggested that the hyperintensity on DWI with corresponding darkness of ADC mapping represented irreversibly ischemic tissue, subsequent studies of multimodal MRI performed before and after thrombolysis have shown that the ischemic zone detected by DWI can disapear with reperfusion therapy [41]. Thus, relying on MRI to identify irreversibly ischemic tissue appears inadequate at this time. However, recent work suggests certain patterns that may predict a lack of response to rt-PA [42]. Conversely, areas of reduced flow on perfusion imaging that are not hyperintense on DWI may identify reversible tissue at risk and may represent a group of patients who are most likely to benefit from reperfusion therapy [42]. Although tailoring reperfusion therapy based on imaging may allow for individualized approaches to intervention and extend the therapeutic window for thrombolysis, such theories need to be tested in carefully designed clinical trials [43].

Conclusions and recommendations

Physicians who treat patients with thrombolytic therapy for acute ischemic stroke should be aware of the risks and benefits of therapy. Hospitals and physicians that provide thrombolytic therapy should follow national guidelines to enhance the quality of care provided [7–10,44]. Although patients with TIA will occasionally be treated with rt-PA, the risk associated with therapy is far outweighed by the overall benefit. Patients with mild stroke symptoms have a reasonable chance for benefit and a low risk from i.v. rt-PA when eligibility criteria are met and guidelines for management followed.

References

1 The National Institute of Neurological Disorders and Stroke rt-PA Stroke Study Group. Tissue plasminogen activator for acute ischemic stroke. *N Engl J Med* 1995; 333: 1581–7.

2 Kwiatkowski TG, Libman R, Frankel MR *et al.*, the NINDS t-PA Stroke Study Group. The NINDS rt-PA stroke study: The effects of t-PA for acute ischemic stroke at one year. *N Engl J Med* 1999; 340: 1781–7.

3 Dyken ML, Conneally M, Haerer AF *et al.* Cooperative study of hospital frequency and character of transient ischemic attacks, I. background, organization and clinical survery. *JAMA* 1977; 237: 882–6.

4 Lyden P, Lu M, Kwiatkowski T *et al.* and the NINDS rt-PA Stroke Study Group. Thrombolysis in patients with transient neurologic deficits. *Neurology* 2001; 57: 2125–8.

5 Werdlin L, Juhler M. The course of transient ischemic attacks. *Neurology* 1988; 38: 677–80.

6 The Study Group on TIA Criteria and Detection. XI. Transient focal cerebral ischemia: epidemiological and clinical aspects. *Stroke* 1974; 5: 277–84.

7 NINDS Proceedings of a National Symposium on Rapid Identification and Treatment of Acute Stroke. December 1996 Website address: http://www.ninds.nih.gov/health_and_medical/pubs/strokeworkshop.htm

8 A Special Writing Group of the Stroke Council, American Heart Association. Guidelines for thrombolytic therapy for acute stroke. A supplement to the guidelines for the management of patients with acute ischemic stroke. *Stroke* 1996; 94: 1167–74.

9 Quality Standards Subcommittee of the American Academy of Neurology. Practice advisory: Thrombolytic therapy for acute ischemic stroke: Summary statement. *Neurology* 1996; 47: 835–9.

10 Albers GW, Amerenco P, Easton JD *et al.* Antithrombotic therapy for ischemic stroke. *Chest* 2001; 119: 300S–320S.

11 Marler JR, Tilley BC, Lu M *et al.* for the NINDS rt-PA Stroke Study Group. Early stroke treatment associated with better outcome. The NINDS rt-PA Stroke Study. *Neurology* 2000; 55: 1649–55.

12 Brott T. Better outcome with early stroke treatment. A pooled analysis of ATLANTIS, ECASS, and NINDS rt-PA Stroke Trials. Presented at the 27th International Stroke Meeting, San Antonio, TX, February 2002.

13 Chiu D, Krieger D, Villar-Cordova C *et al.* Intravenous tissue plasminogen activator for acute ischemic stroke: feasibility, safety, and efficacy in the first year of clinical practice. *Stroke* 1998; 29: 18–22.

14 Tanne D, Bates VE, Verro P *et al.* Initial clinical experience with IV tissue plasminogen activator for acute ischemic stroke: a multicenter survey. The t-PA Stroke Survey Group. *Neurology* 1999; 53: 424–7.

15 Wang DZ, Rose JA, Honings DS *et al.* Treating acute stroke patients with intravenous tPA. The OSF stroke network experience. *Stroke* 2000; 31: 77–81.

16 Katzan IL, Furlan AJ, Lloyd LE *et al.* Use of tissue-type plasminogen activator for acute ischemic stroke: the Cleveland area experience. *JAMA* 2000; 283: 1151–8.

17 Hanson SK, Brauer DJ, Brown RD *et al.* Should use of t-PA for ischemic stroke be restricted to specialized stroke centers. *Stroke* 2000; 31: 313 [Abstract].

18 Kanter D, Kothari R, Pancioli A *et al.* The greater Cincinnati t-PA experience after the NINDS trial: does a longer time to treatment within the current three-hour window reduce efficacy? *Stroke* 1999; 30: 244 [Abstract].

19 Schmulling S, Grond M, Rudolf J *et al.* One-year follow-up in acute stroke patients treated with rtPA in clinical routine. *Stroke* 2000; 31: 1552–4.

20 Albers GW, Bates VE, Clark WM *et al.* Intravenous tissue-type plasminogen activator for treatment of acute stroke: the Standard Treatment with Alteplase to Reverse Stroke (STARS) study. *JAMA* 2000; 283: 1145–50.

21 Hill MD, Woolfendeu A, Teal PA *et al.* Intravenous Alteplase for stroke: the Canadian experience. *The Stroke Interventionalist* 2000; 2: 3–8.

22 The NINDS rt-PA Stroke Study Group. Intracerebral hemorrhage after intra-venous t-PA therapy for ischemic stroke. *Stroke* 1997; 28: 2109–18.

23 Fibrinolytic Therapy Trialists' (FTT) Collaborative Group. Indications for fibrinolytic therapy in suspected acute myocardial infarction: collaborative overview of early mortality and major morbidity results from all randomised trials of more than 1000 patients. *Lancet* 1994; 343: 311–22.

24 North American Symptomatic Carotid Endarterectomy Trial Collaborators. Beneficial effect of carotid endarterectomy in symptomatic patients with high-grade stenosis. *N Engl J Med* 1991; 325: 445–53.

25 Frankel MR, Morgenstern LB, Kwiatkowski T *et al.* Predicting prognosis after stroke, a placebo group analysis from the National Institute of Neurological Disorders and Stroke rt-PA Stroke Trial. *Neurology* 2000; 55: 952–9.

26 Executive Committee for the Asymptomatic Carotid Atherosclerosis Study. Endarterectomy for asymptomatic carotid artery stenosis. *JAMA* 1995; 273: 1421–8.

27 Lyden P, Brott T, Tilley B *et al.* Improved reliability of the NIH Stroke Scale using video training. *Stroke* 1994; 25: 2220–6.

28 Barber PA, Zhang J, Demchuk AM *et al.* Why are stroke patients excluded from t-PA therapy? An analysis of patient eligibility. *Neurology* 2001; 56: 1015–20.

29 The NINDS rt-PA Stroke Study Group. Generalized efficacy of tPA for acute stroke: subgroup analysis of the NINDS t-PA Stroke Trial. *Stroke* 1997; 28: 2119–25.

30 Caplan LR, Mohr JP, Kistler JP *et al.* Should thrombolytic therapy be the first-line treatment for acute ischemic stroke? *N Engl J Med* 1997; 337: 1309–10.

31 Fisher M, Albers GW. Applications of diffusion-perfusion magnetic resonance imaging in acute ischemic stroke. *Neurology* 1999; 52: 1750–6.

32 Sunshine JL, Tarr RW, Lanzieri CF *et al.* Hyperacute stroke: ultrafast MR imaging to triage patients prior to therapy. *Radiology* 1999; 212: 325–32.

33 Schellinger PD, Jansen O, Fiebach JB *et al.* Monitoring intravenous recom-binant tissue plasminogen activator thrombolysis for acute ischemic stroke with diffusion and perfusion MRI. *Stroke* 2000; 31: 1318–28.

34 Albers GW. Expanding the window for thrombolytic therapy in acute stroke. The potential role of acute MRI for patient selection. *Stroke* 1999; 30: 2230–7.

35 Patel SC, Levine SR, Tilley BC *et al.* for the National Institute of Neurological Disorders and Stroke rt-PA Stroke Study Group. Lack of clinical significance of early ischemic changes on computed tomography in acute stroke. *JAMA* 2001; 22: 286.

36 Wildermuth S, Knauth M, Brandt T *et al.* Role of CT angiography in patient selection for thrombolytic therapy in acute hemispheric stroke. *Stroke* 1998; 29: 935–8.

37 Klotz E, Konig M. Perfusion measurements of the brain: using dynamic CT for the quantitative assessment of cerebral ischemic in acute stroke. *Eur J Radiol* 1999; 30: 170–84.

38 Kaufmann AM, Firlik AD, Fukui MB *et al.* Ischemic core and penumbra in human stroke. *Stroke* 1999; 30: 93–9.

39 Christou I, Alexandrov A, Burgin WS *et al.* Timing of recanalization after tissue plasminogen activator therapy determined by transcranial doppler correlates with clinical recovery from ischemic stroke. *Stroke* 2000; 31: 1812–6.

40 Alexandrov A, Masdeu JC, Devous MD *et al.* Brain Single-Photon Emission CT With HMPAO and Safety of Thrombolytic Therapy in Acute Ischemic Stroke. Proceedings of the Meeting of the SPECT Safe Thrombolysis Study Collaborators and the Members of the Brain Imaging Council of the Society of Nuclear Medicine. *Stroke* 1997; 28: 1830–4.

41 Moseley M. Pathophysiologic basis of diffusion and perfusion-weighted imaging. In: 25th International Stroke Conference, New Orleans, LA; February 10–12, 2000.

42 Parsons MW, Barber PA, Chalk J *et al.* Diffusion and perfusion weighted MRI response to thrombolysis in stroke. *Ann Neurol* 2002; 51: 28–37.

43 Warach S. Thrombolysis in stroke beyond three hours. Targeting patients with diffusion and perfusion MRI. *Ann Neurol* 2002; 51: 11–3.

44 Alberts M. Recommendations for the establishment of primary stroke centers. *JAMA* 2000; 283: 3102.

45 Tanne D, Demchuk AM, Kasner SE. Intravenous thrombolysis in acute ischemic stroke: The Phase IV data. *Sem Cerebrovasc Dis* 2001; 1: 130–40.

PART IV

Surgical and Interventional Treatments and Cost-Effectiveness

CHAPTER 17

Surgery for Stroke Prevention

Larry B. Goldstein

Although risk factor modification is widely applicable to patients with transient ischemic attack (TIA) and medical interventions can reduce the likelihood of subsequent stroke in diverse populations, only highly selected patients benefit from surgery. The assessment of an individual patient's potential benefit and risk associated with a surgical procedure intended to prevent stroke can be challenging, but is critical for rational decision making. The primary surgical procedures considered for patients with symptomatic cerebrovascular disease include carotid endarterectomy (CEA), extracranial–intracranial bypass, and procedures for the so-called moyamoya syndrome.

Carotid endarterectomy

CEA is the most commonly employed surgical intervention for patients at risk of hemispheric ischemic stroke. Although often performed as a prophylactic procedure in asymptomatic patients with stenosis of a cervical carotid artery, the present discussion focuses on patients with symptoms (either TIA or nondisabling ischemic stroke) referable to an ipsilateral high-grade extracranial carotid artery stenosis. The efficacy of carotid endarterectomy in these types of patients has been established based on the results of prospective randomized clinical trials. Despite the availability of data from these clinical trials, surgical decisions can be ambiguous because many patients do not precisely meet the criteria used in the controlled studies and because some information required for individual risk–benefit analyses, particularly assessment of perioperative surgical risk, can be either lacking or subjective.

Extracranial carotid artery stenosis is most commonly the result of atherosclerosis. Other conditions that may cause narrowing in these vessels include spontaneous or traumatic arterial dissection, fibromuscular dysplasia, and inflammatory conditions. Endarterectomy has not been studied in controlled trials for these other types of conditions. The commonest symptoms of carotid artery disease are related to distal ischemia as discussed elsewhere in this volume.

There have now been five randomized controlled trials of CEA for patients with symptomatic extracranial carotid artery stenosis [1–5]. The first, the Joint Study of Extracranial Arterial Disease, was published more than three decades ago [1]. The surgical techniques and medical therapies employed in this study are not comparable to those used in the more recent trials. In addition, the study included a high proportion of patients with vertebrobasilar rather than carotid artery distribution symptoms. A second early trial was halted prematurely because of high perioperative morbidity in the surgical group [2].

The three remaining studies, the North American Symptomatic Carotid Endarterectomy Trial (NASCET) [3,6], the European Carotid Surgery Trial (ECST) [4], and the VA Cooperative Symptomatic Carotid Stenosis Trial (VACS) [5] had many similarities, but also differed in several ways. The qualifying symptom(s) (ipsilateral hemispheric TIA, nondisabling stroke or amaurosis fugax) had to occur within 120 days for NASCET and the VACS, but could have occurred up to 6 months earlier in patients randomized in ECST. The VACS was restricted to males. Initially, patients needed to be < 80 years of age for NASCET (this age limit was removed for the latter part of the trial), but there were no age restrictions for inclusion in the other studies. Patients with uncontrolled diabetes or hypertension, unstable angina, a myocardial infarction within 6 months, progressing stroke, contralateral CEA within 4 months or major surgery within 30 days were temporarily excluded from NASCET, but could later be included if the qualifying symptoms occurred within 120 days of surgery. Those with atrial fibrillation were also excluded because a high frequency of cardio-embolic stroke would confound outcome analyses. Reasons for medical exclusion from ECST included uncontrolled diabetes or hypertension, renal failure, chronic obstructive pulmonary disease, emergent medical conditions, and patients deemed unreliable or those requiring concomitant use of oral anticoagulants.

The degree of carotid artery stenosis was determined based on catheter angiography. However, the methods and criteria used to measure the stenosis also varied among the studies [7–11]. Similar methods were used in NASCET and VACS which calculated the percent stenosis of the carotid artery by dividing the residual lumen diameter by the luminal diameter of the distal portion of the same vessel in an area where the vessel walls were parallel. In contrast, ECST measured percent stenosis by dividing the residual lumen diameter by the estimated normal diameter of the artery at that level. Because of this difference in methodology, 48% of patients classified as having > 70% stenosis by ECST criteria would be reclassified as having a more moderate stenosis using NASCET criteria [7,8].

All patients, regardless of whether randomized to surgery or no surgery, received best medical therapy. However, all patients enrolled in NASCET were recommended to receive 1300 mg of aspirin daily whereas those in the VACS were given 325 mg daily. The use of aspirin was not required for patients in the ECST.

Because surgical benefit is highly dependent on risk, NASCET required that individual centers provide evidence that the operation could be performed with acceptable morbidity and mortality. To participate in NASCET, surgeons had to demonstrate a 30-day perioperative stroke and death rate of < 6% for the last 50 CEAs performed within the prior 24 months [12]. The VACS set out criteria for both centers and individual surgeons. Centers were required to have performed 25 or more of the operations annually in the 3 years prior to the study with perioperative morbidity and mortality rates of < 6%; individual surgeons had to perform more than 10 endarterectomies annually within the same criteria [5]. The ECST did not require demonstration of an explicit level of either center or surgeon competence.

The studies also differed in specified primary outcome measures. Stroke or death were primary outcomes for NASCET. For ECST primary outcomes were disabling stroke, fatal stroke, or perioperative death (nondisabling stroke lasting more than 7 days was a secondary outcome measure). Primary outcomes for VACS were stroke, death, or crescendo TIA.

Despite these methodological differences, NASCET [3,12], ECST [4,8], and VACS [5] each show that, when performed with acceptable rates of morbidity and mortality, CEA improves outcomes in selected patients with 70–99% stenosis as defined using the criteria as described for NASCET. Thus, it is important to use this method of measurement when applying the results of these trials. When the data from the three studies were combined in a meta-analysis [13], there was a significant decrease in the estimate of the frequency of stroke or death in the surgically treated patients with a combined risk ratio estimate = 0.67 [95% confidence interval (CI) 0.54, 0.82]. For NASCET and ECST, there was a significant overall benefit of surgery compared with no surgery therapy for these combined endpoints. For the VACS, the overall difference between medical and surgical therapy was not significant; however, the study had limited power.

The reviewed results apply to patients with high-grade (70–99%) symptomatic carotid artery stenosis. The initial report of ECST found no benefit of endarterectomy in patients with < 30% stenosis of the ipsilateral carotid artery [4]. ECST subsequently provided results for patients with moderate stenosis with a mean 6 years of follow-up [14,15]. The study found that although patients might derive some benefit from surgery over the very long term, there was no benefit over a period of 4–5 years in patients with 50–69% stenosis, nor over 6–7 years in patients 30–49% stenosis. Table 17.1 groups ECST results with the approximate corresponding NASCET

Table 17.1 Efficacy of carotid endarterectomy for moderate grade stenosis—ECST

ECST Stenosis Approximate NASCET stenosis	60–69% 30–49%		70–89% 50–69%		90–99% 70–99%	
	CEA	Cont	CEA	Cont	CEA	Cont
N	232	137	482	329	104	60
Major stroke, death, %	35.3	35.0	38.8	42.6	37.5	51.7
Crude annual rate, %	5.9	5.8	6.5	7.1	6.3	8.6
NNT (6 year)	–		26		7	

Data from [15].

Table 17.2 Efficacy of carotid endarterectomy for moderate grade stenosis—NASCET

NASCET stenosis	30–49%		50–69%		70–99%	
	CEA	Cont	CEA	Cont	CEA	Cont
N	678	690	430	428	325	331
Ipsilateral stroke, %	14.9	18.7	15.7	22.2	13.0	26.0
Crude annual rate, %	3.0	3.7	3.1	4.4	2.6	5.2
P	0.16		0.05		< 0.001	
NNT (5 year)	26		15		8	

Reproduced with permission, from Goldstein LB. Extracranial carotid artery stenosis. *Stroke* 2003; 34: 2767–73.

stenosis for the outcome of major stroke or death. Table 17.2 summarizes the overall results of NASCET by degree of stenosis for the outcome of any ipsilateral stroke [6]. Based on these data, there is a mild benefit in favor of CEA for patients with moderate-grade stenosis (50–69% based on degree of stenosis as measured in NASCET).

After the completion of these three studies, Rothwell and colleagues remeasured the angiograms from ECST for uniformity with the other two trials. The data were then pooled for these 6092 patients with 35 000 patient-years of follow-up [16]. This analysis found that CEA was highly beneficial for patients with > 70% stenosis without near-occlusion (16.0% absolute risk reduction at 5 years). For patients with 50–69% stenosis, the absolute risk reduction was < 1% per year (4.6% at 5 years), which many vascular neurologists would consider clinically not meaningful. CEA was not beneficial for patients with < 50% stenosis. In patients with near-occlusion, in which the vessel distal to the stenosis is collapsed, there was not a benefit at 5 years.

Table 17.3 Efficacy of carotid endarterectomy for moderate grade stenosis—NASCET

| | Post hoc *subgroup analysis* | | | | | |
	Medical	*Surgical*	*RR*	*RRR*	*NNT*	*P*
Men	24.8%	16.7%	8.1%	33%	12	0.04
Women	15.1%	13.8%	1.3%	9%	77	0.94
Diabetics	34.6%	26.7%	7.9%	23%	13	0.51
Nondiabetics	19.2%	12.4%	6.8%	35%	15	0.04
Stroke	9.7%	2.2%	7.5%	77%	13	0.01
TIA	5.1%	3.4%	1.7%	33%	59	0.91

Reproduced with permission, from Goldstein LB. Extracranial carotid artery stenosis. *Stroke* 2003; 34: 2767–73.

Gender-based differences in efficacy?

The NASCET investigators point out that the mild benefit of endarterectomy for patients with 50–69% symptomatic stenosis is not uniform. As shown in Table 17.3, men, those without diabetes and those with mild stroke benefited whereas women, diabetics and those with TIA did not. The lack of benefit in women with 50–69% stenosis may have occurred because of their low stroke risk (15% for women vs. 25% for men after 5 years). This difference in benefit between men and women is not present for patients with symptomatic high-grade stenosis. The meta-analysis previously reviewed also compared outcome rates for endarterectomy among patients with 70–99% stenosis based on sex for patients enrolled in NASCET and the ECST (total of 1006 men and 441 women) [13]. There were no significant sex-based differences in individual event rates between the trials and no differences between men and women when the rates were combined.

Subgroup analyses

Despite these data, surgical decisions often remain ambiguous because many patients do not precisely meet the criteria used in the trials and some information required for individual cost–benefit analyses are lacking or subjective. There have been a plethora of secondary publications based largely on *post hoc* analyses of the primary trial data. It must be recognized that clinical decisions based of these secondary analyses are tenuous (i.e. they essentially represent Level III–V data) [17]. Yet these data do have implications for the application of the primary trial results (efficacy) to daily clinical practice (effectiveness). Details of these studies undoubtedly influence how the procedures are used in clinical practice [18].

Although already candidates for endarterectomy, in *post hoc* analyses the NASCET investigators found that patients with ulcerative plaque in addition to high-grade stenosis were at particularly high stroke risk [19]. In addition, patients having hemispheric TIA may be at greater stroke risk compared with those having amaurosis fugax [20]. The 2-year risk of ipsilateral stroke in patients with retinal vs. hemispheric TIA were as follows in NASCET: 75% stenosis, 11.2% vs. 37.4%; 85% stenosis, 17.8% vs. 60.0%; 95% stenosis, 28.9% vs. 96.3%. Although the risk of ipsilateral stroke remains elevated in patients presenting with amaurosis fugax, the risk appears higher in those presenting with hemispheric TIA and similar degrees of carotid stenosis. In contrast, the presence of angiographically defined collaterals is associated with a lower risk of stroke and TIA, both perioperatively and over the long term [21].

Approximately 40% of NASCET patients had so-called 'lacunar' syndromes. Although traditionally thought to be due to intracranial 'small-vessel' disease, this syndrome may have a variety of causes [22], and those with ipsilateral high-grade carotid artery stenosis are considered candidates for the operation. NASCET investigators subsequently compared the benefit of endarterectomy in patients with 50–99% stenosis among those with nonlacunar and lacunar syndromes [23]. The rate of ipsilateral stroke was reduced with CEA from 25% to 10% (66% risk reduction, $P = 0.002$) in those with nonlacunar syndromes vs. a reduction from 16% to 8% (53% risk reduction, $P = 0.22$) in those with possible lacunar syndromes vs. a reduction from 26% to 17% (35% risk reduction, $P = 0.53$) in those with probable lacunar syndromes. Because of sample size limitations and because this represents a *post hoc* analysis, patients with lacunar syndromes need to be investigated for ipsilateral carotid stenosis if they are otherwise surgical candidates. However, the benefit of endarterectomy in these patients may be relatively less as compared to those with nonlacunar syndromes.

The value of CEA in individuals with high-grade tandem lesions (e.g. high-grade ipsilateral intracranial atherosclerotic disease) is considered minimal, and these patients were excluded from NASCET. Intracranial atherosclerotic disease was detected on angiography in one-third of patients in NASCET with the infraclinoid portion of the vessel affected seven times more frequently than the supraclinoid portion or the proximal anterior or middle cerebral arteries [24]. Table 17.4 gives the 3-year risk of ipsilateral stroke and numbers needed to treat to prevent one stroke in patients with or without mild to moderate intracranial atherosclerotic disease. Based on this *post hoc* analysis, the presence of nonhigh-grade intracranial atherosclerosis appears to increase further the risk of stroke in patients with ipsilateral carotid artery stenosis. The numbers needed to treat appear to decrease with increasing degrees of extracranial stenosis and with the presence of ipsilateral intracranial disease, suggesting that CEA is of benefit even in the setting of a noncritical intracranial tandem lesion.

Table 17.4 Endarterectomy vs. medical therapy based on presence of ipsilateral intracranial atherosclerotic disease—NASCET [24]

	Medical RxCEA		*NNT*			
Intracranial atherosclerotic disease	−	+	−	+	−	+
ICA stenosis						
50–69%	14.7%	19.4%	10.5%	11.8%	26	12
70–84%	23.5%	28.8%	10.1%	6.1%	7	5
85–99%	25.3%	45.7%	10.0%	8.6%	6	3

Three-year risk of ipsilateral stroke.
Reproduced with permission, from Goldstein LB. Extracranial carotid artery stenosis. *Stroke* 2003; 34: 2767–73.

Of the 2885 NASCET patients, 3.1% had an unruptured intracranial aneurysm [25]. One of the 25 patients having endarterectomy ipsilateral to the unruptured aneurysm had a subsequent subarachnoid hemorrhage 6 days later and died. However, the site of bleeding was not identified at post mortem evaluation despite the presence of two small ipsilateral aneurysms. None of the 23 patients with an unruptured small aneurysm ipsilateral to carotid stenosis who were treated medically had a subarachnoid hemorrhage. Although the numbers are quite small, it was concluded that the decision regarding endarterectomy should generally not be influenced by the presence of a small unruptured aneurysm in patients with symptomatic carotid artery stenosis.

There are several issues to consider when contemplating CEA in the elderly. Initially, NASCET (but not ECST or VACS) was limited to patients under 80 years of age [3]. The patients enrolled in NASCET and the VACS had a median or mean age of about 65 years [3,5]; those in the ECST were 'aged about 60' [4]. Patients randomized in the VA asymptomatic study had a mean age of 64–65 years [26]. Therefore, data from randomized controlled studies regarding the efficacy of CEA in symptomatic patients over age 79 are limited. A meta-analysis of 36 published studies found that age over 75 years was associated with a 36% increased perioperative risk of stroke or death (found in 10 studies; odds ratio 1.36; 95% CI 1.09, 1.71; $P < 0.01$) [27]. However, at least one study has reported that endarterectomy can be safely performed in even octogenarians [28]. Clinical judgement remains essential when considering any octogenarian for surgery.

Timing of surgery

Consideration of CEA is appropriately delayed after large hemispheric strokes to determine the patient's level of recovery and to avoid the possible further surgery-related injury that was found in studies performed in the 1960s. However, the timing of the operation after a smaller nondisabling stroke remains uncertain. Another NASCET subgroup analysis compared 42 patients with 70–99% carotid stenosis and a nondisabling stroke operated between 3 and 30 days with 58 patients operated after 30 days (range 33–117 days) [29]. Patients operated later more frequently had abnormalities on initial computed tomography (CT) scan (64% vs. 41%, $P = 0.02$), but the groups were otherwise similar. The perioperative stroke rate was 4.8% in the early group vs. 5.2% in the delayed group ($P = 1.00$) with no perioperative deaths. Although the results might be subject to selection bias based on the presence of CT abnormalities, event rates were higher in those with abnormal scans undergoing delayed surgery (5.4%) vs. those with abnormal scans having early surgery (0%). The authors' conclusion was that there is no reason to delay surgery in the setting of a small stroke.

Perioperative platelet anti-aggregants

A further *post hoc* analysis of NASCET data for patients with 70–99% stenosis found the risk of perioperative stroke or death was 1.8% for those taking 650–1300 mg of aspirin vs. 6.9% for those taking ≤ 325 mg daily, suggesting a benefit with higher aspirin doses [30]. The potential danger of *post hoc* analysis was underscored by the Aspirin and Carotid Endarterectomy (ACE) trial that randomized 2849 patients to receive 81, 325, 650 or 1300 mg of aspirin daily following CEA for 90 days [31]. The primary analysis compared the two high-dose groups with the two low-dose groups. Table 17.5 gives the overall results and indicates lower 30-day

Table 17.5 High- vs. low-dose aspirin after carotid endarterectomy—ACE [30]

	Low dose n = 1395	High dose n = 1409	P
30 days			
Stroke, MI, or death	5.4%	7.0%	0.07
Stroke or death	4.7%	6.1%	0.11
Ipsilateral stroke or death	4.2%	5.7%	0.05
3 months			
Stroke, MI, or death	6.2%	8.4%	0.03
Stroke or death	5.7%	7.1%	0.12
Ipsilateral stroke or death	4.9%	6.5%	0.07

Reproduced with permission, from Goldstein LB. Extracranial carotid artery stenosis. *Stroke* 2003; 34: 2767–73.

rates of stroke, myocardial infarction or death in those given lower doses of aspirin. There was no significant difference in the risk of bleeding complications among the groups. It should be noted that longer-term effects of these different aspirin doses were not examined. None of the other available platelet antiaggregants has been tested in the perioperative period following endarterectomy.

Endarterectomy risk

The benefit of CEA in comparison with medical therapy alone is highly dependent on surgical risk [7,31–34]. Postoperative complication rates significantly higher than 4–6% in patients with high-grade symptomatic stenosis would eliminate the benefit of the operation. Observed perioperative mortality is often higher when performed outside of the setting of a clinical trial, even in centers that participated in randomized studies [35]. Although the 30-day death rate following CEA based on Medicare claims data fell from approximately 3% in 1985 to 2.3% in 1991, the combined mortality and stroke rates were estimated to range between 5% and 11% for all Medicare patients in 1991 [36]. Several surgical series report perioperative complication rates of approximately 3% [31,37–39], but community-based surveys have reported combined morbidity and mortality rates of 6–20% [40–46]. Although a variety of preoperative patient-related factors may affect the risk of CEA, surgical volume [35,47–50] and the skill of the surgeon are critical [51–54]. Therefore, knowledge of a surgeon's complication rates is a critical part of the decision to proceed with surgery. Despite the central role of complication rates for surgical decisions, a recent survey found that < 20% of physicians knew their hospital's perioperative complication rates for CEA [55]. A second study surveyed the surgery program directors of medical centers in the USA with an accredited surgery residency program [56]. Approximately one-fifth of those responding to the survey indicated that their programs were not systematically monitoring CEA complication rates. Specific complication rates were unknown in 40% of the programs that were monitoring complications. Ongoing audits of surgical complication rates need to be carried out to provide these essential data [57].

Stroke prevention after endarterectomy

Finally, it is important to recognize that 20% of patients undergoing endarterectomy for symptomatic disease subsequently have strokes related to other etiologies [58]. CEA represents only one mode of reducing stroke risk in patients with TIA or nondisabling stroke. Therefore, these patients need to be fully evaluated for other potential treatable causes of stroke [59].

Extracranial–intracranial bypass

Patients with carotid artery occlusions and those with occlusions or high-grade stenosis above the level of the skull base cannot be approached with CEA. A landmark randomized clinical trial tested the efficacy of anastomosis of the superficial temporal artery to the middle cerebral artery in patients with symptomatic stenosis or occlusion of the trunk or major branches before the bifurcation or trifurcation of the middle cerebral artery, stenosis of the internal carotid artery above the level of the C-2 vertebral body, or occlusion of the internal carotid artery [60]. There was no benefit associated with the operation overall or in any subgroup. Although a variety of issues were subsequently raised and addressed [61–63], the procedure was largely abandoned based on the results of this trial.

It has been suggested that extracranial–intracranial bypass might be of value in a subgroup of patients with carotid occlusions who have a particularly high risk of subsequent stroke. Positron emission tomography (PET) can be used to assess the brain's regional metabolic status. One group found that patients with a previous stroke or TIA in the territory of an occluded carotid artery having ipsilateral increased oxygen extraction as measured by PET had an overall six-fold increased risk of stoke and seven-fold increased risk of ipsilateral stroke over 48 months of follow-up [64]. Similar results were found in a second study [65]. A clinical trial evaluating the efficacy of extracranial–intracranial bypass in high-risk patients with carotid artery occlusion is now planned [66]. However, at this point there remain no proven indications for the operation.

Surgery for moyamoya disease

Moyamoya disease has been described as 'a non-atherosclerotic, non-inflammatory, non-amyloid vasculopathy characterized by chronic progressive stenosis or occlusion of the terminal internal carotid artery and/or middle cerebral arteries'. [46] Arteriographically, the process is also characterized by a puff of smoke appearance of the vessels at the base of the brain. Moyamoya disease refers to the idiopathic form of the condition, whereas the term moyamoya syndrome is used when it results from a defined underlying condition [46]. Most commonly presenting in childhood or in the young adult age group with cerebral ischemia, moyamoya can present with intracerebral hemorrhage in adults. It may have a more benign course in Western compared with Asian populations, where it was first described [46].

Although prospective data comparing medical and surgical therapy for moyamoya are limited [46], a variety of cerebral revascularization procedures have been employed for the treatment of symptomatic disease. These include indirect revascularization such as with encephalo-myo-synangiosis in which temporalis muscle is applied directly to the pial surface, and encephalo-duro-arterio-synangiosis in which the superficial temporal artery and an attached piece of galea are similarly placed, and omental transplantation [67]. Direct superficial temporal to middle cerebral artery bypass procedures are also employed. Although reports of the effectiveness of these various procedures in both children [68] and adults [69] are favorable, the choice of a specific surgical approach and its impact on the ultimate course of the disease remain controversial.

Conclusion

Surgical procedures are of clear benefit in selected patients with TIA. However, the relative benefits vary depending on the particular indication and patient characteristics. Knowledge of the surgeon's complication rates is critical.

References

1 Fields WS, Maslenikov V, Meyer JS *et al.* Joint study of extracranial arterial occlusion. *JAMA* 1970; 12: 1933–2003.

2 Shaw DA, Venables GS, Cartlidge NEF *et al.* Carotid endarterectomy in patients with transient cerebral ischaemia. *J Neurol Sci* 1984; 64: 45–53.

3 North American Symptomatic Carotid Endarterectomy Trial Collaborators. Beneficial effect of carotid endarterectomy in symptomatic patients with high-grade carotid stenosis. *N Engl J Med* 1991; 325: 445–53.

4 European Carotid Surgery Trialists' Collaborative Group. MRC European carotid surgery trial: interim results for symptomatic patients with severe (70–99%) or with mild (0–29%) carotid stenosis. *Lancet* 1991; 337: 1235–43.

5 Mayberg MR, Wilson E, Yatsu F *et al.* Carotid endarterectomy and prevention of cerebral ischemia in symptomatic carotid stenosis. *JAMA* 1991; 266: 3289–94.

6 Barnett HJM, Taylor DW, Eliasziw M *et al.* Benefit of carotid endarterectomy in patients with symptomatic moderate or severe stenosis. *N Engl J Med* 1998; 339: 1415–25.

7 Barnett HJM, Warlow CP. Carotid endarterectomy and the measurement of stenosis. *Stroke* 1993; 24: 1281–4.

8 Rothwell PM, Warlow CP. The European Carotid Surgery Trial (ECST). In: Greenhalgh RM, Hollier LH, eds. *Surgery for Stroke.* London: W.B. Saunders, 1993: 369–81.

9 Rothwell PM, Gibson RJ, Slattery J *et al.* Equivalence of measurements of carotid stenosis: a comparison of three methods on 1001 angiograms. *Stroke* 1994; 25: 2435–9.

10 Rothwell PM, Gibson RJ, Slattery J *et al.* Prognostic value and reproducibility of measurements of carotid stenosis: a comparison of three methods on 1001 angiograms. *Stroke* 1994; 25: 2440–4.

11 Eliasziw M, Smith RF, Singh N *et al.* Further comments on the measurement of carotid stenosis from angiograms. *Stroke* 1994; 25: 2445–9.

12 North American Symptomatic Carotid Endarterectomy Trial (NASCET) Steering Committee. North American Symptomatic Carotid Endarterectomy Trial. Methods, patient characteristics, and progress. *Stroke* 1991; 22: 711–20.

13 Goldstein LB, Hasselblad V, Matchar DB *et al.* Comparison and meta-analysis of randomized trials of endarterectomy for symptomatic carotid artery stenosis. *Neurology* 1995; 45: 1965–70.

14 European Carotid Surgery Trialists' Collaborative Group. Endarterectomy for moderate symptomatic carotid stenosis: interim results from the MRC European carotid surgery trial. *Lancet* 1996; 347: 1591–3.

15 Farrell B, Fraser A, Sandercock P *et al.* Randomised trial of endarterectomy for recently symptomatic carotid stenosis. Final results of the MRC European Carotid Surgery Trial (ECST). *Lancet* 1998; 351: 1379–87.

16 Rothwell PM, Eliasziw M, Gutnikov SA *et al.* Analysis of pooled data from the randomized controlled trials of endarterectomy for symptomatic carotid stenosis. *Lancet* 2003, 361: 107–16.

17 Sackett DL. Rules of evidence and clinical recommendations on the use of antithrombotic agents. *Chest* 1989; 95 (Suppl.): 25–45.

18 Gross CP, Steiner CA, Bass EB *et al.* Relation between prepublication release of clinical trial results and the practice of carotid endarterectomy. *JAMA* 2000; 284: 2886–93.

19 Eliasziw M, Streifler JY, Fox AJ *et al.* Significance of plaque ulceration in symptomatic patients with high-grade carotid stenosis. *Stroke* 1994; 25: 304–8.

20 Streifler JY, Eliasziw M, Benavente OR *et al.* The risk of stroke in patients with first-ever retinal vs hemispheric transient ischemic attacks and high-grade carotid stenosis. *Arch Neurol* 1995; 52: 246–9.

21 Henderson RD, Eliasziw M, Fox AJ *et al.* Angiographically defined collateral circulation and risk of stroke in patients with severe carotid artery stenosis. *Stroke* 2000; 31: 128–32.

22 Millikan C, Futrell N. The fallacy of the lacune hypothesis. *Stroke* 1990; 21: 1251–7.

23 Inzitari D, Eliasziw M, Sharpe BL *et al.* Risk factors and outcome of patients with carotid artery stenosis presenting with lacunar stroke. *Neurology* 2000; 54: 660–6.

24 Kappelle IJ, Eliasziw M, Fox AJ *et al.* Importance of intracranial atherosclerotic disease in patients with symptomatic stenosis of the internal carotid artery. *Stroke* 1999; 30: 282–6.

25 Kappelle LJ, Eliasziw M, Fox AJ *et al.* Small, unruptured intracranial aneurysms and management of symptomatic carotid artery stenosis. *Neurology* 2000; 55: 307–9.

26 Hobson RWI, Weiss DG, Fields WS *et al.* Efficacy of carotid endarterectomy for asymptomatic carotid stenosis. *N Engl J Med* 1993; 328: 221–7.

27 Rothwell PM, Slattery J, Warlow CP. Clinical and angiographic predictors of stroke and death from carotid endarterectomy: systematic review. *Br Med J* 1997; 315: 1571–7.

28 O'Hara PJ, Hertzer NR, Mascha EJ *et al*. Carotid endarterectomy in octogenarians: early results and late outcome. *J Vasc Surg* 1998; 27: 860–9.

29 Gasecki AP, Ferguson GG, Eliasziw M *et al*. Early endarterectomy for severe carotid artery stenosis after a nondisabling stroke: results from the North American symptomatic carotid endarterectomy trial. *J Vasc Surg* 1994; 20: 288–95.

30 Taylor DW, Barnett HJM, Haynes RB *et al*. Low-dose and high-dose acetylsalicylic acid for patients undergoing carotid endarterectomy: a randomised controlled trial. *Lancet* 1999; 353: 2179–84.

31 Whisnant JP, Sandok BA, Sundt TM Jr. Carotid endarterectomy for unilateral carotid system transient cerebral ischemia. *Mayo Clin Proc* 1983; 58: 171–5.

32 Committee on Health Care Issues. Does carotid endarterectomy decrease stroke and death in patients with transient ischemic attacks? *Ann Neurol* 1987; 22: 72–6.

33 Matchar DB, Pauker SG. Endarterectomy in carotid artery disease. A decision analysis. *JAMA* 1987; 258: 793–8.

34 Easton JD, Wilterdink JL. Carotid endarterectomy: trials and tribulations. *Ann Neurol* 1994; 35: 5–17.

35 Wennberg DE, Lucas FL, Birkmeyer JD *et al*. Variation in carotid endarterectomy mortality in the Medicare population: trial hospitals, volume, and patient characteristics. *JAMA* 1998; 279: 1278–81.

36 Dyken ML. Controversies in stroke: past and present. The Willis Lecture. *Stroke* 1993; 24: 1251–8.

37 Nunn DB. Carotid endarterectomy: an analysis of 234 operative cases. *Ann Surg* 1975; 182: 733–8.

38 Muuronen A. Outcome of surgical treatment of 110 patients with transient ischemic attack. *Stroke* 1984; 15: 959–64.

39 Ojemann RG, Crowell RM, Roberson GH *et al*. Surgical treatment of extracranial carotid occlusive disease. *Clin Neurosurg* 1975; 22: 214–63.

40 Fode NC, Sundt TM Jr, Robertson JT *et al*. Multicenter retrospective review of results and complications of carotid endarterectomy in 1981. *Stroke* 1986; 17: 370–6.

41 Dyken ML, Pokras R. The performance of endarterectomy for disease of the extracranial arteries of the head. *Stroke* 1984; 15: 948–50.

42 Brott TG, Labutta RJ, Kempczinski RF. Changing patterns in the practice of carotid endarterectomy in a large metropolitan area. *JAMA* 1986; 255: 2609–12.

43 Easton JD, Sherman DG. Stroke and mortality rate in carotid endarterectomy: 228 consecutive operations. *Stroke* 1977; 8: 565–8.

44 Winslow CM, Solomon DH, Chassin MR *et al*. The appropriateness of carotid endarterectomy. *N Engl J Med* 1988; 318: 721–7.

45 Tu JV, Hannan EL, Anderson GM *et al*. The fall and rise of carotid endarterectomy in the United States and Canada. *N Engl J Med* 1998; 339: 1441–7.

46 Yilmaz EY, Pritz MB, Bruno A *et al*. Moyamoya. Indiana University Medical Center experience. *Arch Neurol* 2001; 58: 1274–8.

47 Fisher ES, Malenka DJ, Solomon NA *et al*. Risk of carotid endarterectomy in the elderly. *Am J Public Health* 1989; 79: 1617–20.

48 Cebul RD, Snow RJ, Pine R *et al*. Indications, outcomes, and provider volumes for carotid endarterectomy. *JAMA* 1998; 279: 1282–7.

49 Hannan EL, Popp AJ, Tranmer B *et al*. Relationship between provider volume and mortality for carotid endarterectomies in New York State. *Stroke* 1998; 29: 2292–7.

50 O'Neill L, Lanska DJ, Hartz A. Surgeon characteristics associated with mortality and morbidity following carotid endarterectomy. *Neurology* 2000; 55: 773–81.

51 Sundt TM Jr, Sandok BA, Whisnant JP. Carotid endarterectomy: complications and preoperative assessment of risk. *Mayo Clin Proc* 1975; 50: 301–6.

52 Riles TS, Imparato AM, Jacobowitz GR *et al*. The cause of perioperative stroke after carotid endarterectomy. *J Vasc Surg* 1994; 19: 206–16.

53 Sieber FE, Toung TJ, Diringer MN *et al*. Preoperative risks predict neurological outcome of carotid endarterectomy related stroke. *Neurosurgery* 1992; 30: 847–54.

54 McCrory DC, Goldstein LB, Samsa GP *et al*. Predicting complications of carotid endarterectomy. *Stroke* 1993; 24: 1285–91.

55 Goldstein LB, Bonito AJ, Matchar DB *et al*. U.S. National survey of physician practices for the secondary and tertiary prevention of stroke: design, service availability, and common practices. *Stroke* 1995; 26: 1607–15.

56 Chaturvedi S, Femino L. Are carotid endarterectomy complication rates being monitored? *Neurology* 1998; 50: 1927–8.

57 Goldstein LB, Moore WS, Robertson JT *et al*. Complication rates for carotid endarterectomy. A call for action. *Stroke* 1997; 28: 889–90.

58 Barnett HJM, Gunton RW, Eliasziw M *et al*. Causes and severity of ischemic stroke in patients with internal carotid artery stenosis. *JAMA* 2000; 283: 1429–36.

59 Wolf PA, Clagett PA, Easton JD *et al*. Preventing ischemic stroke in patients with prior stroke and transient ischemic attack. *Stroke* 1999; 30: 1991–4.

60 The EC/IC Bypass Study Group. Failure of extracranial–intracranial arterial bypass to reduce the risk of ischemic stroke. *N Engl J Med* 1985; 313: 1191–200.

61 Sundt TM. Was the Interational Randomized Trial of Extracranial-Intracranial Arterial Bypass representative of the population at risk? *N Engl J Med* 1987; 316: 814–6.

62 Goldring S, Zervas N, Langfitt T. The Extracranial-Intracranial Bypass Study. *N Engl J Med* 1987; 316: 817–20.

63 Barnett HJM, Sackett D, Taylor DWHB *et al*. Are the results of the Extracranial-Intracranial Bypass Trial generalizable? *N Engl J Med* 1987; 316: 820–4.

64 Grubb RLJ, Derdeyn CP, Fritsch SM *et al*. Importance of hemodynamic factors in the prognosis of symptomatic carotid occlusion. *JAMA* 1998; 280: 1055–60.

65 Derdeyn CP, Videen TO, Simmons NR *et al.* Count-based PET method for predicting ischemic stroke in patients with symptomatic carotid arterial occlusion. *Radiology* 1999; 212: 499–506.

66 Adams HP, Powers WJ, Grubb RL *et al.* Preview of a new trial of extracranial-to-intracranial arterial anastomosis: the Carotid Occlusion Surgery Study. *Neurosurg Clin North Am* 2001; 12: 613–24.

67 Piepgras DG, Ueki K. Moyamoya disease. In: Anonymous. *Neurosurgery.* New York: McGraw-Hill, 1996: 2125–9.

68 Houkin K, Kuroda S, Nakayama N. Cerebral revascularization for moyamoya disease in children. *Neurosurg Clin North Am* 2001; 12: 575–84.

69 Srinivasan J, Britz GW, Newell DW. Cerebral revascularization for moyamoya disease in adults. *Neurosurg Clin North Am* 2001; 12: 585–94.

CHAPTER 18

Angioplasty and Stenting

Alex Abou-Chebl, Jay S. Yadav

Introduction

The days of therapeutic nihilism in the treatment of stroke patients are over. Newer therapies are evolving rapidly and patients who develop transient ischemic attacks (TIA) or stroke secondary to arterial disease can now be offered definitive medical and surgical therapies. Endovascular therapy for cerebrovascular occlusive disease is perhaps the most exciting of the new and still developing therapies. Endovascular therapy involves the percutaneous use of balloon dilatation (angioplasty, PTA) catheters and/or stents to recanalize stenotic vessels. The vessels treatable in this manner include all of the great vessels of the aortic arch, neck, and even intracranial vessels, specifically: the brachiocephalic and subclavian arteries, common carotid arteries (CCA), internal carotid (ICA) and vertebral arteries (VA) both the cervical and intracranial portions, middle cerebral artery trunk (MCA) as well as the basilar artery (BA). This method is appealing because it is less invasive compared with conventional surgery, e.g. carotid endarterectomy (CEA) or extracranial–intracranial bypass, and it can potentially treat lesions that would otherwise be surgically untreatable [1]. As with most of the new emerging therapies for cerebrovascular disease there are many unresolved issues regarding the indications for endovascular therapy: the optimal techniques, the efficacy and safety, and finally the long-term outcomes and durability of the treatment [1–3]. To date there has been only one randomized trial reported of endovascular therapy compared with surgery which has been published and which included at least 100 patients [4]. Much of the data regarding endovascular techniques are derived from series of patients reported by single centers that are little more than case reports, although a few large series, especially of carotid angioplasty and stenting (CAS), have been reported. In this chapter we will attempt to summarize the available published data on endovascular therapy and to discuss issues of patient selection and peri-procedural medical management. Finally, the ongoing clinical trials will be described and future directions suggested.

Cervical carotid and vertebral artery angioplasty and stenting

Internal carotid artery atherosclerosis at its origin is the most common cause of TIA and stroke of arterial origin. Carotid endarterectomy has been shown to be the treatment of choice in patients with symptomatic stenoses measuring > 70% luminal narrowing [5–8]. In the North American Symptomatic Carotid Endarterectomy Trial (NASCET) CEA was superior to medical therapy in patients with > 70% stenosis, reducing the ipsilateral stroke rate from 26% to 9% at 2 years [5]. Patients with 50–69% luminal narrowing benefited from surgery to a lesser extent, with a decrease in 5-year ipsilateral stroke rates from 22.2% to 15.7%. This is the gold standard therapy against which newer therapies must be measured. CEA is not ideal, however, as it is counterbalanced by significant drawbacks. The margins for benefit in NASCET were dependent on a low perioperative stroke and death rate of 5.8%. Higher surgical complication rates reduce the benefit from surgery. The NASCET results do not accurately reflect the real population of symptomatic patients with ICA atherosclerosis for two major reasons. First, the low perioperative complication rates attained by the specialized centers involved in the trial are much lower, by as much as a factor of three, than those obtained in everyday practice [9]. Second, the patients enrolled in the trial were highly selected and did not include in significant numbers those with major medical comorbidities such as renal, pulmonary, and especially coronary artery disease (CAD) as well those with contralateral ICA occlusion or patients age ≥ 80 years. In addition to the risk of stroke and death noted in NASCET, there was a 7.6% incidence of cranial neuropathy and an 8.9% incidence of surgical wound hematoma or infection.

Carotid angioplasty and stenting is an attractive alternative to CEA for several reasons [10]. It is potentially less risky to perform in patients with medical comorbidities, especially those with CAD, since it is performed without general anesthesia (Fig. 18.1) [3,11,12]. CAS is a less invasive procedure and does not carry a risk of cranial nerve palsies or surgical wound hematomas and infection, the frequency and clinical significance of which are not minor [5,6]. CAS may also be applied to patients at particularly high risk of complications from CEA, including patients who have major medical comorbidities, those who have had prior CEA or neck exploration, neck irradiation, as well as individuals who have high carotid bifurcations, contralateral carotid occlusion, or tandem stenoses (Fig. 18.2) [12–26]. Early investigators performed ICA angioplasty only and later used stents only as a rescue if a dissection developed [13,15,16,27,28]. As stent technology improved it became possible to deliver stents into the ICA with a significant improvement in acute outcomes compared with angioplasty alone [10]. Currently, stenting following PTA of the ICA is the standard

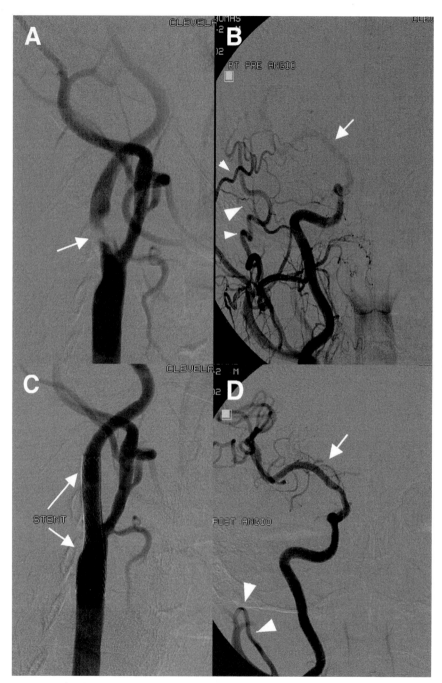

Fig. 18.1 Fifty-five-year-old male with severe ischemic cardiomyopathy who was on the waiting list for a heart transplant developed recurrent amaurosis fugax in the right eye. By computed tomography he was found to have silent borderzone infarcts in the deep white matter of the right hemisphere and on cerebral angiography he had a nearly occlusive, eccentric and ulcerated stenosis of the right internal carotid artery (arrow in A), seen here in the AP plane. (B) The AP intracranial view shows delayed and poor filling

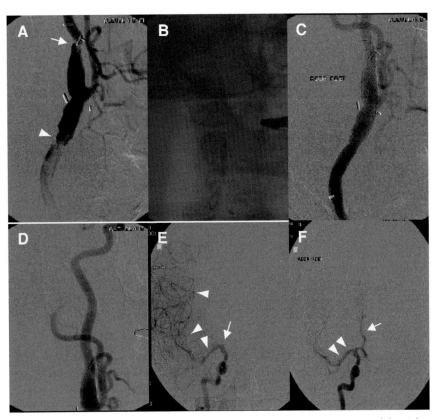

Fig. 18.2 A 76-year-old man with a prior history of carotid endarterectomy of the right internal carotid artery (ICA) for an asymptomatic stenosis 13 years previously, presented with recurrent vision loss in the right eye and tingling of the left arm. A carotid duplex showed the right ICA peak systolic velocity to be 530 cm/s and the ICA/common carotid artery (CCA) ratio to be 10. An ipsilateral oblique angiogram (A) shows an ulcerated, severe (> 95%) stenosis of the ICA at the distal end of the previous endarterectomy site (arrow) as well as a tandem stenosis of the CCA at the proximal end (arrowhead) both consistent with clamp injury. (B) The predilatation balloon inflated in the ICA as well as an umbrella type emboli capture device deployed in the distal cervical ICA. (C,D) The completion angiograms, which reveal the complete resolution of the stenoses proximally, and distally using two separate nitinol stents. The prestent intracranial angiogram (E) shows slow flow into the right middle cerebral artery (MCA) (arrowheads) and no filling of the ACA (arrow), which filled from the left ICA. The poststent angiogram (F) shows improved opacification of the MCA (arrowheads) as well as filling of the ACA (arrow).

Fig. 18.1 Opposite. of the middle cerebral artery (MCA) (arrow), consistent with a high-grade proximal stenosis; note the prominent flow in the external carotid branches (arrowheads). A 10 × 36 mm stainless steel stent was successfully deployed in the internal carotid artery and distal common carotid artery (C) with a 0% residual stenosis. Following stent deployment, the intracranial injection in the AP plane (D) shows a normal filling pattern with MCA (arrow) opacification prior to filling of the ECA branches (arrowheads).

practice [11]. Carotid angioplasty and stenting has also been successfully used to treat a variety of conditions other than atherosclerosis that can affect the internal carotid arteries and cause ischemia including: spontaneous and traumatic dissection, pseudoaneurysms, and fibromuscular dysplasia (Fig. 18.3) [25,29–34].

Endovascular treatment of the other cervico-cranial vessels is less controversial than CAS. This is because these other vessels are less frequently implicated in causing cerebral ischemia and their surgical repair is much more involved and complicated than CEA. The surgical approach to the brachiocephalic, subclavian, and common carotid artery origins requires a thoracotomy (Fig. 18.4). Extracranial VA lesions can be treated with endarterectomy or transposition of the VA to the carotid artery; in either case both techniques require expertise that is not widely available and there are no definitive studies proving the value of these surgical procedures. Endovascular treatment can be performed much more quickly and easily than can surgery (Fig. 18.5). Safety and outcomes are even less well delineated than is CAS, however, and the available data are limited to those obtained from small series and case reports [32,34–52].

Extracranial angioplasty and stenting: technical issues

The first report of carotid artery angioplasty was published in 1981 and was followed by sporadic reports of small series of patients over the following decade [13,15,27–30,35,36,53–57]. It was not until the introduction of intravascular stents, however, that endovascular treatment became a viable approach [3,49,58]. The first large series of CAS was published in 1996 and included 126 procedures performed on 107 patients who were at high risk of CEA [10]. Many other reports have been published in recent years [14,18,20–22,24,34,49,59–79]. The results of many of these series are quite encouraging and suggest that CAS may be an alternative to CEA. These results must be interpreted with caution, however, since these studies are quite heterogeneous in patient selection, endovascular technique and equipment used, as well as in outcome measures. In addition the majority of the procedures reported in these series were performed without emboli capture devices, which have the potential to revolutionize PTA and stenting of the cervico-cranial vessels. Almost all of the reported series to date included both symptomatic and asymptomatic patients and only a small number evaluated outcomes based on the symptomatic status of the ICA. The following discussion therefore will include outcomes of both groups of patients and where possible subgroup results of symptomatic patients will be highlighted.

Appropriate patient selection is the first and most crucial step in ensuring success. Patients who have severe peripheral vascular disease and poor arterial access or those with a very tortuous or steep aortic arch may be

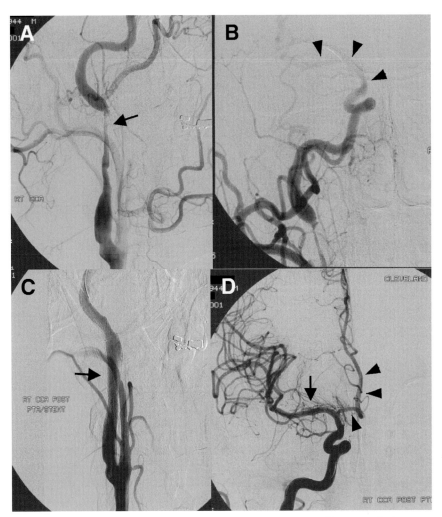

Fig. 18.3 A 57-year-old man with hypertension, coronary artery disease, and a long-standing type B aortic dissection developed a depressed mental status and left-sided hemianopsia and hemiparesis that fluctuated with changes in blood pressure. Urgent angiography revealed (A) spontaneous dissection (arrow) of the right internal carotid artery (ICA) with (B) poor flow intracranially (arrowheads). A single stent measuring 7 × 40 mm was deployed in the right ICA (arrow in C) resulting in normal filling of the middle cerebral artery (MCA) (arrow) and ACA (arrowheads) (D). The patient's fluctuating symptoms resolved and he improved moderately, although he was left with a moderate sized MCA infarct.

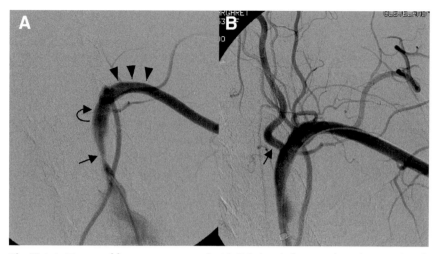

Fig. 18.4 A 47-year-old woman presented with lightheadedness and vertigo associated with left arm claudication. A subclavian steal was suggested by duplex evaluation and confirmed by angiography. An AP plane angiogram (A) of the left subclavian artery shows a severe stenosis of the proximal vessel (arrow) with no filling of the vertebral artery (VA) (curved arrow) and in fact shows retrograde flow into the subclavian from the VA [note the washout of contrast (arrowheads) in the apex of the artery]. After stenting (B) there is a resolution of the stenosis with normal anterograde flow into the VA (arrow). The patient was asymptomatic following the procedure.

difficult or impossible to treat endovascularly. Similarly, patients with renal insufficiency or a history of anaphylactic reaction to angiographic contrast may not be appropriate candidates, although alternatives to conventional contrast do exist. Platelet inhibition has been shown to be important in preventing acute thrombus formation at the site of PTA or stenting in the coronary arteries [80–82]. As a result, all extracranial interventions are performed with platelet inhibition with aspirin, ticlopidine and or clopidogrel and there is little to no disagreement about their use [82,83]. We prefer clopidogrel to ticlopidine for its low risk of side-effects. Patients who have contraindications to the use of aspirin, clopidogrel, or ticlopidine or who are noncompliant or who continue to smoke and live an unhealthy lifestyle may have higher restenosis risks or even acute postprocedure thrombosis [84]. A relative contraindication to endovascular repair is the need for major surgery within 30 days that would necessitate the discontinuation of antiplatelet agents, although there have been some reports of combined CAS and coronary artery bypass graft surgery [85,86]. Platelet glycoprotein IIb/IIIa receptor (GPIIa/IIIa) antagonists have been used by some investigators in high-risk patients undergoing cervico-cranial endovascular repair [23,87–90]. The role of such agents has yet to be

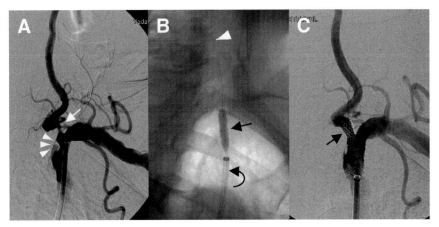

Fig. 18.5 A 69-year-old man with a history of hypertension and smoking developed a left cerebellar hemisphere infarct and was treated with warfarin. He then developed recurrent (2–3/week) spells of hemiparesis and loss of consciousness. Angiography revealed an occluded right vertebral artery (VA) at its origin and (A) a severe stenosis of the left VA origin (arrow) with a moderate, ulcerated stenosis of the proximal subclavian artery (arrowheads). The VA was primarily stented. (B) Note the stent being deployed by an inflated balloon (arrow), the guidewire in the VA (arrowhead) and the guide catheter in the subclavian (curved arrow) can be seen. The subclavian artery was also stented because of the proximity of the stenosis and ulcer to the VA origin and because there was a blood pressure gradient of 40 mmHg across the stenosis suggesting that it was hemodynamically significant. Following stenting (C) the VA ostium is widely patent (arrow). The patient had no further spells of hemiparesis or loss of consciousness.

defined by controlled studies, but one possible role is their use for patients undergoing urgent interventions without prior adequate oral antiplatelet therapy or patients with long stenoses who will be treated with multiple stents.

Advances in percutaneous coronary artery revascularization have served as helpful models for endovascular cervico-cranial procedures. Stents have been shown to improve patency both short term and long term in the coronary arteries [91,92]. The causes of acute failure of PTA include elastic recoil, dissection and intimal flap formation, vasospasm, and thrombotic occlusion (platelet and/or fibrin). Stent deployment decreases the incidence of acute closure or thrombosis secondary to elastic recoil or dissection [3,10,93–96]. Stents may also decrease the risk of late restenosis. In the extracranial cervico-cranial vessels, there is almost universal agreement on the use of stents especially in heavily calcified lesions and at the ostia of the great vessels where elastic recoil is greatest [97] (Fig. 18.6).

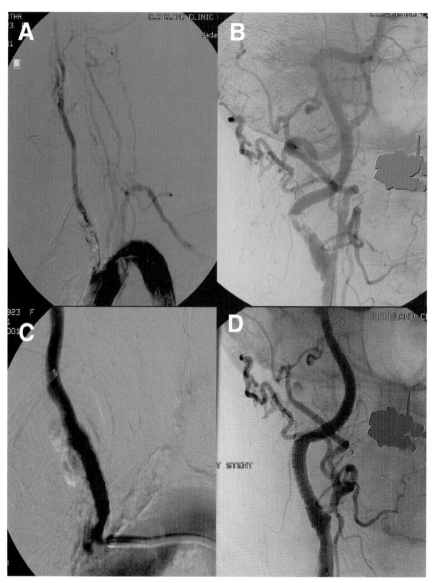

Fig. 18.6 A 78-year-old woman with extensive peripheral and coronary artery disease
had a right middle cerebral artery (MCA) territory transient ischemic attack (TIA).
Carotid duplex revealed severe bilateral internal carotid artery (ICA) stenoses. An
aortic arch angiogram shows severe atherosclerosis of the aortic arch (arrowheads) and
a severely calcified (short arrows), subtotal occlusion of the innominate artery (long
arrow) and occlusion of the right subclavian artery (curved arrow). An ipsilateral
oblique angiogram of the right common carotid artery (CCA) bifurcation (B) shows a
complex, ulcerated, calcified and subtotal occlusion (arrow) of the ICA. Angioplasty of
the innominate artery was carried out with multiple high-pressure inflations and only
after balloon expandable stent deployment and repeat dilatation was an adequate
result obtained (arrow in C). The ICA was successfully treated with a nitinol self-
expanding stent without any residual stenosis (arrow in D).

Angioplasty and stenting are appealing because they are less invasive and may be safer than conventional surgical approaches, but they are not without risks. Risk factors for complications of CAS include age > 80 years, symptomatic status, length of stenosis (> 10–11 mm), heavy ring-like calcification at the ICA bulb, and the presence of intraluminal thrombus [3,85,98]. Several series have found differences in complication rates between symptomatic and asymptomatic patients [75,99]. A study of 111 patients by Qureshi *et al.* suggested that symptomatic patients may have an increased risk of perioperative stroke compared with asymptomatic patients [98]. These results are supported by those obtained in a large multicentre survey of 36 centres that evaluated outcomes in 4749 patients [100]. In that study symptomatic patients had a combined stroke and procedure-related death rate of 5.76%, while asymptomatic patients had a 3.38% complication rate. No statistical values were reported with these figures, but with such a large series it is likely that those numbers represent a clinically significant difference. Risk factors that are of unclear significance include the severity and complexity of the stenosis and recent stroke < 3 weeks [3,20,75,98]. One characteristic that has not been correlated with complications is sex, which is in contradistinction to the increased risk of complications in women reported in the Asymptomatic Carotid Atherosclerosis Study (ACAS) [5,75]. Hypotension and bradycardia are common during interventions on the ICA bulb but are usually transient and mild [101]. Complications of endovascular procedures not specific to cerebral interventions include access site hematomas, allergic reactions to contrast, heart failure, and renal toxicity, the incidences of which are similar to those of cerebral angiography.

The most feared complication of carotid stenting is cerebral ischemia. The most common mechanism of ischemia with endovascular therapy is distal embolization, but acute vessel occlusion due to dissection, vasospasm, or thrombosis are other potential mechanisms. These other mechanisms are fortunately quite rare, especially with the current practice of stent deployment in almost all patients and the aggressive use of antiplatelet agents. Embolization remains the limiting factor in widespread acceptance of PTA and stenting, especially [84]. Emboli as detected by transcranial Doppler ultrasonography (TCD) have been shown to occur in virtually all patients undergoing endovascular treatment of the ICA, especially at the time of balloon inflation and deflation [102–104]. Embolization as detected by TCD is not unique to CAS but also occurs during CEA and has been correlated with the risk of ischemic complications in both CAS and CEA [95,103–105]. Emboli capture devices have the potential to limit distal embolization during CAS (Fig. 18.7). Clinical experience with such devices is limited outside of the ongoing clinical trials [57,106–109]. We feel, as do most experts in the field, that such devices will greatly reduce the risk of distal embolization during CAS and several

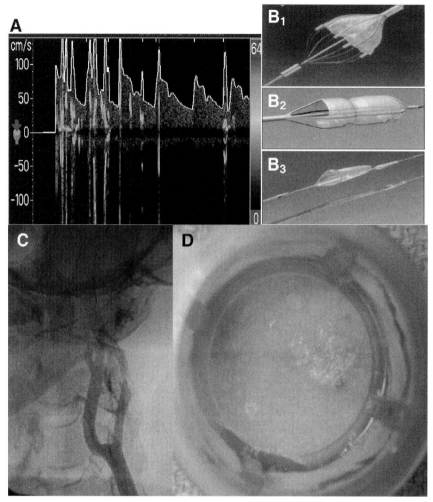

Fig. 18.7 High-intensity transient signals, some of which presumably represent emboli are readily seen by transcranial Doppler ultrasonography following balloon deflation in a patient undergoing carotid angioplasty and stenting (A). Several filter types or 'umbrella' emboli capture devices have been developed (B$_{1-3}$). One such device (Angioguard™, B$_1$) is shown in (C) deployed in the high cervical internal carotid artery (ICA) (arrow) prior to balloon dilatation and stent deployment. Particulate material is frequently seen after the emboli capture devices are removed. In this case (D) the magnified view shows white particles that were trapped on a filter. The particles were hydrophobic and 'greasy' to the touch and probably represented cholesterol and lipid particles from the ICA plaque.

ongoing clinical trials, as will be discussed shortly, include the use of such devices [3]. Intracranial hemorrhage is another possible complication of cervicocranial revascularization, especially CAS. Possible causative mechanisms include embolization and hemorrhagic conversion of the infarcted region, the use of heparin and potent antiplatelet agents, and cerebral hyperperfusion syndrome. The latter is well described after CEA but has rarely been reported following CAS [110,111]. Patients at risk of this complication can be identified preoperatively. Risk factors include perioperative hypertension, revascularization of a severe stenosis with poor collateral blood flow, or the presence of bilateral severe stenoses or contralateral occlusion.

Outcomes and conclusions

There have been more than 25 series and one randomized study of CAS published to date that had a combined total of 2606 patients, 69% of whom were symptomatic. In many of these series there was no mention of outcomes based on symptom status. In addition, Wholey *et al.* surveyed the major centers that perform CAS and obtained global experience data on 4757 patients which they published in 2000 [100]. Of those patients, 63% were symptomatic. As discussed above, these series reflect quite a heterogeneous group of patients and techniques (Table 18.1). Of all of the differences listed in Table 18.1, operator experience is perhaps the most critical, as many studies have shown improved outcomes with increased experience [75,77,100]. In the aforementioned 25 series the technical success rate was 96.3% (range 71.4–100%). In this same group of patients, complications within 30 days included TIAs in 4.4% (range 0–17.6%) and strokes of all severities in 4.3% (range 0–13.3%), while 1.15% (range 0–5.9%) of patients died. For comparison the cohort of major centers surveyed by Wholey had lower complication rates of 2.82%, 3.84%, and 0.86%, respectively [100]. Follow-up of at least 12 months was reported in 84% of the patients in this series and revealed a 2.3% 6-month restenosis rate and a 12-month restenosis rate of 3.4%. The 30-day combined stroke or death rate in symptomatic patients was 5.76%. At 12 months, only 1.4% of patients had had an event, defined as a TIA, stroke, or stroke death. These rates are comparable to those obtained in the NASCET trial of CEA for symptomatic patients [5]. The 30-day event rate in that trial was 6.5%. Considering that many patients treated in major centers were considered high risk for CEA, the retrospective results suggest that CAS may be at least equivalent to CEA and may in fact be safer if surgery-specific complications are considered (e.g. cranial neuropathies or neck hematomas). In asymptomatic patients, however, the complication rate of 3.38% is higher than that obtained in the surgical arm of the Asymptomatic Carotid Atherosclerosis Study, although the stent patients

Table 18.1 Differences between studies of carotid angioplasty and stenting (CAS)

Patient characteristic
  Symptomatic vs. asymptomatic
  High vs. low risk for carotid endarterectomy
  Retrospective vs. prospective data collection

Technical issues
  Experience of interventionalist
  Balloons and stents used
  Use of emboli capture device
  Antiplatelet regimen
  Post-operative management

Outcomes measures
  Inclusion/exclusion of transient ischemic attack
  Definition of stroke
  Definition of stroke severity
  Perioperative mortality
  Evaluation by neurologist
  Definition of technical success
       (Residual stenosis < 70, < 50, < 30%)

Follow-up
  Duration
  Method (US vs. angiography)

---

were typically at higher surgical risk than the patients in ACAS [112]. The results of endovascular treatment of other cervical vessels are promising but the available data are nothing more than anecdotal case series. Given that for many such patients there is no surgical alternative or what alternatives exist are quite invasive, endovascular treatment must be considered on a case by case basis and should be performed by highly experienced interventionalists.

The only study published to date that directly compared endovascular treatment and CEA in a randomized fashion was the CAVATAS study conducted in Europe and Australia [4]. The study enrolled NASCET eligible patients, 90% of whom were symptomatic (37% had had TIA) in the prior 6 months. The 30-day outcomes for stroke and death in the 251 endovascular patients and the 253 CEA patients were 10% and 9.9%, respectively. Although these results were almost double the NASCET results, they showed clinical equipoise between the two therapies. At 1 year there was a statistically significant ($P < 0.001$) increased rate of restenosis (> 70%) in the endovascular group (14%) compared with CEA (4%); however, the stroke rate at 3 years was similar in both groups. Local complications such as cranial nerve injury and hematomas were higher in the surgical group.

Table 18.2 Summary of major ongoing and upcoming clinical trials of carotid stenting

Study name	No. of patients	High risk	Symptom status (stenosis severity)		Randomized	Status
			Symptomatic	Asymptomatic		
ARCHER	398	Yes	Yes (> 50%)	Yes (> 80%)	No (Registry)	Enrolling since 3/2001
CABERNET	380	Yes	Yes (> 50%)	Yes (> 80%)	No (Registry)	Pending
CREST	2500	No	Yes (> 50%)*	No	Yes	Enrolling since 8/2001
SAPPHIRE	900	Yes	Yes (> 50%)	Yes (> 80%)	Yes†	Enrolling since 8/2000
SECURITTY		Yes	Yes (> 50%)	Yes (> 80%)	No (Registry)	Pending
SHELTER	480	Yes	Yes (> 50%)	Yes (> 80%)	No (Registry)	1/2002

*More than 50% angiographic stenosis or > 70% stenosis by Duplex US.
Patients are randomized unless they are deemed inoperable by the surgeon, in which case they are enrolled into a registry of stenting.

In CAVATAS only 26% of patients were treated with a stent, which may explain the very high rate of recurrent stenosis and may even have contributed to the high perioperative event rate.

There are several ongoing clinical trials that will hopefully definitively determine which procedure is superior, CAS or CEA. Table 18.2 lists the major ongoing trials as well as planned trials that will begin enrollment shortly. Only two of the trials are randomized, SAPPHIRE and CREST. The aim of the Stenting and Angioplasty with Protection in Patients at High Risk for Endarterectomy (SAPPHIRE) study is to show efficacy and safety of CAS in a high surgical-risk patient population. The study utilizes a stent that is optimized for the carotids along with an umbrella type of emboli capture device (Angioguard™; Cordis Corp., Miami, FL, USA; Fig. 18.7). The study has recently been presented in abstract form. The Carotid Endarterectomy vs. Stenting Trial (CREST) is an NIH and industry-sponsored trial of a stent specifically designed for the carotids but in a NASCET eligible population (i.e. low surgical risk). Patients will be randomized to CAS or CEA, but the use of an emboli capture device is optional. Enrollment began in mid 2001 and results will not be available for several more years.

A consensus conference of experts from all disciplines (cardiology, radiology, and surgery) was recently held [3,113,114]. The experts agreed further research is needed before CAS can be adopted universally. They felt that the optimal techniques have not yet been defined and that better equipment and cerebral protection devices are needed. A definitive statement of equipoise or superiority of CAS must therefore await the results of

a clinical trial that directly compares CEA and endovascular therapy performed by experienced interventionalists with state of the art techniques
and equipment specifically designed for the carotids, and performed with
emboli capture devices. For the time being, CAS should be performed only
as part of a clinical trial or under an IDE.

Intracranial artery angioplasty and stenting

Intracranial atherosclerosis causes 8–10% of all ischemic strokes [115].
Patients at particular risk of intracranial stenosis include those who have
diabetes mellitus or hypercholesterolemia and those of African-American,
Hispanic, Asian, or Middle Eastern descent [115,116]. The pathophysiology of most intracranial stenoses is thought to be atherosclerosis. The most
common locations for intracranial atherosclerosis are the petrous ICA, the
cavernous ICA, the clinoid or terminal ICA, the MCA trunk, the distal VA,
the vertebrobasilar junction, and the mid BA [117–119]. The small size of
these vessels, their location within the calvarium, their proximity to delicate brain and cranial nerves, and the presence of small perforators complicate and limit surgical therapeutic options. Surgical bypass has been
used in selected patients but in a randomized trial patients treated with
bypass of MCA stenoses fared worse than medically treated patients [120].
Recent developments in percutaneous or endovascular techniques and
equipment have overcome some of these difficulties and now make it
possible to recanalize the intracranial vessels using PTA and stenting.

The data of the risks of stroke or TIA in patients who have intracranial
atherosclerosis have been obtained from mostly small and retrospective series of patients [121–132]. An accurate knowledge of these risks is
essential if the results of endovascular interventions are to be assessed
critically. There is a great variability in the way patients were identified,
evaluated, treated medically, and the duration for which they were followed
in these series. Annual rates of stroke or TIA recurrence are reported to
be as low as 3% and as high as 22.3% [120,124–126,128–130,132–134].
In most of these series the risk of recurrence was between 6% and 10%
annually. Thijs and Albers found as we did in our own unpublished series
that patients who fail any medical regimen are at a particularly high risk of
recurrent ischemia when compared with patients who are not taking an
antithrombotic medicine at the time of initial presentation [111,135].
There may also be differences in stroke risk based on the vascular territory
and patterns of atherosclerosis [113]. Also the risks of lesion progression
may vary depending on location. Akins et al. have reported that in 21
patients followed with serial angiograms over a mean of 26.7 months,
20% of intracranial ICA stenoses progressed > 10% [136]. Of patients with
MCA or VB stenoses, approximately 60% progressed angiographically.
Approximately 20% of lesions regressed and the remainder were stable.

The risk of TIA or stroke in patients who have incidentally found intracranial stenoses but are asymptomatic is unknown.

Stroke mechanisms and the goals of endovascular therapy

The intracranial vasculature is most similar to the coronary vasculature in size but unlike acute myocardial infarction, platelet and fibrin thrombus formation upon an area of acute plaque rupture is not the only mechanism of ischemia due to intracranial atherosclerosis [136–139]. Hypoperfusion and embolism are the other common mechanisms of ischemia associated with intracranial stenosis [133,140]. It is likely that in many patients a combination of these mechanisms is responsible for ischemia [141]. Improving flow through the stenosis should be the primary aim of any endovascular attempt. Even small changes in diameter will have a great effect on flow through the stenotic segment [118,142]. An angiographic endpoint of a smooth lumen of normal caliber, while desirable, is not necessary to help the patient, and the pursuit of such a goal may lead to a poor outcome.

The indications for endovascular repair of intracranial stenosis are controversial [113,114]. Most neurologists and interventionalists would probably disagree with the point of view that the presence of a symptomatic intracranial stenosis is by itself an indication for endovascular repair [113]. Most clinicians recommend angioplasty and or stenting only to those patients who have failed maximal medical therapy, if at all. What is maximal medical therapy? There is no universally accepted definition, but the most common criterion for failure is recurrent symptoms despite a combination of warfarin and low-dose aspirin, although, as was discussed previously, it may be that failure of any regimen may put a patient at high risk of recurrent stroke [135]. This would suggest that recurrent symptoms on any regimen of anticoagulant or antiplatelet agent should be considered a medical failure.

Intracranial angioplasty and stenting: techniques and results

Sundt and colleagues reported the first intracranial angioplasty in 1980 [143]. They performed PTA on two patients with BA stenosis. Their success encouraged others and to date there have been many published case reports and series of PTA of the major intracranial vessels [55,144–155]. Most of these reports have shown favorable outcomes, but all have been retrospective and are for the most part anecdotal. As was the case for extracranial interventions, these reports also differ significantly in patient selection, location of stenoses, endovascular techniques and adjuvant medical therapy used, as well as in the duration and type of follow-up assessment. Direct comparisons between them are problematic and definitive conclusions about efficacy, safety, and the superiority of particular techniques or equipment cannot be made. Unlike the published series of extracranial interventions, however, most if not all patients reported thus far who have had intracranial interventions have been symptomatic. Nonetheless, several concepts and techniques essential for the safe and successful completion of intracranial angioplasty have been learned from this early experience.

As with extracranial interventions, patient selection is critical, perhaps even more so for intracranial interventions. An important selection criterion is the feasibility of the intervention in terms of vascular access, i.e. the presence of tortuous cervical vessels, proximal stenoses, etc. Accurate measurement of vessel size is essential. Oversizing a balloon or stent may cause vessel rupture. The cerebral vessels are quite thin and do not have an external elastic lamina or adventitia. Patients who are medically unstable, who have a terminal illness or a short expected survival may not live long enough to benefit from an intervention and may have an unnecessary high peri-procedural risk of stroke or death. Recent symptoms, especially if associated with an infarct, may increase the risk of complications, particularly hemorrhagic transformation. Some clinicians have excluded or delayed for 6 weeks or more operating on patients with a large stroke [118,156]. The basis for this approach is anecdotal and in part reflects the common practice of delayed carotid endarterectomy following stroke. This is a reasonable approach and we advocate delaying therapy if there is a large stroke. If there is hemorrhagic conversion then endovascular repair should definitely be delayed. Although in general patients with chronic occlusion of a cerebral vessel are not ideal candidates for endovascular intervention because of the increased risk of dissection, Mori *et al.* have reported two series of patients who had chronic occlusion who were treated with angioplasty [157,158]. There was a higher technical failure rate and a 66.7% restenosis rate in those patients, however, and these factors must all be taken into account when evaluating a potential patient.

As with extracranial interventions, adequate platelet inhibition is critical during intracranial interventions and we use the same regimen as discussed above. The role of GPIIa/IIIa antagonists, e.g. abciximab, in the setting of intracranial endovascular stenting procedures is unknown [159]. While clearly of benefit in the endovascular treatment of the similarly sized coronary arteries, the lack of evidence supporting a beneficial effect and the potential risk of ICH, particularly if there is a wire tip perforation, weigh against the use of GPIIa/IIIa receptor antagonists for intracranial procedures. We feel that the use of GPIIa/IIIa should not be routine in PTA of the intracranial vessels but should be reserved for highly selected patients, in particular patients who were not adequately pretreated with oral antiplatelet agents.

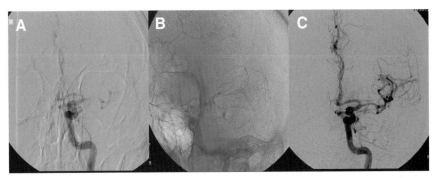

Fig. 18.8 In this patient with recurrent aphasia and poor cerebrovascular reserve by single positron emission computed tomography (SPECT) an AP view (A) of the left middle cerebral artery (MCA) shows a severe mid-MCA trunk stenosis (arrow). Also note the poor filling of the distal MCA territory (arrowheads). In this unsubtracted, ipsilateral-oblique image (B) the support wire (arrow) is seen placed in a proximal M3 branch. After balloon angioplasty (C) there is marked improvement in the luminal diameter (arrow) and filling of the distal branches (arrowheads). The MCA was of small caliber and a stent was not deployed. The patient's symptoms resolved completely.

Whether to deploy a stent or not is controversial, and the experience to date with stenting is limited (Figs 18.8 and 18.9). Most large series of intracranial interventions have not included stenting. A few case reports and small series constitute the current published data on intracranial stenting [96,149,152,159–169]. Some authors advocate stent deployment as a 'bail-out' technique if there is a dissection, slow flow, or elastic recoil after PTA or not at all [118,156,159]. Most authors argue that stents should be deployed whenever possible [96,113,147,149,152,170]. The potential drawbacks of stenting include: added technical complexity, greater difficulty in delivery compared with balloons only, and the potential for occlusion, by the stent struts, of the ostia of small and microscopic perforators off of the MCA and BA.

The first report of an intracranial stent deployment in the BA was published in 1999, which was 19 years after the first report of BA PTA. There are no commercially available stents that have been specifically designed for the intracranial circulation, and coronary stents are used exclusively. In such patients, especially if they have received GPIIb/IIIa receptor antagonists, blood pressure should be maintained in the low normal range. Aspirin and clopidogrel or ticlopidine are continued for 30 days, after which aspirin is continued indefinitely. TCD is a non-invasive and relatively sensitive method of following most ICA siphon, MCA, VA, and BA stenoses and is a convenient and non-invasive method for following patients after an intervention. Acutely, blood flow velocities as measured

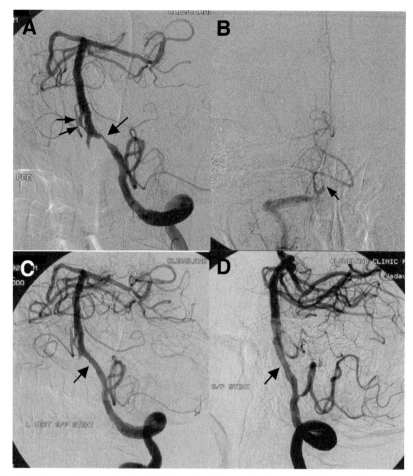

Fig. 18.9 An angiogram in the AP plane of a left vertebral artery (VA) (A) injection in a patient with recurrent brainstem ischemia shows a high-grade stenosis involving the distal left VA (arrow) and a fenestration of the basilar artery (BA) (double arrows). The BA fenestration is a relatively common anatomical variant that was not contributing to his symptoms but did make the endovascular approach more difficult. The right VA (B) is occluded distal to the PICA origin (arrow) and does not contribute flow to the BA. AP (C) and lateral (D) projections show an excellent technical result after angioplasty and stent deployment without any significant residual stenosis in the left VA (arrows in C and D). The patient was cured of the transient ischemic attacks and is currently being treated with one aspirin daily.

by TCD may be elevated and, unless the patient is symptomatic, should rarely be acted upon.

The two most serious and likely complications with intracranial interventions are intracranial hemorrhage and ischemia. Vessel perforation, rupture or dissection with subarachnoid hemorrhage are the most feared complication of PTA and occur with excessive dilatation of the thin-walled cerebral vessels or due to wire tip perforation. In patients who have critical stenoses with poor cerebrovascular reserve as documented by a functional study, e.g. acetazolamide single positron emission computed tomography (SPECT) or TCD, or those who have poor angiographic collaterals, there is a potential risk of hyperperfusion syndrome and intracranial hemorrhage. ICH is the most common cause of death in published reports of intracranial interventions. Few patients will survive a subarachnoid hemorrhage in this setting. Ischemia should be treated with measures to improve perfusion such as blood pressure elevation, hydration and hemodilution, and continuation of antithrombotic agents. Unfortunately in either case, ICH or ischemia, treatments are not ideal and these complications are best avoided.

Outcomes and conclusions

Technical and clinical outcomes have been generally favorable (Fig. 18.10). As yet, however, there have not been controlled, randomized clinical trials and results must be interpreted cautiously. Angioplasty alone has an approximately 78% technical success rate. The stroke and death rates are 13% and 1.6%, respectively. Dissection and arterial rupture occurred in 8.7% of the 259 patients reported in the largest series. Data on restenosis are not available from all of the series and the duration of follow-up varied greatly between the different series. From what data are available, however, the restenosis rate is near 12%. The five series of intracranial stenting published to date include only 58 patients. Although it is not possible to generalize from such a small number of patients, some have suggested that technical success appears to be greater with stenting and complications may be lower [147]. There is, however, a significant case selection bias in favor of stenting, since stents can often not be placed in the most severe and poorly accessible lesions. A review of the combined outcomes of all of the published series reveals that outcomes are not significantly different between angioplasty alone and stenting. Technical success, at 87%, is slightly better with stenting. Stroke and mortality may be higher with stenting, however: 15.6% and 9.8%, respectively. As expected, the rate of dissection or rupture is slightly lower at 6.1%. Restenosis data are even scarcer for patients treated with stenting and no worthwhile conclusion can be made at this time. Many factors may affect the technical and clinical success of intracranial interventions. Operator experience, technical advances, patient selection, lesion characteristics, perioperative antithrombotic

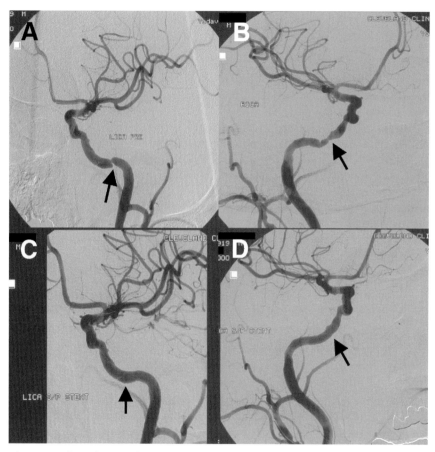

Fig. 18.10 Bilateral internal carotid angiograms in the ipsilateral oblique planes (A and B) demonstrate moderate to severe stenoses in both petrous internal carotid arteries (ICAs) (arrows) in a patient who presented with postural lightheadedness and refractory and lifestyle altering pulsatile tinnitus. The petrous segment of the ICA cannot be approached surgically and is relatively easily treated with angioplasty and stenting because of the lack of perforators and branches. This location has a lower risk of SAH because of the extradural location of the vessels and because the petrous bones limit vessel stretching, making rupture unlikely. In this patient both ICAs were treated with angioplasty followed by stenting with excellent results technically (arrows in C and D) and a significant and immediate decrease in the pulsatile tinnitus. Long-term follow-up is not yet available.

and antiplatelet medical treatment, and the method and duration of follow-up will all affect actual and measured outcomes. There are several ongoing clinical trials, one of which has recently completed enrollment. This study sponsored by Guidant Corporation (SYLVIA: Stenting of Symptomatic atherosclerotic Lesions in the Vertebral or Intracranial Arteries) was aimed at testing the safety and feasibility of using a proprietary balloon and stent (NeuroLink™) delivery system designed specifically for the central nervous system. The study enrolled 60 patients with symptomatic intracranial stenoses or cervical VA lesions that had failed medical therapy. There was no control arm, as this was a feasibility trial and no outcomes or results have been published at the time of writing.

Intracranial angioplasty and stenting are certainly feasible and are appropriate therapeutic options in select patients. They should be reserved for symptomatic patients who have failed medical therapy and not as the primary mode of therapy for intracranial atherosclerosis [113,114]. Intracranial interventions are very complicated procedures and the morbidity and mortality risks associated with these techniques are significant. In particular, intracranial hemorrhage is the most feared complication as it is almost universally fatal. Follow-up and medical management are also critical after interventions are performed. There is a pressing need for prospective clinical trials of intracranial angioplasty and stenting with standardized patient and lesion selection criteria, standardized perioperative medical management, balloons and stents designed for the cerebral vasculature, and comprehensive postoperative management criteria and follow-up.

References

1 Ferguson RD, Ferguson JG, Lee LI. Endovascular revascularization therapy in cerebral athero-occlusive disease. Angioplasty and stents, systemic and local thrombolysis. *Neurosurg Clin N Am* 1994; 5: 511–27.

2 Gomez CR. The role of carotid angioplasty and stenting. [Review] *Semin Neurol* 1998; 18: 501–11.

3 Veith FJ, Amor M, Ohki T *et al*. Current status of carotid bifurcation angioplasty and stenting based on a consensus of opinion leaders. *J Vasc Surg* 2001; 33 (Suppl. 2): S111–S116.

4 Endovascular versus surgical treatment in patients with carotid stenosis in the Carotid and Vertebral Artery Transluminal Angioplasty Study (CAVATAS): a randomised trial. *Lancet* 2001; 357: 1729–37.

5 Anonymous. North American Symptomatic Carotid Endarterectomy Trial. Methods, patient characteristics, and progress. *Stroke* 1991; 22: 711–20.

6 Barnett HJ, Taylor DW, Eliasziw M *et al*. Benefit of carotid endarterectomy in patients with symptomatic moderate or severe stenosis. North American Symptomatic Carotid Endarterectomy Trial Collaborators. *N Engl J Med* 1998; 339: 1415–25.

7 Randomised trial of endarterectomy for recently symptomatic carotid stenosis: final results of the MRC European Carotid Surgery Trial (ECST). *Lancet* 1998; 351: 1379–87.

8 Mayberg MR, Wilson SE, Yatsu F *et al.* Carotid endarterectomy and prevention of cerebral ischemia in symptomatic carotid stenosis. Veterans Affairs Cooperative Studies Program 309 Trialist Group. *JAMA* 1991; 266: 3289–94.

9 Wennberg DE, Lucas FL, Birkmeyer JD *et al.* Variation in carotid endarterectomy mortality in the Medicare population: trial hospitals, volume, and patient characteristics. *JAMA* 1998; 279: 1278–81.

10 Yadav JS, Roubin GS, Iyer S *et al.* Elective stenting of the extracranial carotid arteries. *Circulation* 1997; 95: 376–81.

11 White CJ, Gomez CR, Iyer SS *et al.* Carotid stent placement for extracranial carotid artery disease: current state of the art. *Cathet Cardiovasc Interv* 2000; 51: 339–46.

12 Ouriel K, Hertzer NR, Beven EG *et al.* Preprocedural risk stratification: identifying an appropriate population for carotid stenting. *J Vasc Surg* 2001; 33: 728–32.

13 Numaguchi Y, Puyau FA, Provenza LJ, Richardson DE. Percutaneous transluminal angioplasty of the carotid artery. Its application to post surgical stenosis. *Neuroradiology* 1984; 26: 527–30.

14 Pritz MB, Smolin MF. Treatment of tandem lesions of the extracranial carotid artery. *Neurosurgery* 1984; 15: 233–6.

15 Bergeron P, Rudondy P, Benichon H *et al.* Transluminal angioplasty for recurrent stenosis after carotid endarterectomy. Prognostic factors and indications. *Int Angiol* 1993; 12: 256–9.

16 Ahuja A, Blatt GL, Guterman LR, Hopkins LN. Angioplasty for symptomatic radiation-induced extracranial carotid artery stenosis: case report. *Neurosurgery* 1995; 36: 399–403.

17 Moore WS, Barnett HJ, Beebe HG *et al.* Guidelines for carotid endarterectomy. A multidisciplinary consensus statement from the ad hoc Committee, American Heart Association. *Stroke* 1995; 26: 188–201.

18 Yadav JS, Roubin GS, King P *et al.* Angioplasty and stenting for restenosis after carotid endarterectomy. Initial experience. *Stroke* 1996; 27: 2075–9.

19 Biller J, Feinberg WM, Castaldo JE *et al.* Guidelines for carotid endarterectomy: a statement for healthcare professionals from a special writing group of the Stroke Council, American Heart Association. *Stroke* 1998; 29: 554–62.

20 Mathur A, Roubin GS, Iyer SS *et al.* Predictors of stroke complicating carotid artery stenting. *Circulation* 1998; 97: 1239–45.

21 Teitelbaum GP, Lefkowitz MA, Giannotta SL. Carotid angioplasty and stenting in high-risk patients. *Surg Neurol* 1998; 50: 300–11.

22 Lanzino G, Mericle RA, Lopes DK *et al.* Percutaneous transluminal angioplasty and stent placement for recurrent carotid artery stenosis. *J Neurosurg* 1999; 90: 688–94.

23 New G, Roubin GS, Iyer SS, Vitek JJ. Use of the glycoprotein IIb/IIIa inhibitor eptifibatide in a patient undergoing carotid artery stenting. *J Invasive Cardiol* 2000; 12 (Suppl. D): 23D–24D.

24 Dangas G, Laird JR Jr, Mehran R *et al.* Carotid artery stenting in patients with high-risk anatomy for carotid endarterectomy. *J Endovasc Ther* 2001; 8: 39–43.

25 Koenigsberg RA, Grandinetti LM, Freeman LP *et al.* Endovascular repair of radiation-induced bilateral common carotid artery stenosis and pseudoaneurysms: a case report. *Surg Neurol* 2001; 55: 347–52.

26 Lanzino G, Couture D, Andreoli A, Guterman LR, Hopkins LN. Carotid endarterectomy: can we select surgical candidates at high risk for stroke and low risk for perioperative complications? *Neurosurgery* 2001; 49: 913–23.

27 Brown MM, Butler P, Gibbs J, Swash M, Waterston J. Feasibility of percutaneous transluminal angioplasty for carotid artery stenosis. *J Neurol Neurosurg Psychiatry* 1990; 53: 238–43.

28 Gil-Peralta A, Mayol A, Marcos JR *et al.* Percutaneous transluminal angioplasty of the symptomatic atherosclerotic carotid arteries. Results, complications, and follow-up. *Stroke* 1996; 27: 2271–3.

29 Garrido E, Montoya J. Transluminal dilatation of internal carotid artery in fibromuscular dysplasia: a preliminary report. *Surg Neurol* 1981; 16: 469–71.

30 Belan A, Vesela M, Vanek I, Weiss K, Peregrin JH. Percutaneous transluminal angioplasty of fibromuscular dysplasia of the internal carotid artery. *Cardiovasc Intervent Radiol* 1982; 5: 79–81.

31 Hasso AN, Bird CR, Zinke DE, Thompson JR. Fibromuscular dysplasia of the internal carotid artery: percutaneous transluminal angioplasty. *Am J Roentgenol* 1981; 136: 955–60.

32 Higashida RT, Halbach VV, Tsai FY *et al.* Interventional neurovascular treatment of traumatic carotid and vertebral artery lesions: results in 234 cases. *Am J Roentgenol* 1989; 153: 577–82.

33 Saito R, Ezura M, Takahashi A *et al.* Combined neuroendovascular stenting and coil embolization for cervical carotid artery dissection causing symptomatic mass effect. *Surg Neurol* 2000; 53: 318–22.

34 Malek AM, Higashida RT, Phatouros CC *et al.* Stent angioplasty for cervical carotid artery stenosis in high-risk symptomatic NASCET-ineligible patients. *Stroke* 2000; 31: 3029–33.

35 Theron J, Courtheoux P, Henriet JP, Pelouze G, Derlon JM, Maiza D. Angioplasty of supraaortic arteries. *J Neuroradiol* 1984; 11: 187–200.

36 Courtheoux P, Tournade A, Theron J *et al.* Transcutaneous angioplasty of vertebral artery atheromatous ostial stricture. *Neuroradiology* 1985; 27: 259–64.

37 Higashida RT, Hieshima GB, Tsai FY, Bentson JR, Halbach VV. Percutaneous transluminal angioplasty of the subclavian and vertebral arteries. *Acta Radiol Suppl* 1986; 369: 124–6.

38 Higashida RT, Tsai FY, Halbach VV *et al.* Transluminal angioplasty for atherosclerotic disease of the vertebral and basilar arteries. *J Neurosurg* 1993; 78: 192–8.

39 Mori T, Arisawa M, Honda S, Fukuoka M, Mori K. Percutaneous transluminal angioplasty of supra-aortic arterial stenoses in patients with concomitant

cerebrovascular and coronary artery diseases—report of two cases. *Neurol Med Chir (Tokyo)* 1993; 33: 368–72.

40 Diethrich EB, Gordon MH, Lopez-Galarza LA, Rodriguez-Lopez JA, Casses F. Intraluminal Palmaz stent implantation for treatment of recurrent carotid artery occlusive disease: a plan for the future. *J Interv Cardiol* 1995; 8: 213–8.

41 Brophy DP, Hartnell GG, McEniff NJ. Percutaneous treatment of a symptomatic brachiocephalic artery stenosis with a Palmaz stent. *Cardiovasc Intervent Radiol* 1997; 20: 405–6.

42 Martinez R, Rodriguez-Lopez J, Torruella L, Ray L, Lopez-Galarza L, Diethrich EB. Stenting for occlusion of the subclavian arteries. Technical aspects and follow-up results. *Tex Heart Inst J* 1997; 24: 23–7.

43 Chastain HD 2nd, Gomez CR, Iyer S *et al.* Influence of age upon complications of carotid artery stenting. UAB Neurovascular Angioplasty Team. *J Endovasc Surg* 1999; 6: 217–22.

44 Hadjipetrou P, Cox S, Piemonte T, Eisenhauer A. Percutaneous revascularization of atherosclerotic obstruction of aortic arch vessels. *J Am Coll Cardiol* 1999; 33: 1238–45.

45 Rodriguez-Lopez JA, Werner A, Martinez R, Torruella LJ, Ray LI, Diethrich EB. Stenting for atherosclerotic occlusive disease of the subclavian artery. *Ann Vasc Surg* 1999; 13: 254–60.

46 Ruigrok Y, Cox TC, Markus HS. Positional vertebrobasilar transient ischaemic attacks treated with vertebral angioplasty. *Cerebrovasc Dis* 1999; 9: 171–4.

47 Fukuda I, Mihara W, Sasaki A, Gomi S. Percutaneous vertebral angioplasty before coronary artery bypass grafting. *Ann Thorac Surg* 2000; 69: 924–5.

48 Koenigsberg RA, Dave A, McCormick D *et al.* Complicated stent supported cerebrovascular angioplasty: case analyzes and review of literature. *Surg Neurol* 2000; 53: 465–74.

49 Phatouros CC, Higashida RT, Malek AM *et al.* Endovascular stenting for carotid artery stenosis: preliminary experience using the shape-memory-alloy-recoverable-technology (SMART) stent. *Am J Neuroradiol* 2000; 21: 732–8.

50 Piotin M, Spelle L, Martin JB *et al.* Percutaneous transluminal angioplasty and stenting of the proximal vertebral artery for symptomatic stenosis. *Am J Neuroradiol* 2000; 21: 727–31.

51 Mukherjee D, Kalahasti V, Roffi M *et al.* Self-expanding stents for carotid interventions: comparison of nitinol versus stainless-steel stents. *J Invasive Cardiol* 2001; 13: 732–5.

52 Ziada KM, Roffi M, Yadav JS. Percutaneous stenting of a vertebral artery supplying the entire brain. *Circulation* 2001; 103: E61.

53 Wiggli U, Gratzl O. Transluminal angioplasty of stenotic carotid arteries: case reports and protocol. *Am J Neuroradiol* 1983; 4: 793–5.

54 Tievsky AL, Druy EM, Mardiat JG. Transluminal angioplasty in postsurgical stenosis of the extracranial carotid artery. *Am J Neuroradiol* 1983; 4: 800–2.

55 Tsai FY, Matovich VB, Hieshima GB *et al.* Practical aspects of percutaneous transluminal angioplasty of the carotid artery. *Acta Radiol Suppl* 1986; 369: 127–30.

56 Courtheoux P, Theron J, Tournade A, Maiza D, Henriet JP, Braun JP. Percutaneous endoluminal angioplasty of post endarterectomy carotid stenoses. *Neuroradiology* 1987; 29: 186–9.

57 Theron J, Courtheoux P, Alachkar F, Bouvard G, Maiza D. New triple coaxial catheter system for carotid angioplasty with cerebral protection. *Am J Neuroradiol* 1990; 11: 869–74.

58 Phatouros CC, Higashida RT, Malek AM *et al.* Clinical use of stents for carotid artery disease. *Neurol Med Chir (Tokyo)* 1999; 39: 809–27.

59 Al-Mubarak N, Roubin GS, Iyer SS, Vitek JJ, New G. Techniques of carotid artery stenting: the state of the art. *Semin Vasc Surg* 2000; 13: 117–29.

60 Al-Mubarak N, Roubin GS, Vitek JJ, Gomez CR. Simultaneous bilateral carotid stenting for restenosis after endarterectomy. *Cathet Cardiovasc Diagn* 1998; 45: 11–5.

61 Al-Mubarak N, Roubin GS, Iyer SS, Gomez CR, Liu MW, Vitek JJ. Carotid stenting for severe radiation-induced extracranial carotid artery occlusive disease. *J Endovasc Ther* 2000; 7: 36–40.

62 Al-Mubarak N, Roubin GS, Gomez CR *et al.* Carotid artery stenting in patients with high neurologic risks. *Am J Cardiol* 1999; 83: 1411–9.

63 Al-Mubarak N, Vitek JJ, Iyer S, New G, Leon MB, Roubin GS. Embolization via collateral circulation during carotid stenting with the distal balloon protection system. *J Endovasc Ther* 2001; 8: 354–7.

64 Castriota F, Cremonesi A, el-Jamal B *et al.* The use of coronary angioplasty devices in carotid endovascular interventions: encouraging results in 21 consecutive patients. *G Ital Cardiol* 1999; 29: 391–7.

65 Diethrich EB, Marx P, Wrasper R, Reid DB. Percutaneous techniques for endoluminal carotid interventions. *J Endovasc Surg* 1996; 3: 182–202.

66 Diethrich EB, Ndiaye M, Reid DB. Stenting in the carotid artery: initial experience in 110 patients. *J Endovasc Surg* 1996; 3: 42–62.

67 Dietz A, Berkefeld J, Theron JG *et al.* Endovascular treatment of symptomatic carotid stenosis using stent placement: long-term follow-up of patients with a balanced surgical risk/benefit ratio. *Stroke* 2001; 32: 1855–9.

68 Jacksch R, Schiele TM, Knobloch W *et al.* [Carotid stenting with the new slotted tube stent—prospective multicenter study. Essen experiences]. *Z Kardiol* 2000; 89 (Suppl. 8): 40–6.

69 Jordan WD Jr, Schroeder PT, Fisher WS, McDowell HA. A comparison of angioplasty with stenting versus endarterectomy for the treatment of carotid artery stenosis. *Ann Vasc Surg* 1997; 11: 2–8.

70 Jordan WD Jr, Voellinger DC, Fisher WS *et al.* A comparison of carotid angioplasty with stenting versus endarterectomy with regional anesthesia. *J Vasc Surg* 1998; 28: 397–402.

71 Kaul U, Singh B, Bajaj R *et al.* Elective stenting of extracranial carotid arteries. *J Assoc Physicians India* 2000; 48: 196–200.

72 New G, Roubin GS, Iyer SS, Vitek JJ. Carotid artery stenting: rationale, indications, and results. *Compr Ther* 1999; 25: 438–45.

73 New G, Roubin GS, Iyer SS *et al.* Safety, efficacy, and durability of carotid artery stenting for restenosis following carotid endarterectomy: a multicenter study. *J Endovasc Ther* 2000; 7: 345–52.

74 Robbin ML, Lockhart ME, Weber TM *et al.* Carotid artery stents: early and intermediate follow-up with Doppler US. *Radiology* 1997; 205: 749–56.

75 Roubin GS, New G, Iyer SS *et al.* Immediate and late clinical outcomes of carotid artery stenting in patients with symptomatic and asymptomatic carotid artery stenosis: a 5-year prospective analysis. *Circulation* 2001; 103: 532–7.

76 Shawl FA. Carotid artery stenting: technical considerations and results. *Indian Heart J* 1998; 50 (Suppl. 1): 138–44.

77 Vitek JJ, Roubin GS, Al-Mubarek N, New G, Iyer SS. Carotid artery stenting: technical considerations. *Am J Neuroradiol* 2000; 21: 1736–43.

78 Vitek JJ, Roubin GS, New G, Al-Mubarek N, Iyer SS. Carotid angioplasty with stenting in postcarotid endarterectomy restenosis. *J Invasive Cardiol* 2001; 13: 123–5.

79 Vozzi CR, Rodriguez AO, Paolantonio D, Smith JA, Wholey MH. Extracranial carotid angioplasty and stenting. Initial results and short-term follow-up. *Tex Heart Inst J* 1997; 24: 167–72.

80 Use of a monoclonal antibody directed against the platelet glycoprotein IIb/IIIa receptor in high-risk coronary angioplasty. The EPIC Investigation. *N Engl J Med* 1994; 330: 956–61.

81 Goods CM, al-Shaibi KF, Liu MW *et al.* Comparison of aspirin alone versus aspirin plus ticlopidine after coronary artery stenting. *Am J Cardiol* 1996; 78: 1042–4.

82 Mukherjee D, Roffi M, Kapadia SR *et al.* Percutaneous intervention for symptomatic vertebral artery stenosis using coronary stents. *J Invasive Cardiol* 2001; 13: 363–6.

83 Bhatt DL, Kapadia SR, Yadav JS, Topol EJ. Update on clinical trials of antiplatelet therapy for cerebrovascular diseases. *Cerebrovasc Dis* 2000; 10 (Suppl. 5): 34–40.

84 Yadav JS. Treatment of carotid atherosclerotic disease: carotid endarterectomy or stenting? In: Veith FJ, Amor M, eds. *Current Status of Carotid Bifurcation Angioplasty and Stenting.* New York: Marcel Decker, Inc., 2000: 225–33.

85 Mathur A, Roubin GS, Yadav JS, Iyer SS, Vitek J. Combined coronary and bilateral carotid stenting: a case report. *Cathet Cardiovasc Diagn* 1997; 40: 202–6.

86 Shawl FA, Efstratiou A, Hoff S, Dougherty K. Combined percutaneous carotid stenting and coronary angioplasty during acute ischemic neurologic and coronary syndromes. *Am J Cardiol* 1996; 77: 1109–12.

87 Tong FC, Cloft HJ, Joseph GJ, Samuels OB, Dion JE. Abciximab rescue in acute carotid stent thrombosis. *Am J Neuroradiol* 2000; 21: 1750–2.

88 Qureshi AI, Suri MF, Khan J, Fessler RD, Guterman LR, Hopkins LN. Abciximab as an adjunct to high-risk carotid or vertebrobasilar angioplasty: preliminary experience. *Neurosurgery* 2000; 46: 1316–24.

89 Kapadia SR, Bajzer CT, Ziada KM *et al.* Initial experience of platelet glycoprotein IIb/IIIa inhibition with abciximab during carotid stenting: a safe and effective adjunctive therapy. *Stroke* 2001; 32: 2328–32.

90 Qureshi AI, Ali Z, Suri MF *et al.* Open-label phase I clinical study to assess the safety of intravenous eptifibatide in patients undergoing internal carotid artery angioplasty and stent placement. *Neurosurgery* 2001; 48: 998–1004.

91 Fischman DL, Leon MB, Baim DS *et al.* A randomized comparison of coronary-stent placement and balloon angioplasty in the treatment of coronary artery disease. Stent Restenosis Study Investigators. *N Engl J Med* 1994; 331: 496–501.

92 Altmann DB, Racz M, Battleman DS *et al.* Reduction in angioplasty complications after the introduction of coronary stents: results from a consecutive series of 2242 patients. *Am Heart J* 1996; 132: 503–7.

93 Bergeron P, Chambran P, Hartung O, Bianca S. Cervical carotid artery stenosis: which technique, balloon angioplasty or surgery? *J Cardiovasc Surg (Torino)* 1996; 37 (Suppl. 1): 73–5.

94 Bergeron P, Chambran P, Benichou H, Alessandri C. Recurrent carotid disease: will stents be an alternative to surgery? *J Endovasc Surg* 1996; 3: 76–9.

95 Silver MJ, Yadav JS, Wholey M. Intermediate outcome after carotid stenting: what should we expect? *Semin Vasc Surg* 2000; 13: 130–8.

96 Piotin M, Blanc R, Kothimbakam R, Martin D, Ross IB, Moret J. Primary basilar artery stenting. immediate and long-term results in one patient. *Am J Roentgenol* 2000; 175: 1367–9.

97 Kritpracha B, Beebe HG. Carotid artery stenosis: treatment by angioplasty with or without stent. *Ann Vasc Surg* 1998; 12: 621–4.

98 Qureshi AI, Luft AR, Janardhan V *et al.* Identification of patients at risk for periprocedural neurological deficits associated with carotid angioplasty and stenting. *Stroke* 2000; 31: 376–82.

99 Mathur A, Roubin GS, Gomez CR *et al.* Elective carotid artery stenting in the presence of contralateral occlusion. *Am J Cardiol* 1998; 81: 1315–7.

100 Wholey MH, Wholey M, Mathias K *et al.* Global experience in cervical carotid artery stent placement. *Catheter Cardiovasc Interv* 2000; 50: 160–7.

101 Qureshi AI, Luft AR, Sharma M *et al.* Frequency and determinants of postprocedural hemodynamic instability after carotid angioplasty and stenting. *Stroke* 1999; 30: 2086–93.

102 Benichou H, Bergeron P. Carotid angioplasty and stenting: will periprocedural transcranial Doppler monitoring be important? *J Endovasc Surg* 1996; 3: 217–23.

103 Jordan WD Jr, Voellinger DC, Doblar DD *et al.* Microemboli detected by transcranial Doppler monitoring in patients during carotid angioplasty versus carotid endarterectomy. *Cardiovasc Surg* 1999; 7: 33–8.

104 Manninen HI, Rasanen HT, Vanninen RL, Vainio P, Hippelainen M, Kosma VM. Stent placement versus percutaneous transluminal angioplasty of human carotid arteries in cadavers in situ: distal embolization and findings at intravascular US, MR imaging and histopathologic analysis. *Radiology* 1999; 212: 483–92.

105 Muller M, Reiche W, Langenscheidt P, Hassfeld J, Hagen T. Ischemia after carotid endarterectomy. comparison between transcranial Doppler sonography and diffusion-weighted MR imaging. *Am J Neuroradiol* 2000; 21: 47–54.

106 Theron J, Raymond J, Casasco A, Courtheoux F. Percutaneous angioplasty of atherosclerotic and postsurgical stenosis of carotid arteries. *Am J Neuroradiol* 1987; 8: 495–500.

107 Ohki T, Roubin GS, Veith FJ, Iyer SS, Brady E. Efficacy of a filter device in the prevention of embolic events during carotid angioplasty and stenting: An *ex vivo* analysis. *J Vasc Surg* 1999; 30: 1034–44.

108 Parodi JC, La Mura R, Ferreira LM *et al*. Initial evaluation of carotid angioplasty and stenting with three different cerebral protection devices. *J Vasc Surg* 2000; 32: 1127–36.

109 Al-Mubarak N, Roubin GS, Vitek JJ, New G, Iyer SS. Procedural safety and short-term outcome of ambulatory carotid stenting. *Stroke* 2001; 32: 2305–9.

110 Meyers PM, Higashida RT, Phatouros CC. Cerebral hyperperfusion syndrome after percutaneous transluminal stenting of the craniocervical arteries. *Neurosurgery* 2000; 47: 335–43.

111 Abou-Chebl A, Reginelli J, Bhatt D, Bajzer C, Mukherjee D, Yadov J. Intracranial hemorrhage and the hyperperfusion following internal carotid artery angioplasty and stenting. Poster presentation at American College of Cardiology Annual Scientific Session, March 20th, Atlanta, Georgia.

112 Executive Committee for Asymptomatic Carotid Atherosclerosis Study. Endarterectomy for asymptomatic carotid artery stenosis. *JAMA* 1995; 273: 1421–8.

113 Gomez CR, Orr SC. Angioplasty and stenting for primary treatment of intracranial arterial stenoses. *Arch Neurol* 2001; 58: 1687–90.

114 Chimowitz MI. Angioplasty or stenting is not appropriate as first-line treatment of intracranial stenosis. *Arch Neurol* 2001; 58: 1690–2.

115 Sacco RL, Kargman DE, Gu Q, Zamanillo MC. Race-ethnicity and determinants of intracranial atherosclerotic cerebral infarction. The Northern Manhattan Stroke Study. *Stroke* 1995; 26: 14–20.

116 Feldmann E, Daneault N, Kwan E *et al*. Chinese–white differences in the distribution of occlusive cerebrovascular disease. *Neurology* 1990; 40: 1541–5.

117 Gomez CR. Carotid angioplasty and stenting: new horizons. *Curr Atheroscler Rep* 2000; 2: 151–9.

118 Connors JJ III, Wojak JC. Percutaneous transluminal angioplasty for intracranial atherosclerotic lesions: evolution of technique and short-term results. *J Neurosurg* 1999; 91: 415–23.

119 Hass WK, Fields WS, North RR, Kircheff II, Chase NE, Bauer RB. Joint study of extracranial arterial occlusion. II. Arteriography, techniques, sites, and complications. *JAMA* 1968; 203: 961–8.

120 The EC/IC Bypass Study Group. Failure of extracranial–intracranial arterial bypass to reduce the risk of ischemic stroke. Results of an international randomized trial. *N Engl J Med* 1985; 313: 1191–200.

121 Millikan CH. *Anticoagulant Therapy in Cerebrovascular Disease.* New York: Grune & Stratton, 1965.

122 Whisnant JP, Cartlidge NE, Elveback LR. Carotid and vertebral basilar transient ischemic attacks: effect of anticoagulants, hypertension, and cardiac disorders on stroke occurrence in a community. *Trans Am Neurol Assoc* 1977; 102: 22–4.

123 Whisnant J, Matsumoto N, Elveback LR. Transient cerebral ischemic attacks in a community: Rochester, Minnesota, 1955–1969. *Mayo Clin Proc* 1973; 48: 194–8.

124 Marzewski DJ, Furlan AJ, St Louis P, Little JR, Modic MT, Williams G. Intracranial internal carotid artery stenosis: longterm prognosis. *Stroke* 1982; 13: 821–4.

125 Craig DR, Meguro K, Watridge C, Robertson JT, Barnett HJ, Fox AJ. Intracranial internal carotid artery stenosis. *Stroke* 1982; 13: 825–8.

126 Moufarrij NA, Little JR, Furlan AJ, Leatherman JR, Williams GW. Basilar and distal vertebral artery stenosis: long-term follow-up. *Stroke* 1986; 17: 938–42.

127 Moufarrij NA, Little JR, Furlan AJ, Williams G, Marzewski DJ. Vertebral artery stenosis: long-term follow-up. *Stroke* 1984; 15: 260–3.

128 Caplan L, Babikian V, Helgason C *et al.* Occlusive disease of the middle cerebral artery. *Neurology* 1985; 35: 975–82.

129 Bogousslavsky J, Barnett HJ, Fox AJ, Hachinski VC, Taylor W. Atherosclerotic disease of the middle cerebral artery. *Stroke* 1986; 17: 1112–20.

130 Chimowitz MI, Kokkinos J, Strong J *et al.* The warfarin-aspirin symptomatic intracranial disease study. *Neurology* 1995; 45: 1488–93.

131 Borozan PG, Schuler JJ, LaRosa MP, Ware MS, Flanigan DP. The natural history of isolated carotid siphon stenosis. *J Vasc Surg* 1984; 1: 744–9.

132 Wechsler LR, Kistler JP, Davis KR, Kaminski MJ. The prognosis of carotid siphon stenosis. *Stroke* 1986; 17: 714–8.

133 Hinton RC, Mohr JP, Ackerman RH, Adair LB, Fisher CM. Symptomatic middle cerebral artery stenosis. *Ann Neurol* 1979; 5: 152–7.

134 Pessin MS, Gorelick PB, Kwan ES, Caplan LR. Basilar artery stenosis: middle and distal segments. *Neurology* 1987; 37: 1742–6.

135 Thijs VN, Albers GW. Symptomatic intracranial atherosclerosis: outcome of patients who fail antithrombotic therapy. *Neurology* 2000; 55: 490–7.

136 Akins PT, Pilgram TK, Cross DT 3rd, Moran CJ. Natural history of stenosis from intracranial atherosclerosis by serial angiography. *Stroke* 1998; 29: 433–8.

137 Caplan LR. Intracranial branch atheromatous disease. A neglected, understudied, and underused concept. *Neurology* 1989; 39: 1246–50.

138 Caplan LR. Large-vessel occlusive disease of the anterior circulation. In: *Stroke: A Clinical Approach*. Boston: Butterworth-Heinemann, 1993: 195–236.

139 Chiesa R, Melissano G, Castellano R *et al*. Three dimensional time-of-flight magnetic resonance angiography in carotid artery surgery: a comparison with digital subtraction angiography. *Eur J Vasc Surg* 1993; 7: 171–6.

140 Adams HP, Gross CE. Embolism distal to stenosis of the middle cerebral artery. *Stroke* 1981; 12: 228–9.

141 Caplan LR, Hennerici M. Impaired clearance of emboli (washout) is an important link between hypoperfusion, embolism, and ischemic stroke. *Arch Neurol* 1998; 55: 1475–82.

142 Callahan AS III, Berger BL. Balloon angioplasty of intracranial arteries for stroke prevention. *J Neuroimaging* 1997; 7: 232–5.

143 Sundt TM Jr, Smith HC, Campbell JK, Vlietstra RE, Cucchiara RF, Stanson AW. Transluminal angioplasty for basilar artery stenosis. *Mayo Clin Proc* 1980; 55: 673–80.

144 Mori T, Fukuoka M, Kazita K, Mori K. Follow-up study after percutaneous transluminal cerebral angioplasty. *Eur Radiol* 1998; 8: 403–8.

145 Mori T, Kazita K, Seike M, Nojima Y, Mori K. Successful cerebral artery stent placement for total occlusion of the vertebrobasilar artery in a patient suffering from acute stroke. Case report. *J Neurosurg* 1999; 90: 955–8.

146 Gomez CR, Misra VK, Terry JB, Tulyapronchote R, Campbell MS. Emergency endovascular treatment of cerebral sinus thrombosis with a rheolytic catheter device. *J Neuroimaging* 2000; 10: 177–80.

147 Gomez CR, Misra VK, Liu MW *et al*. Elective stenting of symptomatic basilar artery stenosis. *Stroke* 2000; 31: 95–9.

148 Lanzino G, Fessler RD, Wakhloo AK, Guterman LR, Hopkins LN. Successful intracranial thrombolysis for cerebral thromboembolic complications resulting from cardiovascular diagnostic and interventional procedures. *J Invasive Cardiol* 1999; 11: 439–43.

149 Mori T, Kazita K, Chokyu K, Mima T, Mori K. Short-term arteriographic and clinical outcome after cerebral angioplasty and stenting for intracranial vertebrobasilar and carotid atherosclerotic occlusive disease. *Am J Neuroradiol* 2000; 21: 249–54.

150 Phatouros CC, Higashida RT, Malek AM. Carotid artery stent placement for atherosclerotic disease: rationale, technique, and current status. *Radiology* 2000; 217: 26–41.

151 Rasmussen PA, Perl J 2nd, Barr JD *et al*. Stent-assisted angioplasty of intracranial vertebrobasilar atherosclerosis: an initial experience. *J Neurosurg* 2000; 92: 771–8.

152 Levy EI, Horowitz MB, Koebbe CJ *et al*. Transluminal stent-assisted angiplasty of the intracranial vertebrobasilar system for medically refractory, posterior circulation ischemia: early results. *Neurosurgery* 2001; 48: 1215–21.

153 Alazzaz A, Thornton J, Aletich VA, Debrun GM, Ausman JI, Charbel F. Intracranial percutaneous transluminal angioplasty for arteriosclerotic stenosis. *Arch Neurol* 2000; 57: 1625–30.

154 O'Leary DH, Clouse ME. Percutaneous transluminal angioplasty of the cavernous carotid artery for recurrent ischemia. *Am J Neuroradiol* 1984; 5: 644–5.

155 Higashida RT, Hieshima GB, Tsai FY, Halbach VV, Norman D, Newton TH. Transluminal angioplasty of the vertebral and basilar artery. *Am J Neuroradiol* 1987; 8: 745–9.

156 Marks MP, Marcellus M, Norbash AM, Steinberg GK, Tong D, Albers GW. Outcome of angioplasty for atherosclerotic intracranial stenosis. *Stroke* 1999; 30: 1065–9.

157 Mori T, Mori K, Fukuoka M, Honda S. Percutaneous transluminal angioplasty for total occlusion of middle cerebral arteries. *Neuroradiology* 1997; 39: 71–4.

158 Mori T, Mori K, Fukuoka M, Arisawa M, Honda S. Percutaneous transluminal cerebral angioplasty: serial angiographic follow-up after successful dilatation. *Neuroradiology* 1997; 39: 111–6.

159 Ramee SR, Dawson R, McKinley KL. Provisional stenting for symptomatic intracranial stenosis using a multidisciplinary approach: acute results, unexpected benefit, and one-year outcome. *Cathet Cardiovasc Interv* 2001; 52: 457–67.

160 Malek AM, Higashida RT, Halbach VV, Phatouros CC, Meyers PM, Dowd CF. Tandem intracranial stent deployment for treatment of an iatrogenic, flow-limiting, basilar artery dissection: technical case report. *Neurosurgery* 1999; 45: 919–24.

161 Mori T, Kazita K, Mima T, Mori K. Balloon angioplasty for embolic total occlusion of the middle cerebral artery and ipsilateral carotid stenting in an acute stroke stage. *Am J Neuroradiol* 1999; 20: 1462–4.

162 Gomez CR, Misra VK, Campbell MS, Soto RD. Elective stenting of symptomatic middle cerebral artery stenosis. *Am J Neuroradiol* 2000; 21: 971–3.

163 Al-Mubarak N, Gomez CR, Vitek JJ, Roubin GS. Stenting of symptomatic stenosis of the intracranial internal carotid artery. *Am J Neuroradiol* 1998; 19: 1949–51.

164 Callahan AS 3rd, Berger BL, Beuter MJ, Devlin TG. Possible short-term amelioration of basilar plaque by high-dose atorvastatin: use of reductase inhibitors for intracranial plaque stabilization. *J Neuroimaging* 2001; 11: 202–4.

165 Dorros GJ, Cohn M, Palmer LE. Stent deployment resolves a petrous carotid artery angioplasty dissection. *Am J Neuroradiol* 1998; 19: 392–4.

166 Fessler RD, Lanzino G, Guterman LR, Miletich RS, Lopes DK, Hopkins LN. Improved cerebral perfusion after stenting of a petrous carotid stenosis: technical case report. *Neurosurgery* 1999; 45: 638–42.

167 Lanzino G, Fessler RD, Miletich RS, Guterman LR, Hopkins LN. Angioplasty and stenting of basilar artery stenosis: technical case report. *Neurosurgery* 1999; 45: 404–7.

168 Horowitz MB, Pride GL, Graybeal DF, Purdy PD. Percutaneous transluminal angioplasty and stenting of midbasilar stenoses: three technical case reports and literature review. *Neurosurgery* 1999; 45: 925–30.

169 Morris PP, Martin EM, Regan J, Braden G. Intracranial deployment of coronary stents for symptomatic atherosclerotic disease. *Am J Neuroradiol* 1999; 20: 1688–94.

170 Mori T, Kazita K, Mori K. Cerebral angioplasty and stenting for intracranial vertebral atherosclerotic stenosis. *Am J Neuroradiol* 1999; 20: 787–9.

CHAPTER 19

Cost Effectiveness Issues

Susan L. Hickenbottom

Introduction

In 1998, the American Heart Association estimated the total annual cost for stroke in the USA to be almost US $43 billion (£24 billion) [1]. This figure included US $28.3 billion (£15.9 billion) for direct costs of stroke, including costs for hospital and acute rehabilitation admission, nursing home care, physician and other health professionals' services, drugs, home healthcare and durable medical equipment; and US $16 billion (£9 billion) for indirect costs, attributable to lost patient wages and productivity. In the USA, the estimated lifetime cost for first stroke in 1990 was approximately US $100 000 (£56 200) [2]. The cost of stroke has been analyzed in many other countries [3–10], with some countries reporting annual stroke-related costs compromising up to 4% of their annual healthcare budgets [5,6].

Although these types of studies provide important information about the cost of stroke to society, they do not provide information about which treatments are most efficient in reducing overall disease burden in the setting of economic constraints [11]. In recent years, randomized controlled trials have demonstrated benefit for a multitude of medical and surgical interventions following transient ischemic attack (TIA), many of which have been outlined in previous chapters. Cost-effectiveness analysis (CEA) can provide a means to make comparisons between these interventions. In brief, CEA is a method for evaluating the health outcomes and resource costs of health interventions; the central function of CEA is to show the relative value of alternate interventions for improving health by simultaneously assessing the health effects and costs of those interventions [12,13].

This chapter will review the fundamentals of CEA and examine CEA as it has been applied to TIA and stroke.

Cost-effectiveness analysis

In 1993, the US Public Health Service convened the Panel on Cost-Effectiveness in Health and Medicine [13–16]. The panel members included

Table 19.1 Types of cost analysis

Type	Outcome measure	Example(s)
Cost-minimization	$ vs. $ (outcomes equal)	$ saved
Cost-effectiveness*	$/outcome unit	$/myocardial infarction averted
		$/ER visit avoided for asthma
Cost-utility	$/quality unit	$/quality-adjusted life-year

*Cost-effectiveness is often used as a general term to describe all types of cost analysis.
ER, emergency room.

scientists and scholars with expertise in CEA, ethics, clinical medicine, and health outcomes, who were charged with developing recommendations that would provide a framework for consistent practice in CEA.

The central measure used in CEA is the cost-effectiveness ratio [17]; implicit in the cost-effectiveness ratio is a comparison between alternatives. In general, one alternative is the intervention being studied, while the other is a suitably chosen alternative—'usual care', another intervention or no intervention. The cost-effectiveness ratio is calculated using the following equation:

(Cost 2 – Cost 1)/(Outcome 2 – Outcome 1)

Thus, CEA always provides a relative comparison between two alternatives. The costs included in the numerator are easy to understand; they are the costs of the comparative interventions being evaluated. Outcomes in the denominator of the cost-effectiveness ratio can be defined in various ways, which results in different types of cost-effectiveness analysis [18]. The different types of CEA are summarized in Table 19.1. Cost-minimization analysis is a form of CEA in which the effectiveness of the studied intervention and its comparison are presumed to be equal. In this case, the decision revolves only around cost. In a specific cost-effectiveness analysis, health outcomes units are used in the denominator of the cost-effectiveness ratio. Health outcomes units can include intermediate outcomes, such as disability days averted or number of myocardial infarctions averted, or more distal outcomes, such as lives saved or life years gained. In cost-utility analysis [19], a preference-based system is used, and the outcome measure included in the denominator is most often the quality-adjusted life years (QALYs). The QALY (or other analogous measure) is the most comprehensive measure of outcome used in CEA, as it incorporates both quality and survival information, and it is the preferred outcome measure for CEA [13,14]. Several studies have established patient-based preferences for health states relating to stroke and TIA, allowing for the assignment of QALYs

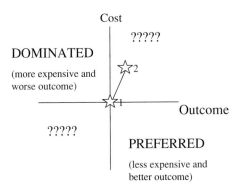

Fig. 19.1 Graphic representation of cost-effectiveness ratios. In this diagram, intervention 2 is the intervention under study and intervention 1 is the alternative (e.g. usual care). Cost of the intervention is represented on the ordinate and the health outcome measure (e.g. myocardial infarctions averted, quality-adjusted life year, etc.) is represented on the abscissa. Interventions with cost-effectiveness ratios falling in the upper left quadrant would be more expensive and less effective than the alternative and thus dominated by the alternative; in the right lower quadrant, they would be less expensive and more effective than the alternative and be dominant, or preferred, over the alternative. In the example shown above, the intervention under study is more expensive and more effective than the alternative. The slope of the line between the two interventions would represent the cost-effectiveness ratio.

for these conditions [20–22]. It should be noted that the term 'cost-effectiveness analysis' is often used to refer to any cost analysis study; this more general usage will be employed in this chapter unless otherwise specified.

Essentially, the cost-effectiveness ratio is the incremental price of obtaining a unit effect (such as dollars per QALY) from a given health intervention when compared with an alternative. When the intervention under study is both less costly and more effective than the alternative, it is described as 'preferred' or said to 'dominate' the alternative (see Fig. 19.1) On the other hand, if the intervention under study is more costly and less effective than the alternative, it is said to be 'dominated' by the alternative. In either of these cases, there would be no need to perform a CEA as the decision about which intervention to choose would be obvious. In general, CEA is most often performed in the circumstances under which the intervention is both more costly and more effective than the alternative, and occasionally when it is less costly and minimally less effective than the alternative. Interventions with a relatively low cost-effectiveness ratio are 'good buys' and would have a high priority for resources [17]. An arbitrary cut-off may be set to delineate what is considered a 'good buy', or cost-effective intervention. For example, most authors consider a

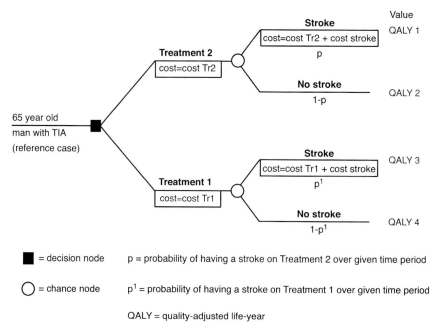

Fig. 19.2 Simplified decision tree for cost-effective analysis.

cost-effectiveness ratio of less than US \$50 000 to \$100 000 (£28 000 to £56 000) per QALY to be cost-effective [11]. The results of a CEA are generated by computer simulation, using decision tree modelling.

A simplified decision model is presented in Fig. 19.2. First, for the question to be answered, the reference case is established for the analysis, for example a 65-year-old man with TIA. For that reference case, probabilities for stroke, complication rates and other pertinent data are gathered from the literature for use in the decision model. A single decision node, represented by the solid square, begins the analysis: to treat with Treatment 2, the intervention under study, or Treatment 1, which could represent no treatment, or treatment with another agent/procedure, often the 'standard of care'. Costs for these treatments are gathered from the literature. More complex models could include more than two options at the decision node, and could also incorporate costs of diagnostic testing and potential complications associated with the treatment options.

The consequences following the decision node could be 'stroke' or 'no stroke', and probabilities for each of these occurring over the course of a set time period, often 1 year, are derived from the literature and incorporated into the chance nodes, represented by the circles. Probabilities at each chance node always sum to 1. The model can then cycle through multiple years, or even for the duration of a patient's life if life table data are incorporated into the model. When the model has been run for the desired time period, cost estimates are produced for each arm of each chance node. Each outcome (e.g. in this model, stroke with Treatment 2, no stroke with Treatment 2, etc.) is then assigned a value based on data from the literature. Using all these data, the model is able to calculate cost-effectiveness ratios for each arm of each chance node, and thereby select the most cost-effective intervention. In order to calculate cost-effectiveness ratios over a broad range of potential costs or probabilities, sensitivity analysis can be performed. In sensitivity analysis, the cost of a treatment such as warfarin, the probability of an outcome such as a stroke, or the probability of a complication such as intracerebral hemorrhage, can be varied across a wide range of potential values and all these values can be incorporated into the model, even simultaneously in very complex models.

Finally, the Panel on Cost-Effectiveness in Health and Medicine established recommendations for the methodological design and reporting of CEA [13–15]. These include establishing a reference case, which includes basic demographic data about the theoretical cohort to be evaluated along with assumptions that the model will make. It was also recommended that CEA studies be performed from the societal perspective, rather than from payor, provider, governmental, individual or other perspectives. While studies performed using one of these alternative perspectives may be appropriate to inform decisions from those particular perspectives, studies based on different perspectives are not comparable. Thus a societal perspective allows for comparisons across interventions and patient groups. In addition, the societal perspective represents the public interest rather than any specific group and allows for maximizing social good under resource constraint. Other recommendations from the panel included what costs should be included in the numerator and denominator of the cost-effectiveness ratio, how to incorporate time preferences and discounting, and handling of uncertainty in CEA. Interested readers are referred to more detailed texts for further discussion of these issues and CEA in general [13–16,23].

Cost-effectiveness studies examining TIA and stroke

While the specific focus of this text is TIA, few CEA studies address TIA specifically. Data from CEA studies specifically using TIA as the reference case will be discussed below where available. Otherwise, results from CEA studies using stroke alone or a combination of stroke and TIA as the reference case will be discussed, with the caveat that the results may not be entirely applicable to the specific population of only TIA patients.

A recent systematic review by Holloway *et al.* summarizes the cost-effectiveness of stroke-related diagnostic, preventive and therapeutic interventions published in 1998 or earlier [11]. This review identified 26 articles that met rigorous inclusion criteria for CEA, including comparison between at least two competing strategies, providing an incremental analysis of cost per effect, and using QALYs as the measured health effect. The review did not include studies that evaluated primary prevention strategies of antihypertensive or lipid-lowering therapy, as systematic reviews of those topics had been previously published, though not specific to stroke prevention [24,25]. Some of the interventions examined in the review are outside the scope of this text, for example, interventions for cerebral aneurysms and subarachnoid hemorrhage [26–34], thrombolytic therapy for acute ischemic stroke [21], screening and management strategies for asymptomatic carotid stenosis [35–39], and postoperative surveillance after endarterectomy [40]. The remaining studies will be discussed below, along with appropriate CEA studies published since the 1999 review.

Antiplatelet therapy for secondary stroke prevention

Three CEA studies regarding the use of antiplatelet therapy for secondary stroke prevention following TIA or stroke have been published [41–43]. One of these studies [43] had methodological flaws, including failure to define the reference case; using the payor perspective; and using 'strokes averted' as its outcome measure (as used in cost-effectiveness analysis), but then applying ratio cut-offs for QALYs (as used in cost-utility analysis) to its outcomes. Thus, this study is excluded from further discussion. The results of the two remaining studies are presented in Table 19.2. The first, a 1994 study [41], compared ticlopidine, 250 mg twice daily, with aspirin, 650 mg twice daily, in a theoretical cohort of 100 high-risk, 65-year-old men and women with recent TIA, transient monocular blindness or minor stroke, followed for 5 years. Much of the ticlopidine data used in the trial

Table 19.2 Cost-effectiveness of antiplatelet therapy

Author	Intervention(s)	Alternative	Reference case	Cost/QALY, $ (£)
Oster [41]	Ticlopidine 250 mg BID	ASA 650 mg BID	65-year-old with recent cerebrovascular event	39 900 (22 400)
Sarasin [42]	ASA 25 mg/ER-DP 200 mg BID Clopidogrel 75 mg QD	ASA 325 mg QD	65-year-old with stroke or TIA	ASA/ER-DP dominates 25 580 (14 360)

ASA, Aspirin; BID, twice daily; DP, dipyridamole; ER, emergency room; QALY, quality-adjusted life year; QD, once daily.

were obtained from the Ticlopidine-Aspirin Stroke Study [44]. The study found that the cost-effectiveness of ticlopidine compared with aspirin ranged from US $31 000 to $55 000 (£17 000 to £31 000) per QALY gained, with the assumption that poststroke utility, or the value assigned to life poststroke, ranged from 0.75 to 0.95, compared with 1.0 for a 'stroke-free' life. At the midpoint of this range, cost per QALY gained was US $39 900 (£22 378). If poststroke utility were lower, e.g. if quality of life poststroke were assessed to be only 0.5 (50%) of prestroke quality of life, the use of ticlopidine would have been even more cost effective.

A 1999 study examined the cost-effectiveness of secondary stroke prevention with three different antiplatelet regimens: aspirin, 325 mg daily; low-dose aspirin, 25 mg twice daily, in combination with extended-release dipyridamole (ER-DP), 200 mg twice daily; and clopidogrel, 75 mg daily [42]. Ticlopidine was not included in the analysis because it was thought likely to be replaced in clinical practice by clopidogrel because of its better hematological tolerance. The reference case for this study was a hypothetical cohort of men and women aged 65 years who had experienced a TIA or nondisabling stroke, and who were followed until death. As in the ticlopidine study above, most of the data for the aspirin/ER-DP and clopidogrel interventions came from single studies: the European Stroke Prevention Study 2 (ESPS-2) [45] and Clopidogrel vs. Aspirin in Patients at Risk of Ischemic Events (CAPRIE) [46] trials, respectively. This CEA study found that treatment with the aspirin/ER-DP combination was both more effective and less costly compared with aspirin alone; thus it was found to be a dominant strategy. The incremental costs incurred by the combination regimen were more than offset by the savings afforded through the avoidance of additional stroke-related costs. Furthermore, only when the additional efficacy of aspirin/ER-DP in preventing both stroke and myocardial infarction was decreased by 50%, or when the cost of therapy was doubled, did this strategy become more costly than aspirin alone. Even then, the cost-effectiveness ratio remained below US $5000 (£2800) per QALY gained. Clopdiogrel was found to be both more costly and more effective than aspirin alone, with a marginal cost effectiveness ratio of US $26 580 (£14 910) per QALY gained. The results of this analysis were sensitive to the efficacy and costs of clopidogrel. The cost-effectiveness ratio exceeded US $50 000 (£28 000) per QALY if the efficacy in preventing recurrent stroke was decreased by half or if the cost of clopidogrel was doubled. The authors concluded that the use of clopidogrel for secondary stroke prevention was cost-effective compared with aspirin in most clinical settings. As there have been no head-to-head clinical trials evaluating the combination of aspirin and ER-DP against clopidogrel for secondary stroke prevention, no direct comparison can be made regarding the cost-effectiveness of these agents compared with each other.

Antithrombotic therapy for atrial fibrillation

Four CEA studies have addressed the issue of anticoagulation in the setting of atrial fibrillation (AF): two in patient cohorts with chronic nonvalvular AF (NVAF) [47,48], one in those with mitral stenosis and AF [49], and one which expanded upon an earlier study using a patient preference-based analysis [50]. Each of these studies analyzed models for primary stroke prevention in the setting of AF, although several did stratify risk for stroke based partly on history of previous stroke or TIA [47,50]. None included analysis specifically for TIA alone; results from these studies are included in this text for completeness, and with the assumption that the results could be generalized to the population of AF patients with a history of stroke or TIA since those patients would be at higher risk of stroke recurrence [51], making any intervention more likely to be cost effective.

The first of the NVAF studies [47] analyzed the reference case of 65-year-old patients considered 'good' candidates for treatment with either warfarin or aspirin, and compared these interventions with the alternative of no therapy, over a 10-year period. Patients were stratified to high risk (NVAF and at least two additional risk factors of stroke, TIA, hypertension, diabetes, or heart disease), moderate risk (NVAF and one additional risk factor), or low risk (no additional risk factors). For high-risk patients, warfarin therapy dominated both aspirin and no treatment, as it was less expensive and more effective than either alternative, even when additional costs for warfarin monitoring and warfarin-induced hemorrhages were included. For moderate-risk patients, warfarin was more cost effective than aspirin, with a cost-effectiveness ratio of US $8000 (£4488)/ QALY gained [range US $200–30 000 (£112–16 800)/QALY gained], and both warfarin and aspirin dominated no treatment. For low-risk patients, warfarin cost US $370 000 (£208 000) per QALY gained compared with aspirin, making aspirin the more cost-effective intervention if a US $100 000 (£56 000) per QALY cut-off were used [11]. However, this analysis was especially sensitive to the recurrent stroke risk for low-risk patients; if the annual rate of stroke were 0.5% higher, warfarin treatment would cost US $66 000 (£37 000) per QALY gained and if the annual rate were 0.5% lower, aspirin would dominate warfarin. The second NVAF study [48] included patients up to the age of 75 in the reference case and compared warfarin with no therapy. This study also found that warfarin dominated no therapy, even with the inclusion of an older reference cohort likely to have higher rates of hemorrhagic complications [52,53].

The study examining rheumatic AF [49] used a reference case of a 35-year-old woman with mitral stenosis and AF, comparing warfarin intervention with the alternative of no therapy, for the duration of the patient's life. In this case, warfarin was found to be a cost-effective therapy, with a cost-effectiveness ratio of US $3700 (£2075) per QALY gained. Finally, the design of the patient preference-based study [50] was slightly different from those discussed above. It built on a previous study by the same authors [47] but used preferences for therapy (warfarin, aspirin, or no therapy) elicited from volunteers with AF [54,55], comparing preference-based therapy with a warfarin-for-all strategy. For high-risk patients with AF, preference-based therapy increased costs and did not improve quality-adjusted survival; thus the warfarin-for-all strategy was considered superior. For moderate and low-risk patients with AF, however, there was a marginal increase in projected quality-adjusted survival and minimal cost savings, leading the authors to recommend that patient preferences for antithrombotic therapy be taken into account for these patients.

Echocardiographic evaluation for cardiac sources of emboli

In 1997, a complex study was performed to examine the cost effectiveness of different diagnostic strategies for cardiac imaging, with the reference case of a 65-year-old patient not on any antithrombotic therapy, in normal sinus rhythm, and with a new-onset first stroke [56]. This study did not specifically include TIA patients. Nine different diagnostic strategies were examined: transthoracic echocardiography (TTE) either in all patients or in a selective population of those with a history of cardiac problems (left ventricular dysfunction or valvular disease); transesophageal echocardiography (TEE) either in all patients or in the above selective population; sequential TTE followed by TEE in patients with a negative TTE in all patients or in the selective population; treating all patients with warfarin without cardiac imaging; and treating no one with warfarin without imaging. Using visualized left atrial thrombus as the only indication for anticoagulation, TEE performed only in patients with a history of cardiac problems cost US $9000 (£5050) per QALY gained. TEE in all patients cost US $13 000 (£7293) per QALY. TTE, either alone or in sequence with TEE, was not cost-effective compared with TEE strategies. The analysis was most sensitive to efficacy of anticoagulation in preventing second stroke and to incidence of intracranial hemorrhage. While the model was reported to be only mildly sensitive to the cost of TEE, it should be noted that only professional and technical costs for echocardiography were included in the analysis. The impact of delay in performing TEE leading to increased length of stay for hospitalized patients was not evaluated; this situation can certainly arise in current medical practice and could affect the cost effectiveness of a TEE imaging strategy.

Carotid endarterectomy

There is conclusive evidence from large randomized trials that carotid endarterectomy (CE) reduces the risk of stroke in symptomatic patients

Table 19.3 Cost-effectiveness of carotid endarterectomy

Author	Alternative(s)	Reference case	Cost/QALY, $ (£)
Kuntz [61]	ASA/best medical therapy	65-year-old-man with angiographically confirmed 70–99% carotid stenosis	4100 (2300)
Nussbaum [62]	ASA	65-year-old-man or woman with TIA with 70–99% carotid stenosis, currently 'well'	Endarterectomy dominates
Matchar [63]	No work-up	65-year-old-man with symptomatic carotid stenosis	38 955 (21 869)

with moderate to severe stenosis of the internal carotid artery [57–59]. Cost effectiveness of CE has also been widely evaluated [60]; as noted in the introductory paragraph of this section, this chapter will focus only on those studies evaluating CE for symptomatic patients (those presenting with TIA or nondisabling stroke). Three studies meet these criteria and are summarized in Table 19.3 [61–63].

The first of these studies [61] evaluated a theoretical cohort of 65-year-old men with angiographically confirmed asymptomatic 60–99% carotid stenosis or symptomatic (TIA or stroke not specified) 70–99% carotid stenosis. For the symptomatic patients, CE was found to be very cost effective compared with best medical management as outlined in the North American Symptomatic Carotid Endarterectomy Trial (NASCET), [57] with a cost-effectiveness ratio of US $4100 (£2300) per QALY gained. The analysis for symptomatic patients was not very sensitive to wide variations in baseline assumptions, including age of patient, cost of CE, persistence of CE benefit, surgical risk reduction, and perioperative stroke risk. For example, even with a perioperative stroke risk as high as 17.4%, the incremental cost-effectiveness ratio was still < US $50 000 (< £28 000) per QALY gained. The second study examined 65-year-old men or women with a prior TIA, presently 'well', with 70–99% carotid stenosis. In the analysis, CE was compared with the alternatives of aspirin therapy or observation alone. CE dominated both these alternative strategies, and as with the first study [61], this model was insensitive to variations in the baseline assumptions, confirming the cost effectiveness of CE in a variety of clinical settings. The third study [63] analyzed a cohort of 65-year-old men with either asymptomatic or symptomatic (TIA or stroke not specified) carotid stenosis, comparing CE with no work-up or treatment. This study also confirmed the cost effectiveness of CE in symptomatic patients, with a cost-effectiveness ratio of US $38 955 (£21 846) per QALY gained. This model was also insensitive to variations in its baseline assumptions.

Two of the three studies evaluating CE outlined above begin assessing costs only at the time of surgery on an already defined operable carotid lesion and do not include costs associated with work-up strategies, [61,62] which may falsely elevate the cost effectiveness of the procedure. However, the one study that does include costs for screening/work-up still finds CE to be cost effective [63]. A final study specifically addresses the cost effectiveness of perioperative imaging strategies for symptomatic carotid stenosis [64]. This study examined four different diagnostic imaging strategies for a hypothetical cohort of symptomatic patients (stroke or TIA not specified) undergoing preoperative evaluation for CE: duplex sonagraphy (DS), magnetic resonance angiography (MRA), conventional angiography (CA), and the combination of DS and MRA supplemented with CA for disparate results (combination strategy). For purposes of analysis, all patients found to have a 70–99% stenosis were managed surgically, while those with 0–69% stenosis or arterial occlusion were managed with best medical therapy as outlined in NASCET [57]. After incorporating costs of testing, surgery, complications and stroke, MRA was not found to be cost effective, as this strategy was dominated by DS. CA was only marginally cost effective with a cost-effectiveness ratio of US $99 800 (£55 971) per QALY gained compared with DS. However, when the diagnostic ability of DS to detect 70–99% carotid stenosis was decreased to a moderately poor level, CA was associated with a favorable cost-effectiveness ratio. For example, if the sensitivity and specificity of DS were reduced to 0.8, CA cost US $32 700 (£18 340) per QALY gained. Analysis for CA was also sensitive to the cost of CA. The combination strategy was found to be cost effective, costing US $22 400 (£12 563) per QALY gained compared with DS alone. The analysis for the combination strategy was most sensitive to the cost of MRA, but even when the cost of MRA increased to US $1000 (£561) (90th percentile cost), the cost-effectiveness ratio for the combination strategy increased only to US $42 000 (£23 555) per QALY gained.

Other interventions

Recent attempts have been made to begin to define the cost effectiveness of diagnostic testing for coagulopathies in patients with ischemic stroke, especially young patients [65–67]. To date, no formal CEA has been performed to evaluate serologic work-up for 'stroke in the young'; current studies indicate that the pretest probability of detecting a coagulopathy is low in the general stroke population, approximately 5% [65,66]. Diagnostic yield of coagulation tests may be increased by using tests with the highest specificities and by targeting patients with clinical or historical features that increase pretest probability, which is postulated to lead to associated cost savings [65].

Diagnosis and management of TIA

While specific guidelines have been developed for the diagnosis and management of patients with TIA, none has included recommendations about hospital admission for evaluation of these patients [68]. Thus, there is currently no 'standard practice' for the evaluation of patients with TIA, although many in the stroke field believe that hospitalization for expedited evaluation would be best. Unfortunately, no CEA studies have been performed to determine the cost effectiveness of differing evaluation strategies for the diagnosis and treatment of TIA (hospital admission, evaluation in an observation unit, outpatient work-up following an emergency department visit, etc.) A 1992 British editorial discusses the issue of the cost-effective TIA work-up, but the authors admit that formal CEA was not performed [69].

A recent study on the short-term prognosis after emergency department diagnosis of TIA may help to set the stage for such an analysis [70]. This study retrospectively examined a cohort of 1707 patients diagnosed with TIA in 16 emergency departments in the Kaiser-Permanente health system in northern California from March 1997 to February 1998. During the 90 days after index TIA, the risk of stroke and other events, including recurrent TIA, death and hospitalization for cardiovascular event was assessed. Strokes occurred in 180 patients (10.5%) within 90 days of TIA presentation, and half of those (91) occurred within 48 h. Strokes were fatal in 38 patients (21%) and disabling in another 115 (64%). Five factors were independently associated with stroke: age over 60 years, a history of diabetes, symptom duration > 10 min, and symptom presentation of weakness or speech impairment. A total of 428 patients (25.1%) had some adverse event (stroke, TIA, death or cardiovascular event) within 90 days. The authors concluded that TIAs are ominous, carrying a substantial short-term risk of stroke and other adverse events.

The determination of short-term prognosis following TIA is an important first step analysing the cost effectiveness of various management strategies for TIA. These data can be used to predict probabilities of stroke or other adverse events in decision analysis. However, more investigation will need to be done into the short-term, early efficacy of diagnostic and management strategies in preventing early recurrent TIA or stroke (expedited carotid and cardiac evaluation, early initiation of antithrombotic or other therapies) before formal cost-effectiveness analysis can be appropriately performed.

Conclusion

Cost-effectiveness analysis is a rapidly growing and potentially useful addition to the medical literature, although its use in the fields of neurology in general and stroke specifically lags behind other areas. Where reliable data are available, CEA can provide valuable information to healthcare organizations and individual practitioners involved in complex decision making in the face of limited resources. Further CEA studies regarding stroke should be undertaken to assist in these decision-making processes.

References

1 American Heart Association (AHA). *1998 Heart and Stroke Statistical Update.* Dallas: AHA, 1998.
2 Taylor TN, Davis PH, Torner JC, Holmes J, Meyer JW, Jacobson MF. Lifetime cost of stroke in the United States. *Stroke* 1996; 27: 1459–66.
3 Smurawska LT, Alexandrov AV, Bladin CF, Norris JW. Cost of acute stroke care in Toronto, Canada. *Stroke* 1994; 25: 1628–31.
4 Terent A, Mrke L, Asplund K, Norrving B, Jonsson E, Wester P. Cost of stroke in Sweden: a national perspective. *Stroke* 1994; 25: 2363–9.
5 Isard P, Forbes J. The cost of stroke to the National Health Service in Scotland. *Cerebrovasc Dis* 1992; 2: 47–50.
6 Haidinger G, Waldhoer T, Tuomilehto J, Vutuc C. Assessment of cost related to hospitalization of stroke patients in Austria for 1992 and prospective costs for the year 2010. *Cerebrovasc Dis* 1997; 7: 163–7.
7 Scott WG. Ischaemic stroke in New Zealand: an economic study. *NZ Med J* 1994; 107: 443–6.
8 Currie CJ, Morgan CL, Gill L, Stott NCH, Peters JR. Epidemiology and costs of acute hospital care for cerebrovascular disease in diabetic and nondiabetic populations. *Stroke* 1997; 28: 1142–6.
9 Jorgensen HS, Nakayama H, Raaschou HO, Olsen TS. Acute stroke care and rehabilitation: an analysis of the direct cost and its clinical and social determinants. *Stroke* 1997; 28: 1138–41.
10 Evers S, Engel G, Arment A. Cost of stroke in the Netherlands from a societal perspective. *Stroke* 1997; 28: 1375–81.
11 Holloway RG, Benesch CG, Rahilly CR, Courtright CE. A systematic review of cost-effectiveness research of stroke evaluation and treatment. *Stroke* 1999; 30: 1340–9.
12 Russell LB, Siegel JE, Daniels N, Gold MR, Luce BR, Mandelblatt JS. Cost-effectiveness analysis as a guide to resource allocation in health: roles and limitations. In: Gold MR, Siegel JE, Russell LB, Weinstein MC, eds. *Cost-Effectiveness in Health and Medicine.* New York: Oxford University Press, 1996: 3–24.
13 Russell LB, Gold MR, Siegel JE, Daniels N, Weinstein MC for the Panel on Cost-Effectiveness in Health and Medicine. The role of cost-effectiveness analysis in health and medicine. *JAMA* 1996; 276: 1172–7.
14 Weinstein MC, Siegel JE, Gold MR, Kamlet MS, Russell LB for the Panel on Cost-Effectiveness in Health and Medicine. Recommendations of the Panel on Cost-Effectiveness in Health and Medicine. *JAMA* 1996; 276: 1253–8.

15 Siegel JE, Weinstein MC, Russell LB, Gold MR for the Panel on Cost-Effectiveness in Health and Medicine. Recommendation for reporting cost-effectiveness analyzes. *JAMA* 1996; 276: 1339–41.

16 Gold MR, Siegel JE, Russell LB, Weinstein MC, eds. *Cost-Effectiveness in Health and Medicine*. New York: Oxford University Press, 1996.

17 Garber AM, Weinstein MC, Torrance GW, Kamlet MS. Theoretical foundations of cost-effectiveness analysis. In: Gold MR, Siegel JE, Russell LB, Weinstein MC, eds. *Cost-Effectiveness in Health and Medicine*. New York: Oxford University Press, 1996: 25–53.

18 Torrance GW, Siegel JE, Luce BR. Framing and designing the cost-effectiveness analysis. In: Gold MR, Siegel JE, Russell LB, Weinstein MC, eds. *Cost-Effectiveness in Health and Medicine*. New York: Oxford University Press, 1996: 54–81.

19 Torrance GW. Designing and conducting cost-utility analyzes. In: Spilker B, ed. *Quality of Life and Pharmacoeconomics in Clinical Trials*. Philadelphia: Lippincott-Raven, 1995: 1105–11.

20 Matchar DB, Samsa GP, Mattthews JR *et al.* The stroke prevention policy model: linking evidence and clinical decisions. *Ann Intern Med* 1997; 127 (8S): 704–11.

21 Fagan SC, Morgenstern LB, Petitta A *et al.* and the NINDS rt-PA Stroke Study Group. Cost-effectiveness of tissue plasminogen activator for acute ischemic stroke. *Neurology* 1998; 50: 883–90.

22 Post PN, Stiggelbout AM, Wakker PP. The utility of health states after stroke. A systematic review of the literature. *Stroke* 2001; 32: 1425–9.

23 Matchar DB. The value of stroke prevention and treatment. *Neurology* 1998; 51 (Suppl. 3): S31–S35.

24 Johannesson M, Jonsson B. Cost-effectiveness analysis of hypertension treatment: a review of methodological issues. *Health Policy* 1991; 19: 55–78.

25 Morris S, McGuire A, Caro J, Pettitt D. Strategies for the management of hypercholesterolemia: a systematic review of the cost-effectiveness literature. *J Health Services Res Policy* 1997; 2: 231–50.

26 King JT, Glick HA, Mason TJ, Flamm ES. Elective surgery for asymptomatic, unruptured, intracranial aneurysms: a cost-effectiveness analysis. *J Neurosurg* 1995; 83: 403–12.

27 Kallmes DF, Kallmes MH, Cloft HJ, Dion JE. Guglielmi detachable coil embolization for unruptured aneurysms in nonsurgical candidates: a cost-effectiveness analysis. *Am J Neuroradiol* 1998; 19: 167–76.

28 Gatetani P, Rodriguez Y, Baena R, Klersy C, Adinolfi D, Infuso L. A cost-effectiveness analysis on different surgical strategies for intracranial aneurysms. *J Neurosurg Sci* 1998; 42: 69–78.

29 Glick H. Economic analysis of tirilizad mesylate for aneurysmal subarachnoid hemorrhage: economic evaluation of a phase 3 clinical trial in Europe and Australia. *Int J Technol Assess Health Care* 1998; 14: 145–60.

30 Kallmes DF. Cost-effectiveness of angiography performed during surgery for ruptured intracranial aneurysms. *Am J Neuroradiol* 1997; 18: 1453–62.

31 Kalmess DF. Routine angiography after surgery for ruptured intracranial aneurysms: a cost versus benefit analysis. *Neurosurgery* 1997; 41: 629–41.

32 Nussbaum ES, Heros RC, Camarata PJ. Surgical treatment arteriovenous malformations with an analysis of cost-effectiveness. *Clin Neurosurg* 1995; 42: 348–69.

33 Porter PJ, Shin AY, Detsky AS, Lefaive L, Wallace MC. Surgery versus stereotactic radiosurgery for small, operable cerebral arteriovenous malformations: a clinical and cost comparison. *Neurosurgery* 1997; 41: 757–66.

34 Jordan JE, Marks MP, Lane B, Steinberg GK. Cost-effectiveness of endovascular therapy in the surgical management of cerebral arteriovenous malformations. *Am J Neuroradiol* 1996; 17: 247–54.

35 Cronenwett JL, Birkmeyer JD, Nackman GB *et al.* Cost-effectiveness of carotid endarterectomy in asymptomatic patients. *J Vasc Surg* 1997; 25: 298–311.

36 Derdeyn CP, Powers WJ. Cost-effectiveness of screening for asymptomatic carotid atherosclerotic disease. *Stroke* 1996; 27: 1944–50.

37 Lee TT, Solomon NA, Heidenreich PA, Oehlert J, Garber AM. Cost-effectiveness of screening for carotid stenosis in asymptomatic patients. *Ann Intern Med* 1997; 126: 337–46.

38 Obuchowski NA, Modic MT, Magdinec M, Masaryk TJ. Assessment of the efficacy of noninvasive screening for patients with asymptomatic neck bruits. *Stroke* 1997; 28: 1330–9.

39 Yin D, Carpenter JP. Cost-effectiveness of screening for asymptomatic carotid stenosis. *J Vasc Surg* 1998; 27: 245–55.

40 Patel ST, Kuntz KM, Kent KC. Is the routine duplex ultrasound surveillance after carotid endarterectomy cost-effective? *Surgery* 1998; 124: 343–52.

41 Oster G, Huse DM, Lacey MJ, Epstein AM. Cost-effectiveness of ticlopidine in preventing stroke in high-risk patients. *Stroke* 1994; 25: 1149–56.

42 Sarasin FP, Gaspoz JM, Bounameaux H. Cost-effectiveness of new antiplatelet regimens used as secondary prevention of stroke or transient ischemic attack. *Arch Intern Med* 2000; 160: 2773–8.

43 Shah H, Gondek K. Aspirin plus extended-release dipyridamole or clopidogrel compared with aspirin monotherapy for the prevention of recurrent ischemic stroke: a cost-effectiveness analysis. *Clin Ther* 2000; 22: 362–70.

44 Hass WK, Easton JD, Adams HP *et al.* for the Ticlopidine Aspirin Stroke Study Group. A randomized trial comparing ticlopidine hydrochloride with aspirin for the prevention of stroke in high-risk paitents. *N Engl J Med* 1989; 321: 501–7.

45 Diener HC, Cuhna L, Forbes C, Sivenius J, Smets P, Lowenthal A. European Stroke Prevention Study 2: dipyridamole and acetylsalicylic acid in the secondary prevention of stroke. *J Neurol Sci* 1996; 143: 1–13.

46 CAPRIE Steering Committee. A randomised, blinded trial of clopidogrel versus aspirin in patients at risk of ischaemic events (CAPRIE). *Lancet* 1996; 348: 1329–39.

47 Gage BF, Cardinalli AB, Albers GW, Owens DK. Cost-effectiveness of warfarin and aspirin for prophylaxis of stroke in patients with nonvalvular atrial fibrillation. *JAMA* 1995; 274: 1839–45.

48 Lightowlers S, McGuire A. Cost-effectiveness of anticoagulation in nonrheumatic atrial fibrillation in the primary prevention of ischemic stroke. *Stroke* 1998; 29: 1827–32.

49 Eckman MH, Levine HJ, Pauker SG. Decision analytic and cost-effectiveness issues concerning anticoagulant prophylaxis in heart disease. *Chest* 1992; 102 (Suppl.): 538S–549S.

50 Gage BF, Cardinalli AB, Owens DK. Cost-effectiveness of preference-based antithrombotic therapy for patients with nonvalvular atrial fibrillation. *Stroke* 1998; 29: 1083–91.

51 EAFT Study Group. Secondary prevention in nonrheumatic atrial fibrillation after transient ischaemic attack or minor stroke. *Lancet* 1993; 342: 1255–62.

52 Hylek EM, Singer DE. Risk factors for intracranial hemorrhage in outpatients taking warfarin. *Ann Intern Med* 1994; 120: 897–902.

53 van der Meer FJM, Rosendall FR, Vandenbroucke JP, Briet E. Bleeding complications on oral anticoagulant therapy: an analysis of risk factors. *Arch Intern Med* 1993; 153: 1557–62.

54 Gage BF, Cardinalli AB, Owens DK. The effect of stroke and stroke prophylaxis with aspirin or warfarin on quality of life. *Arch Intern Med* 1996; 156: 1829–36.

55 Nease RF, Owens DK. A method for estimating the cost-effectiveness of incorporating patient preferences into practice guidelines. *Med Decis Making* 1994; 14: 382–92.

56 McNamara RL, Lima JAC, Whelton PK, Powe NR. Echocardiographic identification of cardiovascular sources of emboli to guide clinical management of stroke: a cost-effectiveness analysis. *Ann Intern Med* 1997; 127: 775–87.

57 North American Symptomatic Carotid Endarterectomy Trial Collaborators. Beneficial effect of carotid endarterectomy in symptomatic patients with high-grade carotid stenosis. *N Engl J Med* 1991; 325: 445–53.

58 Barnett HJM, Taylor DW, Eliasziw M *et al.* Benefit of carotid endarterectomy in patients with symptomatic moderate or severe stenosis. *N Engl J Med* 1998; 339: 1415–25.

59 European Carotid Surgery Trialists' Collaborative Group. Randomised trial of endarterectomy for recently symptomatic carotid stenosis: final results of the MRC European Carotid Surgery Trial (ECST). *Lancet* 1998; 351: 1379–87.

60 Benade MM, Medical MP, Warlow CP. Costs and benefits of carotid endarterectomy and associated perioperative arterial imaging. A systematic review of the health economic literature. *Stroke* 2002; 33: 629–33.

61 Kuntz KM, Kent KC. Is carotid endarterectomy cost effective? An analysis of symptomatic and asymptomatic patients. *Circulation* 1996; 94 (Suppl. II): II194–II198.

62 Nussbaum ES, Heros Erickson DL. Cost-effectiveness of carotid endarterectomy. *Neurosurgery* 1996; 38: 237–44.

63 Matchar DB, Pauk JS, Lipscomb J. In: Moore WS, ed. *A Health Policy Perspective on Carotid Endarterectomy: Cost, Effectiveness and Cost-Effectiveness.* Philadelphia: W.B. Saunders, 1996: 680–9.

64 Kent KC, Kuntz KM, Patel MR *et al.* Perioperative imaging strategies for carotid endarterecomy: an analysis of morbidity and cost-effectiveness in symptomatic patients. *JAMA* 1995; 274: 888–93.

65 Bushnell CD, Goldstein LB. Diagnostic testing for coagulopathies in patients with ischemic stroke. *Stroke* 2000; 31: 3067–78.

66 Bushnell CD, Siddiqui Z, Goldstein LB. Improving patient selection for coagu-lopathy testing in the setting of acute ischemic stroke. *Neurology* 2001; 57: 1333–5.

67 Bushnell C, Siddiqui Z, Goldstein LB. Use of specialized coagulation testing in the evaluation of patients with acute ischemic stroke. *Neurology* 2001; 56: 624–7.

68 Albers GW, Hart RG, Lutsep HL, Newell DW, Sacco RL. Supplement to the guidelines for the management of transient ischemic attacks: a statement from the ad hoc committee on guidelines for the management of transient ischemic attacks, Stroke Council, American Heart Association. *Stroke* 1999; 30: 2502–11.

69 Hankey GJ, Warlow CP. Cost-effective investigation of patients with suspected transient ischaemic attacks [editorial]. *J Neurol Neurosurg Psychiatry* 1992; 55: 171–6.

70 Johnston SC, Gress DR, Browner WS, Sidney S. Short-term prognosis after emergency department diagnosis of TIA. *JAMA* 2000; 284: 2901–6.

CHAPTER 20

Clinical Vignettes

Seemant Chaturvedi

Introduction

Although the clinician strives to be guided by evidence-based medicine, each patient presents a unique clinical scenario. Furthermore, there may not be high-quality data to support clinical decision making in many situations. Therefore, best judgement and the 'art of medicine' are frequently called upon.

Evaluation of patients with transient ischemic attacks (TIAs) or minor stroke has become more evidence-based in the last two decades, although considerable controversy remains in areas such as antithrombotic therapies, indications for carotid endarterectomy (CEA), management of patent foramen ovale (PFO), etc.

In this chapter, we present challenging clinical management dilemmas. Each case presentation is followed by a discussion from one of the cerebrovascular authorities who have authored chapters in this book. Their discussion is meant to be focused and practical and to illustrate the range of treatment practices.

Patient management

1. A 75-year-old-man is admitted to the hospital with dysphasia and right hemiparesis. Subsequent evaluation reveals a left striatocapsular infarct 2 × 2 cm. Carotid duplex is negative. Two-dimensional echo shows an ejection fraction of 15% and moderate aortic stenosis. Follow-up brain magnetic resonance imaging (MRI) 2 days after admission shows significant hemorrhagic transformation with hemorrhage occupying most of the initial infarct volume (not simply petechial hemorrhage). How would you approach this patient in terms of antithrombotic treatment?

Discussant: Patrick Pullicino

This patient has a new-onset striatocapsular infarct and has a low ejection fraction of 15% as an important risk factor for stroke. A third of patients with striatocapsular infarcts have a cardiogenic embolic cause (38% cardiogenic, 20% middle cerebral artery disease), and given the low ejection fraction, the heart is likely to be the source of the stroke in this patient.

If I had seen this patient prior to the finding of hemorrhage on the MRI, the first question would have been whether he should be heparinized. There is an increasing consensus against routine use of intravenous unfractionated or low-molecular-weight heparin in acute stroke, even cardioembolic stroke. There is an increased risk of hemorrhagic transformation of the stroke or of serious non-neurological bleeding coupled with lack of evidence of benefit on outcome, mortality reduction or prevention of recurrent stroke. If the patient was found to have an intracardiac thrombus on echo, however, the very high risk of recurrent stroke would probably have persuaded me to initiate heparin therapy acutely. Without this, I would only have given subcutaneous heparin for prophylaxis against deep vein thrombosis and continued any antiplatelet agent the patient may have been on.

The MRI scan appearance at 2 days of a hemorrhagic transformation of the infarct precludes any antithrombotic treatment. Even without the hemorrhagic change in the infarct, the question that poses itself is: is treatment with warfarin indicated in patients with low ejection fraction? There is really no current answer to this question, but only data from non-randomized or inadequately randomized studies that are insufficient to guide clinical practice. The atrial fibrillation trial results cannot be extrapolated to low ejection fraction patients, because the risk of stroke is lower in heart failure. Numbers needed to treat to prevent a stroke are going to be too high unless (as for atrial fibrillation) we define subgroups at higher risk of stroke. I would therefore only initiate warfarin if the patient had atrial fibrillation in addition to low ejection fraction, and then only after the hemorrhagic change had resolved. If the patient was in sinus rhythm I would probably have initiated aspirin, especially if the patient had ischemic heart disease.

2. A 45-year-old woman has an episode of vertigo, double vision, and right-sided numbness involving face/arm/leg while on vacation. Evaluation with MRI shows a left thalamic infarct. Angiography is negative for stenosis/dissection. Trans-esophageal echocardiography (TEE) shows a moderate-size PFO and aortic valve strands. Skin exam is consistent with livedo reticularis. Blood tests show an anticardiolipin antibody elevation with IgG 36 GPL units and IgM 24 units. All other tests for hypercoagulability are negative. What antithrombotic regimen would you recommend and would you recommend surgical or percutaneous PFO closure or neither?

Discussant: Karen Furie

This young woman has no apparent vascular risk factors and a clinical scenario consistent with a basilar embolus ultimately resulting in a thalamic infarct. She has livedo reticularis and elevated anticardiolipin titers, thus meeting the criteria for Sneddon's syndrome. It would be important to pursue a history of miscarriage or previous episodes of thromboembolism. In addition, a family history focusing on these issues should be solicited. There is no evidence of a large-artery stenosis/occlusion to explain an artery-to-artery embolus. Cardiac testing, however, reveals two abnormalities, a PFO and aortic valve strands.

In the absence of conventional risk factors, the relationship between the elevated anticardiolipin antibody titers and the embolic stroke appears tenable, either on the basis of arterial thrombosis or paradoxical venous thromboembolism. At this point, it would be reasonable to perform studies to look for venous thrombosis in the lower extremities and pelvic veins. The finding of aortic valve strands does not independently increase her risk of recurrent stroke. Valve strands have been observed to be found more commonly in young patients with a recent embolic event than comparably aged healthy controls. Still, up to 15% of healthy young people can have valve strands detected on echocardiography. It would be critical, however, to exclude completely the possibility of nonbacterial thrombotic endocarditis (NBTE), also known as marantic endocarditis. Libman–Sacks endocarditis, NBTE with an associated hypercoagulable state, is associated with lupus and antiphospholipid antibodies. In addition, it would be important that repeat antibody titers should be checked approximately 8 weeks later to ensure that the original finding was valid. I would also use that opportunity to look for other hypercoagulable factors which might predispose to stroke in the young and venous thromboembolism, specifically homocysteine (with B12), activated protein C resistance (with factor V Leiden if abnormal), functional protein C, protein S, and antithrombin III, and the prothrombin gene mutation G20210A.

I would favor treating this patient with warfarin with a target international normalized ratio (INR) of 2.0–3.0. A recent randomized clinical trial in patients with antiphospholipid antibody syndrome failed to show a benefit of high-intensity (INR 3.1–4.0) warfarin therapy. Given her young age and risk of recurrent thrombosis, particularly venous thrombosis, I would favor percutaneous PFO closure to eliminate the possibility of paradoxical embolism, recognizing that she might still require antithrombotic therapy to prevent or treat venous thromboembolism. The concern would be that given the natural vacillation of INRs over time, warfarin alone might be inadequate to prevent recurrent paradoxical embolism.

3. A 65-year-old woman with a history of hypertension and smoking has an episode of transient visual loss in the left eye lasting 5 min. One hour later, while shopping, she has expressive speech difficulty and dragging of the right leg lasting for 45 min. She comes to the emergency room and her neurological exam is normal. BP is 160/80. She is in normal sinus rhythm (NSR). Head computed tomography (CT) is negative. She was not on aspirin previously. She has a soft left carotid bruit. Would you admit her to the hospital? Would you place her on i.v. heparin or an antiplatelet agent? If you would admit her, what tests would you do and how quickly should they be done?

Discussant: James Meschia

This patient has a history and physical examination consistent with TIAs due to artery-to-artery embolism. If she has high-grade stenosis of the cervical portion of the internal carotid artery and she is a good operative candidate, she would need to undergo CEA. The patient is at high risk of an ischemic stroke involving the left anterior circulation. This case should be treated as a medical emergency. Within 24 h (and usually much sooner than this) I would determine whether this patient needs CEA, and if she does need surgery I would refer her immediately to surgeon with a track record in carotid surgery. In general, I would admit a patient like this so that the work-up and surgery could be expedited. There may be exceptions where I would not admit the patient. For example, if an ultrasound of the carotid arteries can be obtained within a reasonable time frame and the ultrasound shows minimal atherosclerosis in the carotid arteries, I would be inclined to treat the patient with antiplatelet agents and follow her as an outpatient. At St Luke's Hospital (Jacksonville, FL, USA), some attending neurologists might obtain an MRI of the brain and a contrast-enhanced MR angiogram as the initial radiographic study of this patient as opposed to the head CT that she had. Such a multimodal MRI would allow more informed triage decisions regarding admission to the hospital. Again, the main point is that I would not discharge the patient from the Emergency Department without first knowing that she has no need for CEA.

I would treat this patient with an antiplatelet agent. Low-dose aspirin has been shown to be superior to high-dose aspirin in the perisurgical period in patients who undergo CEA. In a subgoup analysis of the NINDS heparinoid study known as TOAST, patients did better on intravenous heparinoid if they were found to have a large-vessel type of ischemic stroke. Of course, the usual caveats apply when discussing subgroup analyses. It is possible that the observed benefit was simply the result of the play of chance, but I believe that an independent confirmation of the possible benefit of anticoagulation in patients with large-vessel ischemic strokes is warranted. I am not aware of any reliable randomized controlled trial data supporting the use of heparin or related compounds in patients who present with an acute TIA.

As to the patient's work-up, I would image the cervical carotid arteries. I generally prefer contrast-enhanced magnetic resonance angiography (MRA) as a screening technique. If the results come back as showing 40–69% stenosis, I would obtain a conventional angiogram before making a final decision about CEA. I might not obtain an echocardiogram if the patient has high-grade symptomatic carotid stenosis, because the yield of the echocardiogram would be low in such a case. The stroke work-up and, where necessary, a preanesthesia medical evaluation should be completed within 24 h.

4. A 60-year-old woman is referred from ophthalmology. She had a visual disturbance in the left eye 2 weeks previously and was diagnosed with a quadrant defect in the left eye due to branch retinal artery occlusion. She has a history of hypertension, smoking, and previous coronary artery bypass graft (CABG). She was on aspirin at the time of this event. ECG shows NSR. Carotid duplex shows 50–79% left internal carotid artery (LICA) stenosis with a normal RICA. Two-dimensional echo shows ejection fraction (EF) 50% with no wall motion abnormalities. Conventional angiography shows 60% LICA stenosis (NASCET method) with no ulceration and no distal intracranial stenosis. Would you recommend CEA, carotid stenting, or medical management? If the last hospital audit found the CEA mortality rate to be 1.8% at your local hospital, how would this affect your recommendation if at all?

Discussant: Larry Goldstein

The patient has a moderate-grade (NASCET method 50–69%) stenosis with symptoms and signs of retinal ischemia attributable to that vascular distribution. Overall, the benefit of CEA plus medical therapy compared with medical therapy alone in patients with 50–69% stenosis is moderate (16% vs. 22% risk of ipsilateral stroke or death over 5 years, relative risk reduction 29%, absolute risk reduction 6.5%, number needed to treat = 15 to prevent one event over 5 years). However, based on *post hoc* analyses, the risk and benefit do not appear to be uniform. Those with retinal events are at lower risk of stroke than those with hemispheric events. In addition, the duration of her visual symptoms is not clear from the case description. The benefit among those with moderate stenosis who had TIA is dramatically less than among those with stroke. In addition, the benefit of endarterectomy in women with moderate symptomatic stenosis appears seven- to eight-fold less than the benefit in men. Therefore, I would not recommend an interventional procedure at this point in this patient. She should be vigorously evaluated for other potentially treatable stroke risk factors (dyslipidemia, hypertension, etc.). One might also consider switching to a different platelet antiaggregant, although there are no prospective data available to support this approach. Based on WARSS, there would be no indication for warfarin.

5. A 77-year-old man with a history of hypertension (HTN), diabetes mellitus, and coronary artery disease (CAD) presents with mild left-sided weakness. MRI shows an enhancing, cortical right frontal infarct. His history is notable for previous partial left middle cerebral artery (MCA) infarct. At the time of the current stroke, he is

on ticlopidine. He is also on insulin and diltiazem. Examination reveals moderate cognitive impairment, mild expressive speech difficulty, and mild left hemiparesis. He is in NSR with BP 140/80. Carotid duplex is negative. MRA is negative. TEE shows moderate to severe aortic atherosclerosis in the ascending aorta with no protruding or mobile components. He lives at home with a daughter who is very supportive. What antithrombotic regimen would you recommend? What factors would you consider in deciding to anticoagulate an elderly patient? Is there a role for screening for intermittent atrial fibrillation and if so, how would you do it?

Discussant: Shunichi Homma

The brain imaging finding appears to indicate stroke to be due to embolism. Although there are no mobile, ulcerated or protruding components to the aortic plaque, I would think the 'moderate to severe' plaque would mean a plaque thickness of 4 mm or more which is strongly associated with embolic stroke, particularly of cryptogenic subtype. The mechanism of stroke in patients with large aortic plaques is thought to be due to embolism, as transcranial doppler (TCD) in these patients often document high-intensity transient signals (HITS). This patient was on ticlodipine when the event occurred, so the next reasonable medical regimen would be warfarin. Since the patient appears to have a supportive environment, he should be able to tolerate it. In WARSS (Warfarin Aspirin Recurrent Stroke Study), the rate of major hemorrhage was similar between those on warfarin and aspirin. I would recommend keeping the INR at 2–3. There is no definitive study that has compared an antiplatelet agent with warfarin in stroke patients with aortic plaques. Our PICSS (PFO in Cryptogenic Stroke Study) is investigating this issue and hopefully will provide clarification on this issue.

6. A 62-year-old man with a history of diabetes and hypertension for 20 years each is admitted with right-sided weakness. He has a history of left internal capsule lacunar infarct 3 years previously. He is taking aspirin 325 mg/day at the time of admission. There is no history of CAD or peripheral vascular disease (PVD). Carotid duplex shows 16–49% stenosis bilaterally. Two-dimensional echo is negative. MRI shows 1.0 cm left paramedian pontine infarct with negative MRA. Creatinine is 1.1. Homocysteine is 11.2. He is on insulin, amlodipine, and lovastatin but is not on an ACE inhibitor. He recovers well after a brief rehabilitation stay and is discharged home. What antithrombotic regimen would you recommend? Would you recommend any other tests or medications?

Discussant: Steven Levine

This patient has a new penetrating vessel (paramedian pontine branch syndrome) occlusive process. He has stroke risk factors of age, gender, diabetes, hypertension, prior ischemic stroke (also a lacunar syndrome), and carotid atherosclerotic disease. MRA fails to demonstrate significant large-vessel occlusive disease of the basilar artery. This suggests either that the occlusive process is, indeed, penetrating vessel disease from the stated risk factors, or that the MRA is false negative and there is relevant disease in the basilar artery. Given the risk factor profile, the prior and current lacunar events, it is most likely that this new event is on the basis of arteriosclerosis of a basilar artery branch. Certainly atherosclerosis at the origin (os) of the branch within the basilar artery lumen, with any varying degree of basilar artery stenosis/plaque, cannot be ruled out definitively with an MRA.

I would probably perform a transcranial Doppler ultrasound to look for non-invasive concordance of a nonstenotic basilar artery, and if it was normal or showed only elevated pulsatility/resistance indices (a sign that suggests existing small-vessel disease), I would not pursue conventional angiography. I would want to know about his glucose control as a diabetic and order a hemoglobin A_{1c}. I would more aggressively manage his glucose if there was evidence of significant hyperglycemia (consult an endocrinologist or discuss further diabetic control with his primary care physician). I would also want to know his blood pressure history and would target the more aggressive blood pressure range for diabetics— under 130/85 mmHg. I would probably add an ACE inhibitor if his BP was not at target values. Further tests would also include a lipid panel. I would start vitamin therapy for the homocysteine (cheap, effective, although not yet proven to reduce stroke risk) as risk is directly related to the level, even within the normal range of values. I would inquire about and modify as necessary life style, exercise, weight, diet, cigarette smoking, and regular (at least yearly) diabetic health screenings. As he has had a second stroke on aspirin, his risk of another stroke staying on aspirin may be higher than if he were switched to another antithrombotic regimen. Reasonable choices include (not in any specific order): clopidogrel, ticlopidine (with careful monitoring of hematological function), and lose-dose aspirin + extended release dipyridamole. Combined aspirin plus clopidogrel, while given commonly in clinical practice, has not been shown to date to be more effective than aspirin alone in stroke prevention and the MATCH trial did not demonstrate that clopidogrel + aspirin was more effective than clopidogrel alone for preventing stroke. I would continue to monitor his stroke prevention program and work on continued at least yearly updated stroke risk assessment and prevention ('STRAP') strategies. This would also include education about acute intervention if another event should occur, how to access acute care immediately, and the warning signs and symptoms beyond those he has already suffered from. The choice of any antiplatelet or combination therapy is only a part of the total picture of stroke and cardiovascular disease prevention in this gentleman.

Index

439

Index